LF

WOMEN IN MIDLIFE

WOMEN IN CONTEXT: Development and Stresses

WOMEN IN MIDLIFE

EDITED BY
GRACE BARUCH
Wellesley College
Wellesley, Massachusetts

AND

JEANNE BROOKS-GUNN
Educational Testing Service
Princeton, New Jersey

PLENUM PRESS · NEW YORK AND LONDON

Library of Congress Cataloging in Publication Data

Main entry under title:

Women in midlife.

(Women in context)
Includes bibliographies and index.
1. Middle aged women—United States—Addresses, essays, lectures. 2. Middle aged
women—Addresses, essays, lectures. 3. Middle aged women—Psychology—
Addresses, essays, lectures. 4. Sex role—Addresses, essays, lectures. 5. Middle aged
women—Mental health—Addresses, essays, lectures. I. Baruch, Grace K. II.
Brooks-Gunn, Jeanne. III. Title: Women in mid-life. IV. Series. [DNLM: 1. Women—
Psychology. 2. Middle age—Psychology. HQ 1233 W872]
HQ1059.5.U5W65 1984   305.4   84-3374
ISBN 0-306-41444-9

©1984 Plenum Press, New York
A Division of Plenum Publishing Corporation
233 Spring Street, New York, N.Y. 10013

Printed in the United States of America

To Susannah
G.K.B.

To Rebecca
J.B.-G.

ontributors

ane E. Alington • Centenary College, Hackettstown, New Jersey

salind C. Barnett • Wellesley College Center for Research on Women, Wellesley, Massachusetts

bra Barnewolt • Center for the Comparative Study of Social Roles, Department of Sociology, Loyola University, Chicago, Illinois

ace K. Baruch • Wellesley College Center for Research on Women, Wellesley, Massachusetts

nne Brooks-Gunn • Educational Testing Service, Rosedale Road, Princeton, New Jersey

therine DeLorey • Women's Health Research Institute, Boston, Massachusetts

ia Hay • Wisconsin Family Studies Institute, University of Wisconsin, Madison, Wisconsin

rolyn G. Heilbrun • Department of English, Columbia University, New York, New York

rbara Kirsh • Educational Testing Service, Rosedale Road, Princeton, New Jersey

rgie E. Lachman • Department of Psychology, Brandeis University, Waltham, Massachusetts

ly Long • Department of Sociology, Syracuse University, Syracuse, New York

Helena Z. Lopata • Department of Sociology, Loyola University, Chicago, Illinois

Zella Luria • Department of Psychology, Tufts University, Medford, Massachusetts

Robert G. Meade • Department of Psychology, Tufts University, Medford, Massachusetts

Malkah T. Notman • Department of Psychiatry, Tufts–New England Medical Center, Boston, Massachusetts

Lydia O'Donnell • Wellesley College Center for Research on Women, Wellesley, Massachusetts

Mary Brown Parlee • Graduate Center, City University of New York, Center for the Study of Women and Society, New York, New York

Karen L. Porter • Maxwell School, Health Studies Program, Syracuse, New York

Nancy K. Schlossberg • Department of Education, University of Maryland, College Park, Maryland

Jeanne Spurlock • American Psychiatric Association, Washington, D.C.

Ann Stueve • 23 Hamilton Avenue, Ossining, New York

Jane Traupmann • Family Development Center, Cambridge, Massachusetts

Lillian E. Troll • Department of Psychology, Rutgers University, New Brunswick, New Jersey

Beatrice Blyth Whiting • Graduate School of Education, Laboratory Human Development, Harvard University, Cambridge, Massachusetts

Vivian Wood • School of Social Work, University of Wisconsin, Madison, Wisconsin

Acknowledgments

Hilary Evans, senior editor of the Women in Context series, and Claire Kopp, editor of the series volume, *Becoming Female*, originally proposed this book on midlife women and invited us to co-edit it. Their enthusiasm was infectious, and we have profited greatly from many lively discussions.

As co-editors, we have each relied on our individual support systems while the book was in progress. For Jeanne Brooks-Gunn, Rosemary Deibler and Lorraine Luciano at the Educational Testing Service in Princeton provided assistance on all aspects of manuscript preparation and offered much-needed support and encouragement during editing. Margaret Mahoney and Tom Moloney of the Commonwealth Fund deserve a special thanks for their support during the last year; their thoughts on the special problems of disadvantaged midlife women who are unemployed and/or heads of households were particularly stimulating. Orville Brim and Richard Lerner were partially responsible for the decision to include midlife women in conceptualizations of the timing of female reproductive events and psychological adaptation.

Grace Baruch relied relentlessly on the skills and good will of Kathie DeMarco, who managed the innumerable tasks of a two-city project with patience and precision. The intellectual companionship of Rosalind Barnett is reflected throughout the book. Finally, we are grateful for the patience of our families, especially our husbands, whose support survived lengthy late-night telephone calls that too often occurred on holiday weekends.

Contents

The Study of Women in Midlife

GRACE K. BARUCH AND JEANNE BROOKS-GUNN

To describe the middle years—that relatively long span when one is neither young nor old—as a neglected period may no longer be accurate, given current scientific and popular interest in adult development and aging. But midlife is still too often seen merely as a kind of staging area on the way to old age, when one gathers one's forces and tries to stock up on assets—health, money, relationships—that will be needed for the rigors of the last phase of life. The middle years have been characterized more as a transition period than as a time of growth, satisfaction, and creativity. As this volume will show, although midlife is not without its difficulties, it is, for many women, a time of unexpected pleasure, even power.

MAJOR THEMES

A central theme of this volume is the impact of social change. The influence of economic conditions, of ideology, of the normative timing of such life events as age of marriage and childbearing, are addressed in many chapters from many different perspectives. Social changes are shown to have both negative and positive consequences. On the negative side, for example, the sex differential in life expectancy is a biosocial phenomenon that greatly restricts the availability of sexual partners—or, more precisely, heterosexual partners—for older women. On the positive side, the postponement of marriage and childbearing is related to women's increased commitment to the labor force, which in turn may serve to reduce their poverty in old age. Related to the theme of social change, then, is the question of the extent to which future cohorts of

GRACE K. BARUCH • Wellesley College Center for Research on Women, Wellesley, Massachusetts 02181. JEANNE BROOKS-GUNN • Educational Testing Service, Rosedale Road, Princeton, New Jersey 08541.

1

middle-aged women will resemble their counterparts of today, given the myriad changes over time.

A second theme of the book is the question of the extent, perma nence, and even the reality of improvement in the condition of midlife women. There is convincing evidence of improved mental health—less depression, greater self-esteem—than was so in the 1950s. (Veroff, Dou van, and Kulka, 1981). At the same time, the economy is shrinking discouraging women's employment and increasing the possibility o poverty. It may be that, as life expectancy increases, the penalties o aging are being postponed rather than abolished.

A third theme is that of diversity. In the past, women have too ofter been treated in research and theory as one homogeneous group. This has been especially true for middle aged women. The authors of many chapters emphasize the diversity of experience of midlife women—no only across groups (culture, race, cohort) but within groups. We see the heterogeneity of black women, of women who are returning to school of daughters who are caring for aging parents, of those who enter therapy.

Finally, the need for reassessment and improvement of both thera py and of research design and measurement is emphasized. Assump tions and stereotypes that permeate conceptual models and empirica work perpetuate inaccuracies and gaps in our knowledge. From rigor ous studies employing the latest insights of life-span developmen methodologies to works of fiction portraying patterns not yet discussed by social scientists, new models are being proposed.

TOPICS AND APPROACHES TO THE STUDY OF MIDLIFE

This volume is organized into three sections: Conceptual Ap proaches to Midlife, Roles and Relationships, and Enhancing Well Being.

CONCEPTUAL APPROACHES TO MIDLIFE. In this section, authors ad dress such questions as: What is midlife? How can it be studied? How is it changing?

Jeanne Brooks-Gunn and Barbara Kirsch discuss current perspec tives on the boundaries and events of the middle years, placing these in the context of social and historical changes. The fluidity of boundaries and changes in the timing and patterning of life events, they argue contribute to confusion about midlife, to ambivalence toward it, and to our difficulties in preparing for and adapting to the middle years. They draw on empirical data from a study of two Radcliffe College classes to illustrate incongruities between women's expectations and the realities they later encounter.

Margie Lachman provides a detailed description of how the con
ᴇpts and methodologies of life-span developmental psychology can be
pplied to the study of midlife in women. She analyzes the concept of
ᴇvelopment, arguing that the definition of development is critical to
ᴛudies of the midlife period. Reviewing principles of research design
ɴd measurement, including an analysis of common errors, she proides a framework for approaching a variety of topics relevant to gener
ᴛing a sound data base on women's middle years.

Carolyn Heilbrun draws on both the lives and works of women
ᴠriters, from George Eliot to May Sarton, in her exploration of new
ᴧatterns and models for women's middle years. She argues that inten
ɪty of experiences in these years—energy and delight, creativity and
ᴇnerativity—arise from one's work and from relationships with other
ᴠomen, rather than from the classic erotic plot centering on marriage
ʜat until recently summed up women's adult lives.

Rᴏʟᴇs ᴀɴᴅ Rᴇʟᴀᴛɪᴏɴsʜɪᴘs. Chapters in this section both draw on
ɴd challenge role theory and the literature on women's psychological
ᴠell-being. Authors analyze the economic underpinnings of women's
ꜰe situations and address issues of responsibility and care in a variety of
ᴇlationships.

Helena Lopata and Debra Barnewolt draw on classic theories of
ᴏles and role conflict as background for their empirical study of how
ᴠomen themselves experience their roles. Surveys of Chicago-area
ᴠomen reveal how women in diverse life situations (specifically with
ᴇgard to parenting and work) rank the relative importance of different
ᴏles at present, in the past, and in the future. The authors provide a
ᴛpology of roles and examine such influences on women's perceptions
ᴤ age, cohort, and role involvement.

Judith Long and Karen Porter's chapter critically reassesses the ex
ᴤting literature on roles and role conflict, including the concept of dual
ᴏles. They point out that prior literature assumes the primacy of family
ᴇsponsibilities for women and views paid employment as a deviant
ᴄtivity. Exploring the reasons for women's economic vulnerability, par
ɪcularly in old age, the authors show how women's typical marital and
ᴄccupational "careers" have contributed to their poverty. The public
ᴧolicy implications of traditional views of women are discussed, with
ᴧecial attention given to implications for the Social Security system.

Grace Baruch reviews existing literature about women's psychologial well-being, showing how diversity in the definitions of well-being
ᴇad to inconsistencies in findings. She critically reviews data bearing on
ᴦge and stage theories, including current concepts of the midlife crisis.
ᴠell-being is then examined in relation to women's roles as paid work
ᴇrs, mothers, wives, and daughters. Using data from a study done with

Rosalind Barnett of women aged 35 to 55, she identifies specific at tributes of different roles that may improve or impair well-being. The extent and permanency of changes important for women's pro gress toward equal opportunity are questioned by Diane Alington and Lillian Troll. They provide a brief history of women as students to illus trate how the larger society may exploit as well as simultaneously en courage women. Discouraging turnabouts in social attitudes and blatant barriers remain, but on a more optimistic note the authors argue that the family can promote as well as restrict women's opportunities. Woman as "late bloomer" is portrayed as a repeated and heartening phenomenon

Two chapters focus on the mother – daughter relationship in late life. Ann Stueve and Lydia O'Donnell take the perspective of the daughter, Vivian Wood, Julia Hay, and Jane Traupmann that of the mother. Stueve and O'Donnell ask, how do middle-aged daughters frame their commitments to their elderly parents? Drawing on thei study of daughters with at least one parent over 70, they show the diversity of attitudes and of patterns of responsibility, and analyze these in relation to daughters' age, stage of the family life cycle, and em ployment pattern. Their findings challenge the gloomy picture of the middle-aged woman as inevitably and persistently caught in the middle of onerous duties to parents and children.

In their analysis of the role of mother in later life, Vivian Wood, Julia Hay and Jane Traupmann focus on issues of independence and reciproc ity, which are central values in our society. The maintenance of equity that is, of fairness, in the relationship between parents and children specifically mother–son and mother–daughter, was the major topic o their study of Wisconsin women aged 50 and older. They report on how feelings of being overbenefited or underbenefited in relationships with parents play themselves out in women's relationships with their chil dren.

Jeanne Spurlock's chapter on black women at midlife emphasizes the diversity of experience in what is too often seen as a homogeneous group. She corrects for prior neglect and stereotyping of black middle aged women who, despite their greater poverty compared with white women, are characterized by determination and joy as well as struggle Difficulties in relationships with men are common, but coping capacities are strengthened by the extended family, and the church.

Beatrice Whiting brings the perspective of her studies of other cul tures to her analysis of the lives of American women. Seeking universa dimensions that will permit comparisons across disparate societies, she provides a framework of basic psychological needs and shows, for ex ample, how the need for physical contact goes relatively unmet in olde women in our society. She also points to ways in which men's needs may be frustrated by changes in women's lives, contributing to the potential for backlash.

ENHANCING WELL-BEING. The enhancement of well being can occur in a variety of institutions such as the educational and health-care systems, and in a variety of relationships, including the therapeutic.

Catherine Delorey explores the major threats to women's health, including those from disease and from deficiencies in the health care system. Data from her own study of midlife women and their physicians indicate the persistence of myths and stereotypes about women's health. Overemphasis on, and distortion of, the experience of menopause exemplifies these problems. Delorey describes the progress of the women's self-help health movement and offers recommendations for improvement in an area critical to women's well-being.

Mary Parlee argues in her chapter that studies of the middle years have not yet adequately addressed the interrelation of psychological and biological aspects of midlife changes. Analyzing the reasons for this neglect, Parlee focuses on assumptions embedded in a biological perspective—for example, labeling a depression as "post-partum" rather than "new-mother depression"—and reviews both barriers to and progress in understanding the psychology of menopause.

Diversity is once again the major theme in Nancy Schlossberg's chapter on women as adult learners; older women are now major figures in the population explosion of adult students. She analyzes three kinds of barriers—situational, dispositional, and institutional. Learning is discussed in the context of women's lives within the family, since the phases and transitions they experience there often are the triggers for the pursuit of additonal education. Describing the experiences of women who return to school, she offers suggestions for improving the person–environment fit between the individual woman and the educational institution.

The difficulties and dilemmas women and their therapists face when new roles and old feelings collide are the subject of two chapters on therapeutic issues of today's midlife women. Rosalind Barnett examines how problems women bring to therapy are related to social changes affecting their lives. Old expectations die hard, the departure from familiar patterns is rarely painless, and being different from one's mother is both inevitable and difficult. Too often, women doubt their own perceptions and capacities, and their femininity. Drawing on current research and on case material, Barnett argues that concepts of choice and risk are valuable to both patient and therapist in understanding and resolving psychological problems.

Malkah Notman's chapter continues the process of examining what is new and what is old about issues women currently present to therapists. Realistic limitations on one's life choices exist, and "classic" psychological issues important in the past have not disappeared—anxiety over competition with one's mother, for example. Case material illustrates such persistent problems as well as those arising from new patterns. For example, a mother may pressure her daughter to be more "liberated" than the daughter might wish to be.

Finally, Zella Luria and Robert Meade present a lively, comprehensive, and tough-minded view of the sexual realities of later life. They review the few empirical studies that bear on the sexuality of women in the middle years, placing Kinsey's research in historical context. The implications of men's earlier mortality for older women's sexual choices are explored; they are diverse, varying with such factors as age, race, marital status, and sexual preference. Luria and Meade suggest that such social changes as the sexual freedom of the baby boom generation and the increased power women will derive from occupational advancement mean that current patterns may not apply to the next generation of women reaching midlife.

FUTURE DIRECTIONS

We believe that a combination of social and ideological changes are allowing the study of midlife to flourish, providing a more accurate, less stereotypic and less gloomy picture of these years. An overemphasis on negative images, we would argue, arose from two kinds of bias in theory and research. First, the study of midlife has until recently focused on men (e.g., Levinson, 1978). Major themes in this work involve anguish over mortality and over the inadequacy of one's achievements. The relevance of such themes to the understanding of women's lives is being called into question (Baruch, Barnett, and Rivers, 1983). The large differential in life expectancy between males and females—now nearly years—may well influence the intensity of such concerns. A man of 4 stands at a very different "distance from death" from a woman of the same age. Recent studies suggest she is unlikely to share his sense of imminent mortality or his sense of inadequate accomplishment in the world. For those midlife women who were young adults in the 1940 and 1950s, an era when, far from being held to unattainable standards of professional accomplishment, achievement outside the role of wife and mother was unexpected, almost forbidden, the female version of "too short a time left, too much to do" is often "I have almost too many years left, and the chance to fill them with more than I ever thought I could."

A second source of bias affecting our images of midlife women volves the inordinate attention given to supposedly critical and nega- ve experiences with menopause and "the empty nest." As many chap- rs in this volume emphasize, these are neither central marker events r most women, nor are they main causes of distress. The loss of a uthful appearance also may be little mourned by the healthy middle- ed woman busy with work commitments, and more and more women e in that category. Such predictable changes, especially if they occur n time," rarely prove burdensome.

These two strands of research and theory have caused middle age to viewed with, at best, ambivalence. No wonder that the notion of lping women to anticipate, understand, and prepare for their middle ars has yet to take hold. This volume, we hope, will offer a more lanced and useful view of midlife. The serious and distressing prob- ms that many women face are not neglected, but neither are the op- rtunities for growth and change that we now know are characteristic, t just possible, in adulthood.

We recognize that biases in the study of midlife women are in no ay ancient history. Nevertheless, recent developments in the social iences are yielding valuable new approaches to the study of midlife. rst, the study of adult development within the framework of life-span ychology has called attention to the potential for growth and change roughout the life course. An important by-product of this view has en the development of new conceptual and methodological ap- roaches to the study of midlife that provide a standard for judging old eas and testing new ones. Second, the aging of the members of impor- nt, well-known longitudinal samples, such as the Berkeley and akland growth studies, are providing rich data on the years beyond lolescence in the context of individual life histories (Eichorn, Clausen, aan, Honzik, and Mussen, 1981). Third, we also are benefiting from e aging of many women researchers who, as younger adults, pi- eered new approaches to the study of women, and who are now awn to the study of the middle and later years. Many are represented this volume.

Finally, and perhaps least often acknowledged, social scientists are creasingly having to recognize the influence of the Women's Move- ent, as well as of the social changes it both reflects and catalyzes iele, 1982). New ideas and opportunities, we believe, have changed e nature of the realities women face as they grow older, and mostly in positive direction. The extent to which this is so is debated throughout is volume, but the feeling that one's life is over after 40—that the rimary task as mother is done and the best years past—seems less and less widespread among today's midlife women. New educational and occupational opportunities, although far from adequate, are transforming the midlife experience for many women.

REFERENCES

Baruch, G., Barnett, R., & Rivers, C. *Lifeprints: New patterns of love and work for today* *women*. New York, McGraw-Hill, 1983.

Eichorn, D. H., Clausen, J. A., Haan, N., Honzik, M. P., & Mussen, P. H. *Present and past* *in middle life*. New York: Academic Press, 1981.

Giele, J. Z. (Ed.), *Women in the middle years: Current knowledge and directions for research and* *policy*. New York: Wiley, 1982.

Levinson, D. J. *The seasons of a man's life*. New York: Ballantine, 1978.

Veroff, J., Douvan, E., & Kulka, R. *The inner American: A self-portrait from 1957 to 1976*. New York: Basic Books, 1981.

PART I

Conceptual Approaches to Midlife

.ife Events and the Boundaries of
Midlife for Women

ЕANNE BROOKS-GUNN AND BARBARA KIRSH

> The shock . . . of middle age is a threshold shock. A door is closing behind
> us and we turn sorrowfully to watch it close and do not discover, until we are
> wrenched away, the one opening ahead. (Fromm-Reichmann, F., 1959)

he difficulty of studying midlife in women is illustrated dramatically by
ιe above statement. Midlife typically is characterized as a transitory
ιther than as a distinct phase of the life cycle. As a phase defined
rimarily by the end of youth, it is accorded little importance in develop-
ιental conceptualizations, in literature, or in the media. Midlife also is
efined as the time to prepare for old age and death, the time when one
egins to count forward rather than backward (in terms of years to live
ιther than years lived). This view is reflected in research methodologies
ιat relate behavior in midlife to outcomes in old age. Midlife adjust-
ιent, sexuality, satisfaction, and health are considered possible predic-
ιrs of adjustment to old age but are rarely considered outcomes of
ιrlier behavior (see, as a notable exception, the Berkeley and Oakland
rowth studies; Eichorn, Clausen, Haan, Honzik, and Mussen, 1981).

An approach that treats midlife both as an antecedent and as an
ιtcome embeds midlife within the life cycle. Life-span developmental
sychology stresses that no one life phase may be considered without
·ference to other phases and that a developmental orientation may be
ɔplied to the study of adulthood as well as to childhood and adoles-
ɔnce (Brim and Kagan, 1980).

The metaphor of a door opening as well as closing also alludes to

ANNE BROOKS-GUNN AND BARBARA KIRSH • Educational Testing Service, Rosedale
ɔad, Princeton, New Jersey 08541.

the importance of change and the multidimensional and multidirec tional nature of change. As Brim and Kagan (1980) state:

> Growth is more individualistic than was thought, and it is difficult to find general patterns. The life span development view is sharply opposed to the notion of adult stages, arguing that stages cast development as undirectional, hierarchical, sequenced in time, cumulative, and irreversible—ideas not supported by commanding evidence. The facts instead indicate that persons of the same age, particularly beyond adolescence, and the same historical period are undergoing different changes; one person may show an increase in certain attributes while another shows a decline in the same aspects of behavior and personality.

In addition, midlife, if viewed as embedded within the life cycle rather than as the beginning of the end, may be characterized as mor· than preparation for death, retirement, loss of relationships, and illness Instead, it may be portrayed in terms of generativity, satisfaction, an· competence, as many of the chapters in this volume suggest.

In this chapter, midlife is discussed in terms of the life events tha· often occur at this time and are often considered markers of midlife, an· of the boundaries of midlife that may or may not be fluid, depending o· historical changes and individual perceptions. How individuals and so ciety prepare for midlife—given that some life events associated wit· midlife are normative while others are not, that boundaries of midlif· are fluid, and that midlife is sometimes not accepted as a life phase—wi· be considered. Finally, why so many individuals are ambivalent abou· midlife will also be discussed.

BOUNDARIES OF MIDLIFE

The life-span developmental approach, by stressing the multid· mensional and multidirectional nature of change, makes clear that th· boundaries of any life phase may be more fluid than rigid (Brim an· Baltes, in press). It follows that an individual may not be readily class· fied as to a particular life phase (if, indeed, such categorization we· even desirable).

However, the need to classify life stages seems to be universa· throughout history, life phases have been outlined, with chronologic· age boundaries often given. In current Western society, midlife is ofte· thought to *begin* at age 35. Yet this is the point in which one-half of one· life is *over*, in terms of male life-expectancy norms. If "middle" is th· halfway point between two times, then 35 would be men's mid-poin· not the beginning of middle age for men, who have a life expectancy · 78, and 39 would be women's midpoint.

While the boundaries seem quite fixed in people's minds, they are reality quite fluid. With the historical changes that have occurred for omen in midlife from the 1920s to the present, it seems that the defini- on of midlife may have been shifted upward. The boundaries may be onstructed by the society and the individual and may be less tied to ironological age. There are several possible reasons for the upward iift. First, young adulthood is more protracted: Education is pro- nged, marriage and childbearing are delayed, and career decisions are ade more cautiously. Consequently, many individuals in their 30s port that they have not entered midlife yet. When they are queried, e typical response is that they have not bought a house, begun a mily, or been married for any length of time, have just separated or vorced, are in the midst of changing jobs, or are embarking on retrain- g activities. Implicit in these statements is the construction of midlife s-à-vis its embeddedness in a series of life events, as discussed in the receding section.

Second, the health of the midlife woman, especially those in the iddle class, is relatively good. The belief that midlife ushers in ill ealth, or at the very least fatigue, aches, and pains, may not be corrobo- ted by experience. Instead of inferring that midlife does not neces- rily result in health-related problems, women infer that they have not t reached midlife. The adage "You're only as old as you feel" is indica- re of this view.

Third, midlife may be a time of enhanced sexuality for many wom- (see Luria and Meade, Chapter 17 of this volume). Greater enjoyment d comfort with one's own sexuality are not expected by many midlife omen. Again, the inference is that midlife has not been reached rather an that midlife may mark increased sexual enjoyment for many.

Fourth, midlife typically is believed to coincide with the time at hich active parenting ends, when children leave their parents' home. more women have children later, and as more reblended families are rmed, women may have children and adolescents in their home roughout their 40s and 50s. Again, a woman's perception of herself as ing in midlife may be postponed.

Fifth, the change in life expectancy alters the boundaries of midlife. hen life expectancy was in the 60s, being 50 or 55 had a very different eaning than it does today, when life expectancy is in the 70s and nost in the 80s. Perhaps the upper boundary of midlife remains elastic cause the length of old age has remained fixed. In other words, if old e is defined as the last 15 years of life, then the increase in life expec- ncy would lengthen midlife but not old age.

Finally, being old carries a stigma in the United States. A recent say in the *New York Times* (1982) begins: "I am old. These hateful

words are all but forbidden in these United States. The simple declara
tion marks the worst kind of deficit. Such a stamp is applied by a natio
addicted to the mindless worship of youth."

In order to avoid the appellation of old age, the term *middle age* i
expanded upward. While middle age may not be perceived as positivel
as youth, it is still preferable to old age. The old age stereotype encom
passes notions such as senility, incompetence, illness, and debilitatior
If these terms define old age, and a 55- or 60-year-old woman does nc
possess these traits (or perceive herself to possess them), then the terr
middle age would be offered to distinguish one from other similar-age
individuals who possess these undesirable traits. Strangely enough, th
majority of 55- and 60-year-olds do not "fit" the stereotype, remainin
healthy, competent, independent, and active. The pervasiveness of be
liefs about old age may underline the necessity to counteract them b
expanding the upward boundary of middle age.

Markers of Midlife

One of the major problems in conducting research on midlife, e:
pecially for women, is that many different markers or life events hav
been used to delineate this period; these multiple life events overla
conceptually, methodologically, and descriptively. Not only do the
overlap but they are taken from different disciplines, making cros
discipline comparisons difficult. Within any particular field, this pleth
ra has not been problematic, however, because little interdisciplinar
research has been conducted on midlife. Notable exceptions include th
attempt to relate the onset of menopause to changes in the parentin
role and/or the employment role. For example, the early work on th
"empty nest" syndrome demonstrated that for many midlife wome
hospitalized for depressive symptoms, the primary problem was loss (
their major role (in this case that of parent with dependent childrer
rather than a decline or change in circulating hormones (Bart, 1970). I
any case, as researchers from different fields begin to review eac
other's work and to collaborate, the discrepancies between their marke
will become more jarring and the failure to consider life events simu
taneously more untenable.

Another problem is that even within a field or subspecialty, whi
consensus may exist as to the type of marker deemed most appropriat
individual variance in the experience of life events makes generalizatic
difficult and research designs problematic.

At least six different markers of midlife may be found in the liter
ture. While some focus on physical, psychological, or social life event
others combine all three aspects.

The first and simplest marker is chronological age. Age typically presents physical, psychological, and sociocultural indices of changes. r example, even though age is clearly a physical marker, women who main very active physically may be physiologically similar to women 5 ars younger than they are. In addition, cultural differences may make e use of age as a marker problematic. Spurlock (Chapter 10) has ar- ed that midlife begins earlier for black women due to their relatively orer health and nutrition, limited access to medical care, earlier child- aring, and shortened life expectancy compared to whites. Finally, storical changes in age as a marker may have occurred, partially as a nction of changes in health status and longevity.

Second, parenting status is almost always considered a relevant arker. For women, midlife has been characterized as the middle stages parenting (i.e., being parents of older children, teenagers, or young ults). Research on women's midlife crises focused on the end of active ild-rearing. However, the assumption that midlife will coincide with a ecific stage of parenting is no longer viable. First, a significant number parenting careers are either earlier or later than the norm. In the white iddle class, a number of women have chosen to begin childbearing in eir 30s, so that midlife may coincide with early stages of parenting. At e other extreme are teenage parents, who will have grown adult chil- en before they are 40. Indeed, if teenage pregnancy does perpetuate elf within families (and there is limited evidence that this is the case), enage mothers will be grandmothers before they are 40. Second, using ildbearing as a marker omits those women who remain childless. ildless women, teenage parents, and older parents may constitute e-third of all women in America today.

The more relevant use of child-rearing as a marker encompasses the ncept of off-time and on-time life events. Neugarten (1979) has dis- ssed the concept of a life clock in which major events occur in a more less systematic and time-ordered fashion. Teenage pregnancy typ- lly is defined as an event that is unplanned and/or unanticipated, an ent that places the women off time vis-à-vis the norm for child-rear- g. However, the perception of being off time or on time regarding e's cohort may be more important than one's actual status vis-à-vis e societal norm. In black urban America today, having a child at 17 to is not perceived as being out of phase, although having one at age 15 (Furstenberg, 1976). Similarly, in segments of middle-class society, ving a firstborn after age 30 is typically not perceived as off time by the other (although it may be perceived as off time by the grandmother). rceptions of timeliness may affect life satisfaction, adjustment, and pectations more than actual timeliness, as is suggested by research on bertal girls. Although the mean age of menarche is about 12½ in

America today, great individual variations occur. Girls who begin t menstruate prior to seventh grade or after eighth grade are defined, b most researchers, as early or late, respectively (Brooks-Gunn and Rubl 1982, 1983). However, when girls are asked about whether or not the are early, late, or on time, 20% are classified differently than their actu status would suggest; in other words, some girls who are off time b lieve they are on time and vice versa (Tobin-Richards, Boxer, and P tersen, 1983). In addition, their perceptions of timeliness are mo strongly associated with self-esteem than are actual physical indices pubertal status (Tobin-Richards *et al.*, 1983). Thus, with regard to midli and parenting, perceiving oneself to be in phase may be more importa than being in phase normatively.

The next most important marker, in terms of the research literatur is change in work life events. Since employment and child-rearing ofte covary, especially in earlier cohorts, it is often difficult to treat en ployment as an independent variable. At the same time, for certai subgroups of women, employment may be a relevant dimension, e pecially for those groups who alter their employment situations at mi life—entering the work force for the first time, reestablishing work pa terns after children enter school, moving from part time to full time, moving to a higher position. These four work life events may occur i midlife, with the first three being much more likely to occur in midli women than men (see Long and Porter, Chapter 5, this volume). A women's employment histories seem to be more fluid and less line than men's employment histories, employment's usefulness as a mark for midlife may not be as great.

A more profitable approach might be to identify certain clusters women for whom work-life events were altered during midlife. Lopa and Barnewolt (Chapter 4, this volume) describe groups of women terms of the importance of family and employment to them. Sever subgroups of women are identified, each of which has distinguishir characteristics. Another approach would be to look at those women wh change their employment patterns at midlife versus those who do no One might expect those women who are in flux to show different pa terns of physical adjustment, life satisfaction, role negotiations, an power within the family from those of the women whose patterns r main fairly stable over time.

Fourth, the activities that women engage in during midlife as well the mix of these activities have been considered significant life events midlife. It has been assumed that during midlife, child-rearing deman decrease while other demands (employment, community, and oth family members) increase. At the same time that child-rearing deman decrease, other relational demands may be placed on the woman, parti rly those of older parents, grandchildren, and husband. In general, e literature using these markers has placed the responsibility upon the men herself. Demands of parents, grandchildren, and children are sumed to be the responsibility of the midlife woman rather than the dlife man. Midlife men seem to be perceived as having some control er the amount of time these demands place upon them, while the dlife woman is not perceived to have much control, being required to ke on additional relational requests. Whether employed women are owed to be "excused" from these tasks, to provide support through ancial remuneration, or to request additional time from husbands, her than being expected to add these responsibilities, is under study rody, 1980). Given that older parents expect their midlife daughters to more responsive than their sons and that midlife daughters (and ughters-in-law) provide more support than do sons (Wood *et al.*, apter 8), one might expect employed women and their older parents to perience some difficulty adjusting to such demands.

Fifth, hormonal changes are occurring at this time and may or may t be a significant life event. Hormonal changes precede the onset of enopause, are gradual, and vary greatly across individual women. ue indication of these gradual changes is the greater incidence of infer-ty in midlife women than in younger women. Such infertility is a nificant and often unanticipated life event for midlife women who anned their child-rearing careers for their 30s and 40s.

Since the experience of life events may not be normative during dlife, research needs to focus on (a) the appropriate referent group (or ups), rather than comparing individuals to societal norms that may t be salient to the individual (as in the example of urban teenage thers); (b) women's perceptions of the timeliness of specific events, ich may differ from the actual timeliness vis-à-vis specific referent ups; (c) the importance of others' beliefs about timeliness in deter-ning an individual's reaction to a life event (as in the example of the ther who wishes to have a grandchild earlier than her daughter wish-to have a child); and (d) the relationship of differing measures of eliness to an individual's life satisfaction and feelings of effectance d self-worth. In addition, discrepancies in the timeliness of life events ed to be examined; for example, one may feel on time with regard to ild-rearing but off time with regard to employment. Is it more disrup-e to the individual to be off time with regard to certain life events than others, or is the notion of off time more cumulative?

In sum, many of the life events associated with midlife are associ-d only in a probabilistic sense, in that all individuals do not experi-ce them, or experience them at different times or in a different se-ence. The variability of midlife markers and the lack of cohesion among them makes it difficult, if not impossible, to discuss transitions midlife. How one prepares for a transition that is so fluid as to make tl term *transition* possibly untenable will be discussed later.

HISTORICAL CONTEXT OF MIDLIFE EVENTS

The transition to midlife may be more or less fluid, depending the historical context within which it is embedded. Some of the moval markers that determine the elasticity of boundaries are entrance into a progress through educational institutions, age at marriage, movi away from the nuclear family, age of parenting, and widowhood. Wh these events are experienced by the individual, societal changes infl ence the probability that a number of individuals will experience a l event at a particular time (Riley, 1973). Important variables in a cohor movement through life include mortality, fertility, marital status, r tionality (immigration), rural–urban residence, and education.

Rossi (1980) suggests that our models of adult development aro out of a specific historical period, that of perhaps the most stable tir (1950s and 1960s) in the past century. Patterns of predictable life ever are predicated on this model. Instead of using as the normative gro those adults who experienced the Great Depression as children or ad lescents, World War II as adolescents or adults, and the return to lar, families and low labor force participation by women in the 1950s, o needs to compare them to other cohorts. Indeed, some demographe have stopped talking about the rapid and surprising decline in the bir rate through the late 1960s and 1970s and instead have focused on tl rapid rise in fertility rates immediately following World War II.

Other sociologists have discussed the importance of historical co text in defining life phases and interpreting life events. Hareven (197 suggests that three aspects of life-course analysis are particularly re vant: (1) the synchronization of individual with family transitions, the interaction between life-course transitions and historical change and (3) the cumulative impact of earlier life-course transitions on subs quent ones. Analyzing historical changes in definitions of life phase Uhlenberg (1978) finds three somewhat universal age strata—childho (0–15), adulthood (15–60), and old age (60+). Although he believes th social conceptions have changed over the century, the

context of each age category has persisted over this period: Children are expected to live with parents, attend school, and be socialized into the culture; young adults are expected to establish families and take on adult work responsibilities; middle-aged adults are expected to complete the rearing of their children and maintain stability in their occupations; and the elderly are

expected to progressively relinquish various roles and complete the life
course by dying. (p. 67)

It is interesting that although Uhlenberg does not differentiate be-
reen young and midlife adult phases in his three strata, he does so in
s discussion of the context of the categories. In other conceptions,
ung and midlife adults are usually separate, as are childhood and
lolescence.

Uhlenberg (1978) outlines a typology of five family life courses
omen typically follow into midlife. These are that (1) women marry,
ar children, and are still alive and married at the age of 50 (the nor-
atively expected); (2) women die before they reach 50; (3) women
ver marry and survive to 50; (4) women are married without children
id reach 50; and (5) women bear children and survive to 50, but their
arriages are not intact because of death or divorce. Uhlenberg com-
red these life courses for cohorts born in 1870, 1890, 1910, and 1930.
ie most dramatic changes over time have been in (1) increasing life
pectancy, so that more women in the later cohorts reach midlife and
ore reach midlife with their spouses; (2) increasing rates of marriage,
that fewer of the 1930 cohort are single compared to the older groups;
) declining age at marriage; and (4) changes in childlessness and never-
arried status. Childlessness increased dramatically from the 1870 co-
rt (9%) to the 1890 cohort (14%) and the 1910 cohort (16%), who were
ung adults during World War I and the Depression. Women born in
30 had the lowest childlessness rate (4.5%), bearing their children
iring the late 1940s to the early 1960s. Declines in early widowhood
er the 1870–1930 period have been matched by higher divorce rates,
t women tend to remarry after divorce, so that families are more likely
be intact in midlife for the 1930 cohort than they were for the older
omen. Uhlenberg's conclusion is that the rates of conformity with the
rms of women's role performance increased from the 1870 cohort to
e 1930 cohort. He predicted in 1974 that women would enter midlife
m subsequent birth cohorts with far less conformity to these family
les because of divorce and because of norms allowing voluntary child-
ssness and nonmarital status.

One of the more fascinating aspects of Uhlenberg's analysis is the
vious omission of employment as a marker of status. By concentrating
the family life course, the notion is reinforced that women follow a
nited life script. That women are defined by marriage and children
eans that most of their script is written by the end of young adulthood.
iey are going to experience significant life events only in terms of
vorce, remarriage, or the death of a spouse. As an example, one of the
ost popular and often quoted statements from the teenage pregnancy

literature suggests that for the young unmarried mother, 90% of her lif script is written, most of it dismal. Such a view does not allow fc changes, for resilience, or for growth, all of which have been found i studies of teenage parents (Furstenberg, 1976). Given this subtle bt farily prevalent belief, it is no wonder that the study of midlife wome has languished. The movement from young to middle adulthood i considered a nonevent.

In addition, it is doubtful that a similar analysis would be unde. taken for men, even though most men could be classified within the fiv life-course categories. The cohorts of men born in 1870, 1890, 1910, an 1930 also experienced the changes in age of marriage, childlessness, lif expectancy, divorce, and remarriage. However, discussions of men midlife courses concentrate on work life (Levinson, 1978; Vaillant, 1977

It is a common experience for the baby boom cohort (born betwee 1946 and 1964) to seek markers of age status and not find firm enoug passage rites to convince them of changed status. For example, whe large numbers of baby boomers left home for college, a passage rit occurred, removing them from the nuclear family; but the enormot numbers of the cohort encouraged the formation of a new stage—th youth culture of the 1960s and early 1970s—rather than the expecte move into adulthood. The age of 21 had been a legal marker of adu status, but the law shifted downward to 18 with the population explc sion, giving full legal rights to vote, join the military, drink (in mo: states). This fluctuating marker reduced the legal coming-of-age to or celebrated more for the adolescent pleasures of driving and drinkir than for the responsibility of being a full citizen.

Other markers continue to shift—protracted education, high rate of premarital sex and cohabitation, divorce and remarriage, and chang ing values whereby women can delay or decline marriage and still de rive high levels of life satisfaction. (Although this was probably alway the case for individuals, societal beliefs seem to be more accepting these alternatives than ever before.) Marriage and the end of educatic have become less salient markers of attainment of adult status.

Some former midlife markers have changed, and others are new fc women and are still being defined. What existed as clear age boundarie for former generations (or at least appear clear in retrospect) often fac or blur as other cohorts approach them, partly because of changir characteristics of those younger cohorts. The upper limit of middle ag as discussed earlier, was probably 55 to 60, with the years beyond tha classified as old age. Yet the large number of people beyond 55 who d not feel "old" alter the upper boundary of midlife.

The older members of the baby boom generation currently are wi ness to some unexpected changes in their parents' life-style and attitud

anges, new love relationships after divorce or death of a spouse,
rther education, new hobbies, career switches, geographic moves—all
pendent of course, on financial stability and health. It is difficult for
ople in their 30s and 40s to feel middle-aged when their parents exhib-
"youthful" rather than elderly behavior.

The high divorce rate has had an impact on markers surrounding
iddle age. Abrupt changes in life-style usually accompany divorce,
isettling women economically, geographically, and emotionally. A di-
rced 45-year-old woman may well lead a life similar to that of a 35- or
en 25-year-old unmarried woman—wear the same clothing styles,
end the same singles events, live in the same apartment complexes
nce their incomes could well be comparable). They may both be single
rents of children still at home, and be searching for a better job and
od love relationships.

Finally, the tremendous recent emphasis on physical fitness oc-
rred as the baby boom generation reaced "middle age." This may be
erpreted as a conscious effort to continue young adulthood in ap-
arance, activities, and values (Jones, 1980).

EPARATION FOR MIDLIFE

In general, preparation for life events or transitions occur for those
ents that are anticipated. Two approaches to the issue of preparation
 life events have been suggested, each of which involves the distinc-
n between anticipated and unanticipated life events. Brim and Ryff
79) have hypothesized that a taxonomy of life events characterized by
ee properties might be useful for examining anticipatory socializa-
n. The three properties of life events that they believe to be relevant
 (1) age-relatedness, or the relationship of an event to chronological
e, (2) the social distribution of an event, or if an event occurs, the
mber of persons who will experience it, and (3) the likelihood of
currence for an individual, or the probability of an event occurring to
y given person. From this three-dimensional classification system,
ht types of events may be generated. For some of these events, antic-
tory socialization occurs and for some it does not. Events that are
died typically are those for which preparation does take place—those
ents that are highly age-related, are shared by many, and are likely to
ur to any given individual. These are the events studied by so-
logists and psychologists, as they are normative, age-graded, and
ll labeled. At the other extreme are events for which preparation does
 take place—events that are not likely to occur to an individual, are
 predictable in terms of timing, and are not common enough to allow
 shared experiences with many others (Brim & Ryff, 1979). However,

many life events are not so clear-cut: They may have some relationshi to age or there may be a moderate likelihood of occurrence, as in the cas of divorce. Many of the examples of events in the middle given by Brin and Ryff are midlife events—death of a father or husband, children' marriages, becoming a grandparent, "topping out" in one's career. Th individual may not prepare for such events, given their weak rel: tionship with the three dimensions discussed earlier. These events con trast with many of those in young adulthood, which are more normativ and age-graded. Children and adolescents are overtly taught how t perform familial and occupational roles in preparation for youn adulthood. This preparation has predominantly meant becoming a wil and mother for women, and husband, father, and economic provider fc men. Once these roles are established in adulthood, however, the e: pectations and socialization for the next stage (midlife) are generall unfocused, at best.

The value of the anticipation of life events is that the individual provided information regarding the event (and the appropriate soci roles and sanctions surrounding it) and is encouraged to seek out info mation. The individual may search for role models who have exper enced the upcoming event or may be contacted by a potential role mod who wishes to "pass on" information to the individual. She may l introduced to or seek out new social referent groups such as profe sional women's organizations, single parents' organizations, paren teacher organizations, and so on. The individual may begin to rehear a new set of behaviors related to the life event. More generally, inform tion gathering may be at a cultural level, where attitudes and beliefs a acquired or at least become more salient, given the anticipated chang With regard to childhood and adolescence, the ways in which sex rol are acquired and changes integrated into one's self-definitions ha' been studied in great detail (Maccoby and Jacklin, 1974; Brooks-Gur and Ruble, 1983). During midlife, little research on anticipatory s cialization has been conducted. In fact, it is not clear (1) whether or n anticipatory socialization takes place, (2) what form it might take (acti seeking, passive reception, active offering), (3) whether or not inc viduals desire more preparation or are at least aware of the lack preparation, or (4) whether or not life events would be experienc differently if anticipatory socialization took place.

Another way to look at anticipatory socialization is in terms of t timing of life events. The notion of an event being on time implies th the event is normative and occurs at the time when it is expected occur. Off-time events, in this framework, are still expected (i.e., ea puberty, late menopause, late parenting) but occur at a time when th are not anticipated. Whether or not the lack of anticipatory socializati

the perception of being out of phase affects an individual's experience
a life event is not well understood. The most information comes from
e study of maturational status in adolescence, vis-à-vis one's peers.
ethodologies comparable to those used for untangling the effects of
·ing early or late, perceiving oneself to be so, and the composition of
e referent group with respect to maturational timing in puberty might
: developed for midlife events; events with biological links (such as
enopause, parenting, and physical changes) might be most amenable
such an approach.

Returning to the concept of unanticipated events, rather than off-
ne events, it is clear that socialization occurs; it is just that it is often
ter the fact. In this case, *post hoc* socialization may occur in the observa-
n of role models, seeking new referent groups, asking friends for
formation, and being offered information, these processes being the
me as an anticipatory socialization. Typically, this is studied under the
bric of adaptation to life changes rather than as socialization. The term
plies that the process is internal, intrapsychic, and individualistic.

Another problem arises when a cohort anticipates one set of experi-
ces, because of the experience of previous cohorts, and then finds
elf in a very different set of conditions. In fact, some have hypoth-
ized that vast changes in major social institutions may be expected
hen the experiences of a cohort contrast sharply with those of the
evious cohort (Ryder, 1965). An example of such contrast is the situa-
n of the generation that grew up with the Depression and World War
followed by their children of the baby boom. In this case, one's
ticipatory socialization may not be adequate. For example, many of
ir female friends lament, as they juggle the responsibilities of children,
ouses, parents, community, and employment, "If mother had only
ld me it would be like this." Of course, mother could not, as she was
uch less likely to have been employed during her childbearing years,
be rearing children alone, or to have parents live well into their 80s.
rhaps the interest in research on role models arose out of the unmet
ed of women researchers themselves for anticipatory socialization
periences.

Another example of inadequate socialization due to the reliance on
periences of the preceding cohort involves more indirect forms of
cialization, specifically cultural awareness of maternal employment.
a national survey of families (*General Mills Family Report*, 1977), 80% of
adults felt that women with young children should not work outside
: home, except in cases of extreme economic need. Clearly, such a
ltural belief could discourage women from seeking information about
inaging young children while employed, even though many women
: available to provide such information.

Even within a cohort, an event may be experienced quite diffe
ently. Elder (1974) has presented a fascinating analysis of the life exper
ences and adjustment of two cohorts who were young during the Grea
Depression. Those who were young children and those who were ente
ing adolescence during the Depression had different experiences an
outcomes. Within the cohort just entering midlife, life courses have bee
quite divergent, even in women from similar backgrounds (Zadel
1975).

Another approach emphasizes personally normative events tha
may be experienced as crises even though they occur for a number of (o
all) individuals. Erikson's conceptualization of life development was in
strumental in the acceptance of this view of adult development. Studie
on midlife men (Vaillant, 1977; Levinson, 1978) are examples. Develop
ment is seen as potentially enhanced by satisfactory coping with suc
events as divorce, death of parents and spouse, and children leavir
home. Although an individual cannot fully prepare for these event
being independent, capable of financial decisions, and open to chang
for adaptation to new experiences and acquaintances would be essenti
for adaptation to these common events.

THE RADCLIFFE STUDY[1]

In order to examine the question of whether or not women a
prepared for midlife and, if so, whether various cohorts perceive the
preparation differently, two cohorts of Radcliffe College graduates a
being examined. This study involves women who finished Radcliffe
1947 and in 1962, years noted for striking contrasts in historical ar
cultural circumstances. Questionnaires completed by these two grou
provide rich information on early influences, college experiences, adt
attitudes toward self and society, and also on the actual roles and a
tivities chosen for each decade of adult life. Each stage of life for tl
Radcliffe alumnae was subject to different historical events and cultu
values, so early influences such as family structure and class bac
ground may interweave in contrasting ways with individual procliviti
and personalities in influencing adult life patterns. Eighty-three wom
from the class of 1947 completed a questionnaire at their 35th reunic
thus, they were in their mid-50s, just finishing midlife. In contrast, tl
Radcliffe class of 1962 was tested at their 20th reunion, when they we
in the early 40s. More than one-half of the 1962 class completed tl
questionnaire.

[1]We wish to thank the Henry A. Murray Center for the Study of Lives, at Radcli
College, for their support of B. Kirsh and for provision of data from their archives.

reparation for Careers

Few of the graduating class of 1947 had assumed they would have
reers; few prepared for them. They had expectations of idyllic married
e, and most of them did marry soon after college (68% by the end of
50). They had more children at younger ages than the class of 1962.
fteen percent of the younger women had given birth after the age of
). In 1982, of the 83 women attending their 35th reunion, 14 had no
ildren, 5 had one child, 17 had two, 20 had three, 16 had four, 7 had
e, 1 had six, and 3 had seven. These highly educated women had
rticipated enthusiastically in the baby boom between 1946 and 1964.
Even with relatively large families, this group had 31 master's de-
ees and 15 doctoral or professional degrees. Only 10 of these 83 wom-
ı attending the reunion were not working; the rest listed a wide variety
occupations, including professor, therapist, librarian, lawyer, writer,
ısiness executive, and clerical worker. Many had started their careers
te in life when child-care responsibilities decreased or when they be-
me single again. About half of the women at the reunion were still
arried to their first husband; 12 had remained single, 6 were widowed,
) were in their second or third marriages, and 9 had divorced and not
married.
More of the 1962 graduates had established careers than had the
47 graduates. The social context had changed in the 15 years between
eir graduations. The earlier class had grown up through the Depres-
ᴏn and World War II and anticipated unlimited domesticity and finan-
al security after college graduation. They hoped for and had large
milies, spending their 20s and 30s at home with children and chores,
doing some volunteer work. They had given scant thought to their
tures beyond these early adult years. Most of them voiced surprise at
ᴏw unprepared they were for midlife. Substantial effort was essential
order to adapt to new life-styles and gain self-knowledge, as changes
fected them both from external, or social, sources and from internal, or
ᴇrsonal, sources. Difficulty in coping with drastically changed circum-
ances was a common theme among the 1947 graduates at the time of
eir 30th reunion.

reparation for Changes in Sexuality

When the Radcliffe graduates from the class of 1947 were surveyed
) years after college about their attitudes toward changing sexual stan-
ards, very few of the women accepted the changed attitudes or behav-
ᴏrs for themselves. Many voiced worry and disapproval as to the nega-
ve consequences they had seen, in terms of broken marriages and

personal unhappiness. A common response was that they had had to learn to accept the changed sexual standards because of conflicts over their children's sexuality, but they said they personally remained "conventional" and "old-fashioned." Several women endorsed the decreas in hypocrisy and sexual double standard but worried about the be wildering choices faced by other women, particularly adolescents, in making choices about sexual behavior.

This cohort of women, now in their 50s, were caught unprepared for social change in the norms regarding sexuality. They grew up in a time when delayed gratification (economically and sexually) was endorsed as a way to get through the Depression and World War II. They married early and produced relatively large families; now, many of them are unexpectedly single because of divorce or widowhood, and those that remain married must reestablish relationships with husbands in new family situations without children's intrusions. They clearly feel the pressure to be more sexual at a time of increasing physical symptoms of aging. One woman complained: "I feel my age. Arthritis spreading from back to knees to ankles. Memory giving me trouble (no one prepared me for this so young!)."

And yet some studies suggest that women's sexuality increase with age in terms of interest and ease of arousability. This is in contrast to a decline of sexuality with age in men. Rubin (1979) found that many of the marriages she studied had been plagued with sexual problems i the early years, but that when sexual norms relaxed and fear of pregnancy faded with age, couples improved their sexual relationships during midlife. Among Rubin's sample, over 60% of the women had been virgins before they were married. Both cultural and life-stage factors have helped improve their sex lives to a point where, according to Rubin roughly 90% of these midlife women have experienced orgasms.

Preparation for Changes in Relationships

Midlife typically entails a reevaluation and renegotiation of many relationships. Long marriages are altered by children leaving home allowing more time for companionship between spouses; at the same time, many women return to work, go to school, or change careers a their children enter adolescence and young adulthood. A new work away from the home generally serves to engender feelings of competence and instrumental orientation in women whose daily lives have been oriented around family and home. Frequently, household chores decision making, and financial matters are areas of negotiation when women feel more independent. There can be strains in a long marriage when the midlife woman moves out into the work world around the

ıme time her husband begins to relax in his occupational role and
ants to appreciate more leisure and home-centered activities.

Relationships between the midlife woman and her parents change,
so. She often has more responsibilities and worries in caring for aging
arents, helping them with decisions and practical matters they had
reviously felt adequate to attend to themselves. Often relationships
etween elderly parents and the midlife child improve and they come to
ppreciate each other in more mature ways. With the death of one
arent, the midlife woman generally has a greater role in the physical
ıd emotional well-being of the remaining parent. Also, the midlife
ıdividual faces mortality of both parent and self as signs of aging and
ness increase (Wood *et al.*, Chapter 9, this volume).

The women in the 1947 Radcliffe class report that they experienced
ears of turbulence with their adolescent children, but now, in their 50s,
ıey have far better understanding of and relationships with their
own children. The women mention areas of disapproval of their chil-
ren's life-styles—particularly in the realms of sexuality and values to-
ard money and career—but they have come to accept their children's
ves as entities separate from their own. This acceptance of separateness
ıhanced the parent–child relationship.

Of course, midlife women who are single experience different sorts
: relationships with men and other women than their married peers.
'omen in the 1947 and 1962 Radcliffe classes reported happy surprise at
ıding romance and fulfilling love relationships in their 30s, 40s, and
)s. These relationships could be characterized as less sex-role-stereo-
ped and more companionate than earlier marriages or relationships.
eliance on women friends, often from college, was strong, especially
nong single women. These friends formed a support network rivaling
' sbustituting for family relationships, particularly for the 1962 cohort.

HE AMBIVALENCE SURROUNDING MIDLIFE

Not only is midlife an ambiguous phase, as illustrated by the fluid-
y of its upper boundary, the lack of consensus on the timing of certain
'e events, the multiplicity of markers used to define the midlife experi-
ıce, and the lack of any conceptual framework embedding midlife in
ıe life cycle, but individuals feel ambivalent about it as well. To become
ı adult is often seen as equivalent to the end of exploration and
:owth. The adolescent perceives the adult world as muted rather than
.vid, dead rather than passionate and alive. This is reflected in the
ıllowing quote:

> To much of the public . . . the mode of authority in America, the mode that
> deals with real experience, the mode that is neither dead (as the adult mode

> seems to be) nor compromised (as the childish world of television seems to
> be), is the adolescent mode—mode of exploration, becoming, growth, and
> pain. (Troll, 1982)

The author is suggesting that even adults agree with the unspoke
premise that to be adult is to be grown up and "mature" in the sense c
having closed all doors to exploration. If popular opinion assigns suc
attributes as aliveness, excitement, and growth to the young, what re
mains for the rest of us—stodginess, inertia, absence of feeling? Eve
though adulthood is perceived this way in literature, the media, an
even research, most individual adults would state that they valu
growth and perceive pain as a measure of progress (Spacks, 1981). How
ever, even if individuals perceive their own lives to be rich and intense
at the same time their general perception of adulthood reflects the nc
tion of "living death." Thus, the private experience of adults may b
very different from the public view of adults. This is why the study c
the midlife experience as embedded in the life cycle is so important, as
illustrates the possibility of growth and change throughout life. Howev
er, popular conceptions of midlife suggest that growth is truncated fc
women but not for men.

It is not surprising that adults may be ambivalent about the onset c
midlife, given that they share the general belief in midlife as a negativ
event or a nonevent, even in the face of contradictory evidence fror
their own and their friends' lives. Direct contradiction to this pessimist
view of adulthood is also being put forth by a variety of authors today
as seen in this volume. Midlife may be a time of great growth, expar
sion, and satisfaction.

A large part of the ambivalence about midlife is probably due to th
feelings and experiences related to physiological changes associate
with aging. Much of the life-course research on adulthood either ignore
or denies these effects, although Rossi (1980) recently has made an ele
quent plea for the inclusion of biological change into our models of adu
development. Not only do physiological events need to be studied wit
regard to co-occurrence with social and psychological events, but won
en's perceptions about such changes need to be explored.

In a study of 68 women aged 33 to 56 and their families, Rossi (198
asked the women what age they would most like to be. Not surprisin
ly, none wanted to be older. One-half wished to be under 30. The mea
desired age was 32 to 33 years, regardless of the current age of th
woman. Rossi found that while chronological age did not predict th
desired age, the actual symptoms of aging did (eyesight, shape of bod
condition of teeth, energy level). In addition, having a large famil
being older when the first child was born, and being less educate
contributed to the desire to be younger. Analyses of the individual cor

ributions of factors such as attractiveness, fatigue, and medical prob-
ems to negative feelings about one's actual age or to the desire to be
ounger would provide needed information about the ambivalence sur-
ounding midlife.

Finally, it is commonly believed that by midlife there is no plot line
eft for women, or that the plot line is completely predicated upon the
woman's marital and parental status. (The plot line is as follows: Leave
ather's home, enter husband's home, rear children; the rest of the plot
emains unfinished.). If women are defined only in relationship to oth-
rs (children and husband), then the end of parenting is the termination
f their plot line. However, with the advent of multiple roles for midlife
women, especially that of employment, a new plot line may be written
hat focuses on achievement and creativity. In fact, Heilbrun (Chapter 3)
rgues that the central theme of midlife for women is achievement,
ather than relationships. Men, she claims, have known about the im-
ortance of achievement for a long time. She advocates that women take
nto account the possibility for enlarging the sphere of work during
midlife. This view may be a reaction to the tacit assumption that midlife
women continue their role as the bearers of responsibilities to the fami-
y, with the additional concerns of older parents taking the place of
arenting. Instead of arguing that midlife offers the possibility of work
atisfaction, one might argue that this possibility exists throughout the
fe-span. The processes by which women are limited in their achieve-
ent of such satisfaction may be similar across the life-span, rather than
eing specific to each stage.

REFERENCES

art, P. B. Mother Portnoy's complaints. *Trans-Action*, 1970, *8*(1–2), 69–74.
im, O. G., and Baltes, P. (Eds.). *Life span developments and behavior* (Vol. 5). New York:
    Academic Press, in press.
im, O. G., and Kagan, J. *Constancy and change in human development.* Cambridge, Mass.:
    Harvard University Press, 1980.
im, O. G., and Ryff, C. *On the properties of life events. Kurt Levin memorial address.* Paper
    presented at the APA Meetings, New York, September 1979.
rody, E. "Women in the middle" and family help to older people. *Gerontologist*, 1981, *21*,
    471–485.
rooks-Gunn, J., and Ruble, D. N. The development of menstrual-related beliefs and
    behaviors during early adolescence. *Child Development*, 1982, *53*, 1567–1577.
rooks-Gunn, J., and Ruble, D. N. The experience of menarche from a developmental
    perspective. In J. Brooks-Gunn and A. Petersen (Eds.), *Girls at puberty: Biological and
    psychosocial perspectives.* New York: Plenum, 1983.
ichorn, D. H., Clausen, J. A., Haan, N., Honzik, M. P., and Mussen, P. H. (Eds.). *Present
    and past in middle life.* New York: Academic Press, 1981.
lder, G. H. *Children of the Great Depression.* Chicago: University of Chicago Press, 1974.

Furstenberg, F. F., Jr. *Unplanned parenthood*. New York: Free Press, 1976. General Mills Company. *General Mills Family Report*, 1977.

Hareven, T. (Ed.). *Transitions: The family and the life course in historical perspective*. New York: Academic Press, 1978.

Jones, L. *Great expectations: America and the baby boom generation*. New York: Coward Press, 1980.

Levinson, D. J. *The seasons of a man's life*. New York: Ballantine Books, 1978.

Maccoby, E. E., and Jacklin, C. N. *The psychology of sex differences*. Stanford: Stanford University Press, 1974.

Neugarten, B. L. Time, age and life cycle. *American Journal of Psychiatry*, 1979, *136*, 887–894.

New York Times. December 18, 1982.

Riley, M. A. Aging and cohort succession: Interpretations and misinterpretations. *Public Opinion Quarterly*, 1973, *37*, 35–49.

Rossi, A. S. Life-span theories in women's lives. *Signs*, 1980, *6*, 4–32.

Rossi, A. S. Aging and parenthood in the middle years. In P. Baltes and O. Brim (Eds.), *Life span development and behavior*. New York: Academic Press, 1981.

Rubin, L. *Women of a certain age*. New York: Harper, 1-79.

Ryder, N. B. The cohort as a concept in the study of social change. *American Sociological Review*, 1965, *30*, 843–861.

Spacks, P. M. *The adolescent idea*. New York: Basic Books, 1981.

Tobin-Richards, M. H., Boxer, A. M., and Petersen, A. The psychological significance of pubertal change: Sex differences in perceptions of self during early adolescence. In J. Brooks-Gunn and A. Petersen (Eds.), *Girls at puberty: Biological and psychosocial perspectives*. New York: Plenum Press, 1983.

Troll, L. *Continuations: Adult development and aging*. Monterey, Calif.: Brooks/Cole, 1982.

Uhlenberg, P. Changing configurations of the life course. In T. Hareven (Ed.), *Transitions: The family and the life course in historical perspective*. New York: Academic Press, 1978.

Vaillant, G. E. *Adaptation to life: How the best and the brightest came of age*. Boston: Little, Brown, 1977.

Zadeh, P. *Radcliffe Alumnae Quarterly*, 1975.

Chapter 2

Methods for a Life-Span Developmental Approach to Women in the Middle Years

Margie E. Lachman

The central thesis of this chapter[1] is that the study of women in midlife can be enriched if it is placed in a change-oriented, life-span framework. This message is conveyed by the title of this book—*Women in Midlife*—which places middle age in the context of the life span. The book's title also conveys a message about the current state of the field of life-span human development. Until recently, researchers have focused primarily on the young and the old. Thus, there is a gap in our knowledge about the middle of the life-span. This neglect of the middle years is particularly true with regard to the study of women, but the situation is slowly being rectified (see Baruch, Barnett, and Rivers, 1983; Eichorn, Clausen, Haan, Honzik, and Mussen, 1981; Giele, 1982; Lowenthal, Thurnher, and Chiriboga, 1975; Rossi, 1980; Rubin, 1979; Stewart and Platt, 1982; as well as this volume).

This chapter suggests an organizing conceptual framework and compatible methodological procedures for the study of women in midlife. First, conceptual features of a life-span developmental view are presented. Second, two measurement topics are discussed: (a) reliability of change and (b) age-related validities. Third, two research topics are presented: (c) multidimensionality of change and (d) research designs

I would like to thank Avron Spiro III and John R. Nesselroade for their helpful comments on an earlier version of this chapter.

MARGIE E. LACHMAN • Psychology Department, Brandeis University, Waltham, Massachusetts 02254.

for the study of development. For each topic, some of the common pitfalls that plague developmental researchers are presented and recommendations for overcoming these problems are proposed. Methodological points are illustrated with examples from research on personality and intellectual functioning in adulthood.

Since only a limited number of issues can be addressed within the confines of a single chapter, this chapter is a selective rather than a comprehensive presentation of developmental research methods. In particular, methodological issues and exemplary topics from life-span developmental psychology are emphasized. For the interested reader, a number of sources provide a broader coverage of developmental methodology (e.g., Achenbach, 1978; Baltes, Reese, and Nesselroade, 1977; Wohlwill, 1973). Although the chapter's content is primarily derived from a psychological perspective, the issues raised should be applicable to those from other disciplines who are interested in the study of women in midlife and in the critical evaluation of research on this subject. One of the advantages of adopting a life-span developmental approach for the study of midlife is that it is a pluralistic and multidisciplinary perspective. Indeed, the life-span perspective, which will be discussed in the next section, has its counterparts in a number of fields other than psychology, including sociology, economics, history, and biology (Baltes, Reese, and Lipsitt, 1980).[2]

LIFE-SPAN DEVELOPMENTAL APPROACH

What features of a life-span developmental approach can be useful for research on women in the middle years? In this section the basic assumptions and characteristics of a life-span developmental approach are presented and applied to the study of women in midlife (Baltes *et al.*, 1980; Brim and Kagan, 1980; Lerner and Ryff, 1978). The goals of life-span research are to examine the nature and course of development and to search for the antecedents and consequences of developmental change. Life-span researchers engage in the description, explanation, and optimization of development. One of the basic assumptions of a life-span view is that development occurs throughout life. This assumption, however, cannot be subjected to empirical scrutiny without specifying a definition of development.

Definition of Development

Within a life-span view, the definition of development is less restrictive than that usually associated with child development perspec-

[2]The descriptive term, *life-course*, rather than *life-span*, has been used in sociology, history, and economics (Elder, 1978; Rossi, 1980).

ves (Lerner, 1976; Harris, 1957). In child development models, evelopment typically is characterized by the presence of stages, an nd-state orientation, structural reorganization, invariant sequences, nd unidirectional and universal changes (Flavell, 1970; Kohlberg, 1969; Vohlwill, 1973). This view has come to be known as the "strong" model f development. In contrast, a "weak" view of development includes ny change that is reliable in its definition of development (Baer, 1970). 1 the most extreme version of the "weak" view, change and development are synonymous.

In a life-span view, development is represented along a continuum f change rather than at either the "strong" or the "weak" extreme 3altes and Nesselroade, 1979). A life-span view imposes fewer retrictions than many child development models for classifying change as evelopment. According to a life-span conception, developmental hanges during adulthood may be characterized by multidirectionality, eversibility, and variability (nonuniversality) across individuals, cultures, and historical time. This broader definition of development may nclude structural reorganization, invariant sequences, and other features that are characteristic of child-oriented viewpoints, but other forms f change are also included (Reese and Overton, 1970; Looft, 1973). ndeed, some researchers have applied stage models to the study of dult personality development (e.g., Erikson, 1963; Labouvie-Vief, 1982; evinson, 1978; Vaillant, 1977). Even when stage models are applied to 1e study of adulthood, however, they may take on forms different from 1ose associated with the structural-cognitive models of child development (e.g., Piaget, Werner). For instance, adult models often include the pecification of an invariant sequence, but not of structural reorganizaon (Levinson, 1978). Others have found that normative stage models re less useful for studying adult development and instead have focused n nonnormative life events as an organizing framework for the study of dult development (Hultsch and Plemons, 1979). The pluralistic concepon of a life-span developmental perspective allows for the possibility of 1ultiple influences and diverse outcomes.

ources of Development

The diverse nature and course of life-span development has its rigins in the interaction of biological (heredity) and environmental (experiential) factors. According to the model developed by Baltes and his olleagues (Baltes, Cornelius, and Nesselroade, 1979; Baltes et al., 1980), eredity and experience are the underlying determinants of three major ets of influences that control development: (a) normative age-graded, ɔ) normative history-graded, and (c) nonnormative.

Normative age-graded influences are those that occur regularly within a culture with respect to timing and duration in the life-span. The menopause is one example of a normative age-graded developmental phenomenon for women in midlife. Normative history-graded events are those that occur in a uniform way for the majority of members of a given cohort.[3] The effects of historical change may be reflected in birth cohort differences. By definition, different cohorts are exposed to different historical/cultural events and they experience the same event at different points in the life-span. The Great Depression, for instance, was found to have long-term (i.e., from childhood to old age) consequences for women (Elder and Liker, 1982) and a differential impact for the 1920 and 1928 birth cohorts (Elder, 1979). Finally, nonnormative events are those that do not follow a regular pattern but rather can occur at any time for any person or group. These events may include rare occurrences, such as diseases (e.g., Parkinson's disease) or an earthquake, as well as more common events when they occur at unexpected or non traditional times in the life-span (e.g., early widowhood or returning to school in midlife). Baltes *et al.* (1980) have speculated that age-graded influences are more salient, relative to other influences, in child development and late old age, whereas during midlife, nonnormative events are expected to be the most important set of influences. However, further research is needed to examine the interactive role of the three primary sources of development and their impact at different points in the life-span.

VARIABILITY AND PLASTICITY IN DEVELOPMENT. It has been proposed that age- and history-graded influences and nonnormative life events interact to produce the differential and normative patterns that are characteristic of life-span development (Baltes *et al.*, 1980). In response to their joint effects, life-span development is characterized by both regularity and variability. Thus, within a life-span view, development during the middle years may reflect a great deal of regularity, but also interindividual (between-person) variability and intraindividual (within person) plasticity (Baltes and Baltes, 1980). Interindividual differences can take on meaning at a number of different levels within a life-span view. One form of interindividual variability can be found at the level of cohort. Between-cohort differences can be a marker of historical-cultural changes. Consider a hypothetical example using the dimension of life satisfaction. In Figure 1A it is shown how two cohorts of women may differ in level of satisfaction and in the direction and course of change Cohort 2 is always more satisfied with life than Cohort 1; moreover

[3]The term *cohort* is used throughout this chapter to refer to birth cohort, that is, those who are born during the same period of time. In general, cohort can refer to any group of individuals that experiences a given event within the same time period.

Figure 1. (A) Between-cohort differences in life satisfaction change over two occasions. (B) Within-cohort differences in life satisfaction by socioeconomic status (SES) over two occasions.

Cohort 2 becomes more satisfied over time, whereas Cohort 1 does not change in level of satisfaction over the life-span.

Another form of interindividual variability can be found at the intra-cohort (within-cohort) level. In Figure 1B we see that for Cohort 1, the middle-class women are always higher in life satisfaction than the lower-class women, and the former group increases in satisfaction as the members get older, whereas the lower-class women become less satisfied as they age. These data illustrate that variability is possible at many levels. Elder (1979) has shown that the personality development of women may vary as a function of their birth cohort, and that within cohorts, patterns of development may be further differentiated according to factors such as social class and educational status.

Although we may be able to obtain an accurate description of age and cohort differences in change, both age and cohort are merely markers or indexes for underlying processes. Identification of age- and cohort-related change does not tell anything about the how and why of development. It is for this reason that several researchers have challenged the role of age and cohort as the primary organizing variables for life-span developmental psychology (Wohlwill, 1970). To go beyond the level of description of cohort differences requires theoretically guided models and explanatory methods. The methods and interpretations will depend on the status that is assigned to the cohort variable (Baltes *et al.* 1979). In psychology, cohort differences are usually considered in terms of limitations on external validity. Are the results found for one cohort applicable to other cohorts? For sociologists, however, cohort usually is a theoretically meaningful variable that requires explanation. Why do cohorts develop differently? Elder (1979) has suggested that one way to shed light on cohort differences is to examine subgroups within cohorts. Analysis of group differences in exposure to various events or experiences can provide useful information about the processes underlying cohort differences.

In addition to differences in change patterns between persons, a life-span view acknowledges and seeks to chart within-individual variability or plasticity (Baltes and Baltes, 1980). There is an emphasis placed on determining the range of potential behaviors that could be achieved and the conditions under which optimal development can be realized (Denney, 1982). To accomplish this, research efforts should be directed at identifying the antecedents of developmental change. Knowledge about various influences on development can have direct implications for intervention and treatment programs. Within a life-span view, a strong emphasis is placed on preventive and optimization, rather than remedial, forms of intervention (Danish, Smyer, and Nowak, 1980; Turner and Reese, 1980).

Life-Span Development and Women in Midlife

Although the origins of a life-span development view have been traced to the 18th century (see Baltes, 1979; Reinert, 1979), its application to the study of women in midlife is a more recent endeavor (Giele, 1982; Neugarten, 1968; Rossi, 1980). One emphasis of a life-span view is on the dynamic nature of middle age. The key factor is *change*, which can occur on a number of levels (e.g., individual, cultural) and in a variety of

ırms (e.g., differential, normative, qualitative, quantitative). In non-
evelopmental views, middle age often is defined in a static way with
xed chronological age boundaries. The most apparent weakness of
ïese latter views is evident just if one considers that the age range
ssociated with middle age varies widely across persons and cultures
ïhannon and Kedar, 1979–80).

A second emphasis suggested by a life-span approach is the com-
lexity of change patterns during midlife. In some nondevelopmental
pproaches, midlife is approached in terms of a series of events (e.g.,
ıenopause, "empty nest," widowhood) without regard to the context
ı which these events occur. A life-span view focuses on the interre-
tionships among different events and areas (e.g., family, work) of life
ïlder, 1978). The empty nest, for example, cannot be fully understood
ınless something is known about other aspects of a woman's life. For
ʌample, we would want to know information about her relationship
ıth her children when they were at home, the quality of her marital
ʌlationship, whether she is working outside of the home, her health
ʌatus, whether she has a sick parent to care for, and other factors.

A third emphasis of the life-span approach is that each period of life
 part of an integrated whole. Thus, middle age cannot be treated as an
ɔlated period. In some cases, early experiences may be transformed by
ter experiences (discontinuity). In other cases, experiences in midlife
ʌay be a direct outgrowth of earlier events (continuity). A fourth em-
ʌasis of a life-span view is on the historical and cultural relativity of
evelopment; development is embedded within a historical context.
ʌhat holds true for a cohort of middle-aged persons in one histor-
ʌl–cultural context may not hold for those in other contexts.

esearch Issues

To summarize, life-span developmental researchers are concerned
ith the description, explanation, and optimization of behavior-change
ɔocesses that occur from birth to death. It is recognized that develop-
ent may be multidirectional, multidimensional, and variable. More-
ʌer, development occurs at both the individual and societal levels. A
ımber of methodological challenges arise in life-span research because
 these features. Four goals for life-span research are considered here.
rst, it is necessary to adopt techniques that enable the reliable mea-
ırement of change. A second task for life-span researchers is to devel-
ɔ and utilize measurement instruments that are valid for the age range
 be studied. Third, it is important to employ designs that can capture
ʌe complexity and diversity of change. A fourth priority is to identify

methods for examining individual and cultural/historical patterns o
change. In the remainder of this chapter, research methods that ca
assist in accomplishing these four objectives will be considered.

Measurement Issues

Researchers have identified two broad classes of measurement: (1
open-ended or unstructured and (2) fixed-choice or structured. Both c
these measurement strategies are potentially useful for the study c
women in midlife. For exploratory work, open-ended questions are gen
erally desirable because they do not limit the respondents' range c
answer choices. Open-ended responses can be usefully applied in deve
oping fixed-choice questions or they can be subjected to an objectiv
coding system in order to quantify the responses. For descriptive an
explanatory hypothesis-testing, structured measurement is usuall
more appropriate. In this format, respondents are given specific choice
from which to select answers. In the domain of personality assessmen
for example, three types of structured data sources have been identifie
(Block, 1977; Cattell, 1965). These are life-ratings (e.g., checklists of dai
activities or moods, behavioral observations), questionnaires (e.g., se
report personality inventories), and objective tests (e.g., experiment;
tasks). Regardless of the particular form of inquiry, there are two mea
surement issues that must be addressed: reliability and validity of mea
surement. The following discussion will focus on issues of reliability an
validity that have particular relevance for developmental research. I
order to address these specific issues, however, it will be useful to beg
by presenting a general overview of the reliability and validity concept

Assessment of Reliable Change

The primary goals of life-span research are the identification and th
explication of change processes. A necessary prerequisite to fulfillin
these goals is to achieve reliable measurement. Measurement reliabili
implies accuracy, precision, and consistency in the assignment of nun
bers to characterize behavior. The assessment of reliability provides a
index of the accuracy of measurement. According to classical measur
ment theory (Lord and Novick, 1968), if a measure is reliable, a respons
or recorded outcome should be repeatable. There are many factors th
can interfere with measurement accuracy, and, in practice, measur
ments always contain some degree of error. It is unsystematic or rando
fluctuations that contribute to unreliability of measurement. For instanc
random variation in measurement may result from extraneous facto
related to the testing conditions, the experimenter, or the subjects (Nu

ally, 1978). These random fluctuations or measurement errors must be istinguished from systematic changes across occasions. The latter, so-illed true changes, are not troublesome in terms of measurement relia-ility and, moreover, are at the very heart of developmental analyses. As 'ill become apparent throughout this discussion, one of the notable tasks iat faces the developmental researcher is the separation of "true" devel-pmental changes from unsystematic or unreliable fluctuations in scores. Iethods for separating systematic and unsystematic changes will be resented after a brief discussion of reliability.

Several methods can be applied to the analysis of measurement ›liability. Each of these forms takes into account different information ›out the sources of random fluctuations (Ghiselli, Campbell, and edeck, 1981). The decision to use a given method should be based on ıe's research goals as well as on the measurement information that is ⁄ailable. The four most common forms of reliability are consistency est–retest), equivalence (alternate forms), homogeneity (internal con-stency), and interrater agreement. Space limitations make it impossible ⟩ go into detail on these aspects of reliability. For those readers who are ıterested in a more in-depth coverage of reliability issues, any of the ıllowing are useful sources: American Psychological Association (1974); nastasi (1968); Ghiselli et al. (1981); Lord and Novick (1968); Nunnally 978).

RELIABILITY VERSUS CHANGE. We will concentrate our discussion on ıe consistency form of reliability because of the unique problem it raises r the developmental researcher. Consistency reliability is frequently ferred to as test-retest reliability, since it is calculated as the correlation ›tween two administrations of the same test. As such, it is an index of ıe degree to which scores remain constant over time. To the extent that measure is consistent, individuals should receive the same score on ·peated administrations over short time intervals (e.g., 1 week, 1 onth).

For the developmental researcher, perhaps the most serious draw-ıck of this form of reliability is that it confounds true change in the easured attribute with error of measurement in the scale. The retest ·rrelation coefficient indicates the degree to which individuals main-in their relative rank ordering over time. In the context of reliability, if e estimate is relatively low, this is taken as evidence that the instru-ent is unreliable. However, such an outcome also could reflect legiti-ate rank-order change in a reliably measured dimension; that is, peo-e may actually change their relative status on a given dimension. To inimize the extent of "true" change in reliability assessments, the easurement specialist usually recommends that the retest coefficient · estimated within a relatively short (e.g., 1-month) period. This strat-

egy will be effective in controlling change in many cases since few di
mensions would be expected to undergo systematic change over such i
short time period. There are, however, some problems that arise with
this strategy. First, if the retest interval is too short, the subjects may
remember their responses and thereby create an illusion of reliability by
recording the same responses from memory. Second, there are instance
(such as when assessing moods or other psychological states) whe
short-term, even daily, changes would be entirely possible and likely
For example, emotional states such as anxiety have been found to un
dergo short-term changes (Nesselroade and Bartsch, 1977). Under such
circumstances, the consistency reliability index makes it difficult to sepa
rate "true" change from measurement error. If a state anxiety inventor
was administered on two occasions over a 2-day period and a relativel
low (e.g., .30) retest correlation was found, this could be a result c
unreliability of the anxiety scale that was used, but it also could b
indicative of change in the mood of anxiety. In situations where short
term developmental changes or mood fluctuations are anticipated, th
use of the test-retest form of reliability assessment is contraindicated
Other forms, such as homogeneity, are usually more appropriate unde
these circumstances.

Stability

To deal with the confounding of measurement error and change
developmental researchers have made a useful distinction between th
reliability of a measure and the stability of a phenomenon (Baltes et al
1977). Reliability refers to whether an instrument is measuring an a
tribute in a repeatable or consistent manner. Stability, however, de
scribes the nature and extent of change in the dimension that is bein
measured. Note that high stability describes the "no change" end of th
continuum, and its opposite, lability, implies change or low stability
    The conceptual distinction between reliability and stability is usefu
since change is viewed as a phenomenon of interest, rather than as
form of error, in developmental research. One operational problem tha
has been noted in developmental analyses is the difficulty in separatin
random from true sources of fluctuations in scores. Test–retest reliabilit
is operationally equivalent to the stability coefficient since both are con
puted as the correlation between performances on the same instrume
on two occasions.
    As an index of change, the stability coefficient reflects the degree
which the individual rank orders in scores have changed over time.
there are changes in rank order, this is indicative of interindividu
differences in change. Consider a case where a scale of life satisfaction

dministered on two occasions at a 1-month interval and the stability orrelation coefficient is .35. If this is the only reliability information that s available, it would be difficult to determine whether people had hanged in their life satisfaction or the assessment of life satisfaction was nreliable. Therefore, we need to obtain a reliability estimate such as the plit-half index of homogeneity, which controls for cross-occasion fluc- uations. Let us assume in this case that the split-half index was .85. his provides evidence that the assessment is fairly reliable according to omogeneity criteria, and, therefore, there is reason to attribute the ifferences in scores to reliable interindividual changes in life satisfac- on over time.

For some time now, researchers have noted the challenges that face ie developmental researcher in separating legitimate change from oise in measurement (Bereiter, 1963). Several sophisticated procedures ave been developed to carry out this task (e.g., Carmines and Zeller, 979; Heise, 1969; Jöreskog, 1979; Wheaton, Múthen, Alwin, and Sum- iers, 1977). While these methods require familiarity with concepts that re beyond the scope of the present chapter, they should be examined y the reader who is interested in learning about techniques for the eparation of unreliability and change.

One simple procedure for aiding the diagnosis of change, the cor- ection for attenuation, will be suggested here. The correction for at- nuation is based on the assumption that reliability of a measure marks ie upper-bound limit for a correlation involving that measure (Ghiselli al., 1981). The correlation between two measures cannot exceed the roduct of the square roots of the reliabilities of the two measures. Thus, nce a stability coefficient is a correlation between the same measure on vo occasions, it is restricted by the measure's reliability. For example, if life satisfaction scale has an internal consistency of .92 at occasion 1 id .90 at occasion 2, the stability coefficient could not exceed .91 ($\sqrt{.92}$ $\sqrt{.90}$). If the stability estimate is .49 in our example, this is indicative f change, since .91 is the upper bound given the reliabilities. An esti- ate of stability is meaningful only when considered in relation to relia- lity. For instance, the same stability of .49 could be indicative of no liable change (high stability) if the internal consistency of the life satis- ction scale at each occasion was .50. Note that the problem with using ily the statistical significance for interpreting change is that even if the ability coefficient is different from zero, it may be indicative of change. the example above, a coefficient of .49, although statistically signifi- int with a sample of 15 or more, should be interpreted as reliable iange if the reliability is high. Indeed, with a stability coefficient of .49, ily 24% of the variance at occasion 2 can be accounted for by occasion 1 ores.

The correction for attenuation is a procedure that places the stability coefficient within the context of measurement reliability (Nunnally 1978). It involves making an adjustment to a correlation, in this case the stability, to compensate for measurement error. The correction for attenuation estimates the stability correlation under the assumption that reliability at both occasions is perfect (i.e., 1.0). To continue with the life satisfaction example in which the reliabilities are .90 and .92, if we had corrected for attenuation, the .49 stability would increase to .54. If the reliability at both occasions had been .50, the stability estimate of .4 when corrected would increase to .98. In general, the lower the reliabilities of the measures, the greater the effects of the correction for attenuation on the correlation coefficient.

Several researchers have pointed out the importance of correcting for attenuation in personality research, where often the reliabilities of measures are relatively low (.30 to .50) (Block, 1977; Epstein, 1979). Without correcting for measurement error, it is possible that the degree of stability will be underestimated, as illustrated in the above example. The goal of such efforts is to get the most accurate measurement possible and at the same time to permit sensitivity to developmental changes. must be noted that stability is always a relative phenomenon, and in isolation the stability coefficient is not a meaningful index (Wohlwill 1973). Reliability of measurement provides a useful standard for the evaluation of stability versus change.

Validity of Measurement

In addition to reliability of measurement, a major goal for researchers is to achieve validity of measurement. Validity refers to the degree to which an instrument measures what it is intended to measure. The relationship between reliability and validity is sometimes overlooked by researchers. Reliability is a necessary, but not a sufficient condition for validity of measurement. If a measure is not accurate or consistent, it cannot be considered valid; however, even if a measure reliable, this does not assure its validity. Before the validity of an instrument can be assessed, its purpose or goals must be specified. Traditionally, discussions of measurement validity have focused on three classical forms—content, criterion-related, and construct validity (American Psychological Association, 1974; Ghiselli et al., 1981; Nunnall 1978).

Developmental Issues of Measurement Validity. Because life span developmental research involves the assessment of behavior across multiple age groups and multiple occasions, a number of special validity concerns arise. These issues are referred to here as age-related lidity and structural validity. Like the traditional forms, they focus on hether a measure is measuring what it is supposed to measure. However, since developmental research involves age and time comparisons, Iditional questions arise as to whether a measure is valid for different ;e groups or on different occasions. Although these aspects of validity e singled out here as of particular concern for developmental research 1 women in midlife, they may be considered special cases of the classi- il validity forms. Thus, to understand fully the nature of age-related 1d structural validities, the reader should be familiar with the tradi-)nal validity forms mentioned above.

Age-Related Validity. One of the challenges facing the researcher of e-span development is how to measure the same construct in multiple ;e groups. If one is interested in how a given phenomenon such as tachment (see Lerner and Ryff, 1978) develops from birth to death, it comes important to determine how to measure the construct in a eaningful way for the entire range of age groups that will be exam- ed. The problem is particularly salient in the study of middle age and ;ing because the majority of measures have been developed and stan- irdized on children and young adult samples; thus, the validities for iddle and older age groups are unknown.

The age-validity problem has been clearly illustrated with the case psychometric intelligence (Baltes and Willis, 1979). Intelligence tests nerally have been carefully developed and standardized for the pur- se of predicting school performance in children and adolescents. Nev- theless, researchers have employed these same instruments to study anges in intelligence in middle and old age, without first determining eir meaning for these age groups (Labouvie-Vief, 1977). Results based the inappropriate use of intelligence tests or other measures may be isleading. If middle-aged adults score lower on a test than college 1dents, does this mean that they have less intelligence or is it an ference based on improper measurement? Rather than continue to ply youth-centered criteria and standards for evaluating intellectual rformance in middle and old age, researchers have begun to ask: hat are the proper criterion measures for middle age (Labouvie-Vief d Chandler, 1978)? For example, Schaie (1977–1978) has suggested at in middle age, the function of intelligence is to integrate long-range als and to solve real-life problems. Thus, measurement instruments ould include content that is related to these aspects of functioning.

Two general strategies can be used to deal with the age-validity oblem. The first is to conduct studies that are aimed at validation of isting measures for age ranges that were not included in initial scale velopment procedures. For example, Costa and McCrae (1980) have amined the usefulness for middle- and old-aged adults of the 16 Per-

sonality Factors inventory originally validated by Cattell, Eber, and Tat
suoka (1970) for young adult samples. In their investigations of the
factor structure of the 16 PF, they found the same personality factors a
all age levels and concluded that the inventory is valid for middle- and
older-aged adults. This procedure, whereby the validity of an extan
measure is determined for multiple age groups, has some drawbacks
First, this strategy does not allow for unique, age-specific dimensions
Second, test items are not always appropriate or predictive for a wid
age range.

An alternative to validating existing scales is to develop new age
specific measures for the constructs of interest (e.g., Lachman, Baltes
Nesselroade, and Willis, 1982). This allows for consideration of cor
structs that may be relevant only for a specific age group. Research b
Clayton and Birren (1980), for instance, has indicated that wisdom is
characteristic that is unique to later life. In the field of intellectual aging
Demming and Pressey (1957) recognized the need for age-specific mea
surement more than two decades ago. More recently, this need has bee
addressed by several researchers in the field of intellectual aging wh
have revived the search for meaningful measurement procedures an
more adequate criteria for evaluating performance in middle and old ag
(Quayhagen, Gonda, and Schaie, 1979; Popkin, Schaie, and Krause
1980; Schaie, 1978). These researchers have directed their efforts to th
development of age-relevant assessment devices in order to constru
measures that are ecologically valid for adults in middle and old age

In addition to not allowing for unique age-specific constructs, ar
other problem with trying to validate existing scales is that the item
may not be appropriate for all age groups. For example, when question
about behavior and habits in school are included in achievement mot
vation questionnaires, they are not likely to be meaningful for middl
aged adults. Achievement motivation can have a different meaning ar
may be manifested in different contexts (e.g., career) for middle-age
groups. This argues for developing age-specific measures for life-spa
research. A concern related to age validity is whether measures are vali
across sexes. Are questions that have been validated on males appropr
ate for females? As has been pointed out with regard to age, there ma
be constructs that are unique for one sex group, or the same variab
may take on different meanings for men and women. Many of th
theoretical constructs and measurement instruments for adult develoj
ment have been standardized on samples of males. One challenge th
faces researchers of women in the middle years is to determine th
validities of these existing theories and concepts for women. Another
to develop new conceptions of development that may or may not l
applicable to men (e.g., Gilligan, 1982).

Two solutions to the age- and sex-related validity problems have en suggested. The researcher is encouraged both to examine the valid-es of extant measures for middle- and old-aged and male and female mples and to develop new age- or sex-specific measures for the unique pects of women's adult development. Even if these two strategies are llowed, there still is a major validity issue that cannot easily be solved either. The problem arises because in many studies researchers are terested in comparing multiple age groups simultaneously. Therefore, e must consider whether the same construct is being measured at all e levels. This question of whether the same psychological measure is lid for multiple age groups is analogous to the pharmacological case, here the same drug may have different benefits or side effects when ministered to different age groups. In the realm of personality re-arch, this issue arises, for example, when a self-report item means mething different to members of different cohort groups. Consider an m from the Extraversion scale of the Eysenck Personality Inventory ysenck and Eysenck, 1963), which asks whether the respondent can go and enjoy gay parties. In my own experience with administering is scale, I have found a striking difference in the responses of college udents and older adults to this item: The majority of college re-ondents have asked for clarification as to the meaning intended by ;ay parties," whereas only one of all the older adult subjects did so. e college students were unclear whether the item referred to jolly rties or homosexual parties. The older respondents seemed to take the rmer interpretation for granted (or else they were more timid about king for clarification). As this example illustrates, the validation pro-ss must take into account that the meaning of an item, or the construct at it represents, may vary with the age or cohort of the respondents.

Cross-age validation requires careful construction and pilot-testing measures. One useful method for testing the age equivalence of mea-res is factor analysis. This procedure permits the assessment of hether measures have the same underlying structure or pattern for all ;es (Labouvie, 1980; Nesselroade, 1977). The confirmatory factor-anal-is method developed by Jöreskog (1979) is particularly applicable since enables the testing of the equivalence of a factor solution simul-neously for multiple groups (Jöreskog and Sörbom, 1978). The same chniques can be adopted for examining whether a measurement struc-re is equivalent for males and females. The multioccasion extension of e age-validity problem is referred to here as structural validity and is scussed in the next section.

Structural Validity. Structural validity or measurement equivalence /er time is another validity problem that commonly arises in life-span velopmental research. When an instrument is administered on multiple occasions in the context of a longitudinal study, the measuremer validity may be subject to change. For example, if the development creativity is studied by asking subjects to think of novel uses of commo objects on several occasions, does this task measure creativity in th same way on each occasion? The definition of creativity in this conte involves novel applications of familiar objects. If subjects are given th same task on repeated occasions, however, the task no longer involve novelty. Thus, the nature of the creativity assessment changes, and th task may become more a measure of memory than of creativity. Even different items (i.e., alternate forms) are used on each occasion, th validity of the task still may change due to the fact that the subjects a asked to "be creative" on more than one occasion.

Structural validity is related to age validity because, with longitud nal designs, people will necessarily be of different ages on each me surement occasion. The major difference is that the structural equi alence problem involves repeated assessment of the same persons and aimed at determining whether retesting changes the validity of a tes This phenomenon of the changing structural or measurement validity tests is similar to the internal validity problem of retesting, which will b discussed later.

In addition to changes in test structure over time, in longitudin research there is also the problem of the "aging of tests" (Gribbin an Schaie, 1977). In Schaie's longitudinal study of intelligence, the origin version of the Primary Mental Abilities (PMA) test (Thurstone an Thurstone, 1948) had been adopted at the first occasion of measuremer in 1959. By the second occasion of a measurement, the PMA had bee revised (Thurstone, 1962). Schaie (1979) noted that the original editio was better suited for the older cohorts but that the new version w more appropriate for the younger cohorts. This was particularly true f the verbal meaning subtest, because there are cohort differences in tl popular word meanings and frequency of word usage. In order to pr serve the longitudinal continuity of measures, Schaie decided to reta the 1948 edition for all subsequent measurement occasions. This dec sion was supported by the results of a study in which both the 1948 ar 1962 versions of the PMA were given to the youngest cohorts in tl longitudinal study (Gribbin and Schaie, 1977). By examining fact structures of the various subtests, the validity of the 1948 edition w found to be acceptable for the youngest cohorts. As mentioned for a validity, factor analysis is one useful method for checking the structur validity of a test. Factor-analysis procedures can be used to determir whether the internal structure of a measure and/or the correlatio among factors remain stable over time (Labouvie, 1980).

Summary

In this section we have discussed several key measurement issues that may confront researchers studying development during middle life. Reliability and validity are crucial in order to ensure accuracy and meaningfulness of one's measurements. Both reliability and validity, however, are sensitive to sampling, testing conditions, and other variable factors. Therefore, it is recommended that the reliability and validity of a measure to be investigated for every intended purpose (Nunnally, 1978). In developmental research, when multiple age groups and testing occasions are investigated, it is particularly important to investigate the reliability and validity of measurement for all groups. For example, it is unreasonable to assume that if a measure of achievement motivation is reliable or valid for college-aged males in 1960, it will be appropriate for middle-aged women in 1980. For this reason, examination of the measurement properties of instruments is critical in life-span developmental research. In the next sections we will focus on research design issues for the study of development in midlife.

RESEARCH DESIGN ISSUES

Multidimensionality of Change

As mentioned earlier, the study of adult development from a life-span perspective involves the description and explanation of intraindividual change and interindividual differences in change (Baltes et al., 1980). In order to gain a full and complete picture of development, it is useful to examine multiple aspects of change. In the following sections, several components of change are considered. Particular attention is devoted to two major categories: quantitative and qualitative changes (Baltes and Nesselroade, 1973). Quantitative change refers to differences in the magnitude or level of change, whereas qualitative change is represented by shifts in pattern or by reorganization of structure.

QUANTITATIVE CHANGE. Developmental studies, traditionally, have been focused on changes in the group average or the mean. There are, however, at least two other indices that are informative with regard to the quantitative description of change. These are the correlational stability index and the variance. Each of these components of change offers unique information, and when considered in concert, they can capture and illustrate the multidimensional nature of change.

In many accounts of adult development, researchers focus only on mean level changes. Although this kind of analysis provides relevant

information, it refers to only one aspect of change. It can indica
whether a group shows more or less of a given trait at different time
Examining change at the group level, however, may mask individu
changes. As can be seen in Figure 2A, it is possible for individuals to
change over time yet to have the mean level remain constant. Examina
tion of only group level changes in this case would obscure change at th
individual level. One way to obtain a more complete picture of indi
vidual change is to compute individual change scores (i.e., Occasion :
score minus Occasion 1 score).

The stability (test-retest) coefficient provides another meaningfu
index of individual changes (see earlier discussion of stability). Specifi
cally, it indicates the extent to which individuals maintain their relativ
rank orders over time. The stability coefficient is sensitive to individu
changes in rank orders; thus, a low stability coefficient is indicative o
interindividual differences in change. In Figure 2A, individuals' posi
tions have fluctuated from the first to the second occasion. This patter
is an example of high negative stability since those with high scores :
Occasion 1 have lower scores at Occasion 2 and those with low scores :
Occasion 1 have higher scores at Occasion 2. The outcome in Figure 2
presents a powerful case for considering multiple aspects of change. :
only the mean were examined, it would appear as if no change ha
occurred, whereas, in fact, at the individual level there was chang

Another picture of change is illustrated in Figure 2B. Here there :
perfect stability—i.e., rank orders are maintained—but the overall grou
mean has increased. Again, a focus on only one dimension would pre
sent a limited view of change versus stability. In Figures 2C and 2D, tw
other combinations are presented: respectively, mean change and lo
stability (rank-order change) and no change in either mean or ran
order. These examples illustrate how consideration of multiple aspec
of change can enrich the study of development and provide a mor
complete picture.

A third component of change is represented by the variance of
measure. The variance is a marker of the extent of individual di
ferences. As such, it allows for comparison of variability across ag
groups and occasions. Several researchers have considered whether in
terindividual variability increases with aging (Baltes et al., 1980; Frie
and Crapo, 1981). The focus of this inquiry has been on comparir
estimates of the variance of a measure for young and old age groups. T
date, the variance has been given very little attention as an index o
change. Moreover, few studies even contain information about the vari
ance (Bornstein and Smircina, 1982).

QUALITATIVE CHANGE. Although most research questions are fo
mulated in terms of quantitative aspects of change, there is another clas

Figure 2. Intraindividual change and interindividual differences in change over two occasions: (A) no average change and high negative stability; (B) average change and high correlational stability; (C) average change and low correlational stability; (D) no average change and high correlational stability. Based on Baltes, Reese, and Nesselroade (1977).

of questions that have as their focus changes in structure or pattern. Th approach to change requires a multivariate approach since it involv consideration of changing relationships among several variables.

The factor-analytic model is one approach that easily lends itself the examination of qualitative change. In a factor-analysis framewor structural changes can be manifested in terms of changes in factor pa terns (e.g., number of factors, patterns of factor loadings) or the fact correlation matrix. For further discussion of qualitative changes with the factor model framework, see Baltes and Nesselroade (1973) Nesselroade (1977).

Research on the integration-differentiation-reintegration hypothes of intellectual development (Reinert, 1970) illustrates the application factor analysis to examine structural change components. This hypot esis states that during the life-span the organization of intellectual abi ties changes from a general, undifferentiated, or global intelligence to more specialized, multidimensional intelligence, and later to a new for where abilities are again more integrated. Baltes, Cornelius, Spir Nesselroade, and Willis (1980) found that the structure of intelligence old age is represented by fewer factors and by higher intercorrelatio between factors than have been found in young adults. The data, the support the hypothesis that, with aging, there are structural chang that are reflective of a reintegration in intellectual functioning.

Structural changes in intelligence and in other domains are an i teresting substantive research focus in their own right. In the "stron conceptions of development, as discussed earlier, development involv structural reorganization of behavior over time (Kohlberg, 1969). Tl investigation of structural change, however, is also desirable from methodological standpoint. It is recommended that structural invarian of a construct be demonstrated prior to examining quantitative aspec of change (Baltes and Nesselroade, 1973). It is necessary to establish th the same construct is being measured at different occasions and/or different groups before examining increments or decrements in th dimension. Empirically, of course, it is possible to have both structur and quantitative changes. However, if there is both structural reorg nization and quantitative change, it is difficult to know how to interpr quantitative increases and decreases in scores (Baltes and Nesselroad 1973). For example, reports of intellectual declines in adulthood must I interpreted with caution if these dimensions are also undergoing stru tural changes. Under these circumstances, the entire nature or structu of intelligence has changed.

In summary, consideration of both quantitative and qualitative a pects of change should enable the researcher to capture the multidime sionality, multidirectionality, and complexity of life-span developmer

though changes in level are the most commonly studied, examination
correlational stability as well as structural aspects may shed additional
ht on midlife development. It is interesting to consider that at differ-
t points in the life span certain forms of change may be more preva-
t. Schaie (1977–78) has proposed a model for the life-span develop-
nt of cognitive functioning in which qualitative changes occur from
late 30s to the early 60s and quantitative intellectual changes occur in
rly and late adulthood. He suggests that the structural changes in
gnitive functioning during the middle years yield a new pattern,
ich facilitates integrating long-range goals as well as solving real-life
oblems with greater flexibility. Some researchers have proposed that
re is structural reorganization in cognitive functioning throughout
adult years (e.g., Labouvie-Vief, 1977, 1982), while others have sug-
sted that there are few or no structural changes in adulthood (Flavell,
70). Use of the methods described here would enable the researcher to
t empirically these various positions on the nature of midlife de-
lopment.

In this section, several forms and indices of change have been dis-
ssed. Since each component adds a unique piece of information about
 nature of change and development, it is useful to examine as many
ms of quantitative and qualitative change as is possible. However,
re are specific design requirements that are necessary in order to
nsider certain change components. For example, the stability coeffi-
nt can be examined only in longitudinal studies since multiple occa-
ns of measurement are required to compute the stability coefficient.
raindividual changes in level, variance, or structure also can be stud-
 only within a longitudinal framework. In cross-sectional studies, it is
ssible to look only at interindividual (age) differences in means, vari-
ces, or structure. Differences across age groups, as will be pointed out
 the next section, can provide only an approximation and sometimes
 inaccurate account of developmental change. Quantitative changes
ch as those described here can be considered in either the univariate
 the multivariate case, whereas qualitative changes, specifically, re-
ire multivariate analysis (see Harris, 1975; Morrison, 1976; or Nessel-
de, 1977, for coverage of multivariate techniques). In the next sec-
n, specific designs for the study of change will be considered.

assical Developmental Research Designs

Given the major focus of life-span developmental research on intra-
lividual changes and interindividual differences in change over time,
 s crucial to employ research designs that permit a direct assessment of
ange. Traditionally, the cross-sectional and longitudinal methods

have been used in developmental research. There are, however, som
major flaws and widespread misunderstandings associated with thes
designs (Baltes *et al.*, 1979). First, the cross-sectional and longitudin
designs will be described and particular attention will be devoted t
their strengths and weaknesses. Then, some alternative designs for de
velopmental research will be specified.

CROSS-SECTIONAL DESIGNS. As mentioned earlier, one goal for life
span developmental research is to identify age-related changes in beha\
ior. The cross-sectional design involves the assessment of multiple san
ples from different age levels at one time. As such, the cross-section:
method provides information about age group differences, but not nee
essarily about age-related changes. As illustrated in Table 1, the cros:
sectional method involves a comparison of samples of different ag
groups who also are from different birth cohorts. For instance, the 2(
year-olds in 1980 were born in 1960 and the 40-year-olds were born i
1940. Thus, any outcome that indicates differences between the 20- an
40-year-olds in 1980 will, by design, reflect birth cohort (1960 vs. 194(
differences as well.

One major weakness associated with the cross-sectional method :
that it provides no direct information about intraindividual changes;
can approximate change only through the observation of group (ag
cohort) differences. For example, questions as to whether the 1960 co
hort when 40 (in the year 2000) will show characteristics similar to thos
of the 40-year-olds from the 1940 cohort cannot be addressed with th
cross-sectional design. Nor can it be determined whether the 1940 co
hort at 20 in 1960 was like their 20-year-old counterparts in 1980. In th
cross-sectional design, age and cohort effects are confounded; grou;
differ not only with respect to age but also with respect to cohort. B
cause cohorts may differ in the way they were reared and in the set
historical events that they experienced as they were growing up, we ca
expect to find differences in their patterns of life-span developmen

Table 1. *Cross-Sectional and Longitudinal Methods[a]*

Time of measurement	Cohort			
	1960	1940	1920	1900
1980	20	40	60	80
1960				60
1940				40
1920				20

[a]Entries are age levels. Horizonal rectangle is cross-sectional method. Vertical rectangle is longitudinal method.

Other problems associated with the cross-sectional method become parent when considered within a quasi-experimental design framework (Campbell and Stanley, 1963; Labouvie, Bartsch, Nesselroade, and ltes, 1974; Schaie, 1977). The classical cross-sectional design does not ve experimental design status because (a) the independent variable, e, cannot be directly manipulated, and (b) respondents cannot be ndomly assigned to age groups. As such, there are several threats to e internal validity of the cross-sectional design, and, as a consequence, e cannot be certain that age is the factor responsible for any differences tween groups. Campbell and Stanley (1963) have discussed eight factrs that threaten the internal validity of preexperimental and quasiperimental research designs: maturation, history, selection, experiental mortality, testing, instrumentation, statistical regression, and lection by maturation interaction. These factors will be addressed here potential sources of invalidity for the cross-sectional and longitudinal signs. Note, however, that not all of these factors pose threats for velopmental research designs. In fact, maturation, rather than being a urce of invalidity, is the major variable of interest for developmental search (Baltes et al., 1977). Other factors such as history and selection n also provide a meaningful focus for developmental study and thus ed not always be considered design threats.

One threat to the internal validity of cross-sectional designs is selecn bias. Those middle-aged and older adults who are available for search tend to be positively selected relative to others from their corts. Cross-sectional comparisons, then, can underestimate age diffences because the older groups are likely to be positively biased with ;ard to such factors as intelligence and health. Moreover, it is difficult find different age-cohort groups who are equivalent on all variables. horts often differ on variables (e.g., education and socioeconomic tus) that are known to be related to psychological outcomes (Krauss, 30). Such differences between cohorts should be taken into consideran when selecting research samples. When these differences between norts cannot be controlled, it may be more appropriate to conduct thin-cohort analyses (Krauss, 1980). Examination of differences in deopmental outcomes within a cohort may reveal something about the cesses associated with between-cohort differences.

Another problem of selection in the cross-sectional design is that :h cohort has a unique life history and there are no controls for the ditions that existed prior to the research. Baltes (1968) has referred to s as a problem of generation effects. In his research on the Great pression, Elder (1979) has illustrated that the timing of historical nts has had a differential impact on the development of cohorts. us, any differences found between age groups could also reflect dif-

ferences in cohort-related histories. Indeed, cohort differences have
been found in a number of domains, including intelligence (Baltes *et al.*
1979; Schaie, 1979) and personality (Elder, 1979; Nesselroade and Baltes
1974). These cohort differences in performance could be due to differen
tial patterns in the timing of major events (e.g., the Great Depression) o
the regular course of cultural change (e.g., exposure to television, com
puters, or lifelong education).

Another problem that threatens the internal validity of cross-sec
tional designs is instrumentation. The interview conditions, test forma
or test administrator may vary across age groups and be responsible fo
differences in behavioral responses. For example, 20-year-olds are likel
to be interviewed in the context of a school setting, such as an introdu
tory psychology course for academic credit, whereas older persons ma
be tested in a senior center or in the home. Any differences between ag
groups could reflect these conditions, rather than true age difference:

As already discussed, there are several problems with the cros
sectional design that place limitations on its usefulness for life-spa
developmental research. However, the cross-sectional design is widel
used because of its economy with regard to time. Researchers cann
always wait for their subjects to grow older in order to study adu
development. Thus, the cross-sectional method is more practical tha
long-term longitudinal designs because multiple age groups can be e:
amined with only one occasion of measurement. Despite this advar
tage, it is rarely the case that cross-sectional results can be unquestior
ably interpreted as age changes. Only if all age cohorts have bee
selected from the same parent population and have experienced th
same life histories, and, therefore, differ only with respect to age, a:
cross-sectional age differences interpretable as average intraindividu
age changes (Baltes and Nesselroade, 1979). This assumption, howeve
is difficult to test and is unlikely to occur due to rapid changes in histo
ical–cultural conditions and the selective sampling issue already men
tioned. Thus, in most cases the cross-sectional method can only provic
an approximation to intraindividual (age) change. Nevertheless, cros
sectional findings can be suggestive of developmental trends. The r
sults can then be followed up to determine whether the same patterr
can be replicated over time.

LONGITUDINAL DESIGNS. The longitudinal method is often consi
ered the *sine qua non* of developmental research (McCall, 1977). The ter
longitudinal implies there are multiple assessments of the same perso
over time (Baltes and Nesselroade, 1979).[4] This design is illustrated

---

[4]Procedures that involve the sampling and measurement of independent groups or par
from the population at different times also have been included in the definition of longi
dinal studies (Schaie and Hertzog, 1982).

'able 1. Notice that the 1900 birth cohort is followed from 1920 to 1980, uring which time they age from 20 to 80 years. Because of its direct ɔcus on intraindividual change, the longitudinal method is usually con- idered more appropriate than the cross-sectional method for the study f development. Although in a longitudinal study the same people are ɔllowed over time and behavior changes can be charted across different ges, this method does not always offer a clear-cut assessment of age- ʔlated change. Since there are a number of threats to the internal valid- y of longitudinal designs, it is not always possible to isolate age as the 'causal'') factor responsible for differences. The major sources of inva- dity for the longitudinal design are history, instrumentation, testing, ɔortality, and statistical regression.

In the single-cohort longitudinal design, history rather than age ʌay be the factor that is responsible for the results. A given outcome ʌay be due to environmental events that occurred over the period of ɪvestigation. This would imply that the same results would have oc- ɪrred for other age-cohort groups had they been included in the de- gn. As an example, consider a hypothetical 5-year longitudinal study f depression in a cohort of women during the transition to midlife. If epression was found to increase in these women over this 5-year peri- ɪ, it would not be clear whether the change could be attributed to the ʌidlife transition or to environmental events. For example, it could be ʌat changes in the economy and unemployment conditions led to the ʌanges in depression. If several age cohorts had been followed over the ʌme period, all, regardless of age, might have shown similar increases ɪ depression.

Instrumentation effects, similar to those mentioned for cross-sec- ɔnal research, also can jeopardize the internal validity of longitudinal ʔsigns. For example, the conditions of test administration can vary eatly across occasions and thereby distort the results. In addition, ʌere is the problem of retesting. The same questions are usually asked peatedly, so that responses may change due to familiarity with the ʌestions or to participation in the study, rather than to aging. Posttest- ʌly control groups can be added to determine the extent of retest ef- cts (Nesselroade and Baltes, in preparation).

Another design threat involves the mortality or selective attrition of ʌbjects from one occasion to the next. Anyone who has done longitudi- ʌl research, even over a short period of time, knows how rare it is to aintain all the members of one's sample over time. For many reasons .g., illness, lack of interest, death), people may drop out of the sample. ʌe internal validity problem arises when there is an interaction be- ʌeen maturation and attrition, that is, if those who remain in the study ʔvelop in a way that is different from those who drop out. For instance, we are interested in whether introversion increases over the adult life-

span, we must determine whether those who drop out are more intro
verted. If so, we could get a false picture of decreasing introversion (i.e.
increasing extraversion) with aging.

A final threat to the internal validity of longitudinal designs is statis
tical regression. Because of measurement unreliability, extreme score
tend to regress toward the mean over time (Cronbach and Furby, 197C
Furby, 1973). Since it is rare to achieve error-free measurements (se
earlier discussion of measurement reliability), regression to the mean i
a common threat in longitudinal research. The problem of statistica
regression is that extreme scores (either high or low) are often the resul
of unique patterns of random error that will not occur in the same wa
twice. Therefore, scores will change in a predictable way; that is, the
will approach the mean. This phenomenon of regression is manifeste
when high scores decrease and low scores increase from the first to th
second occasion (Baltes, Nesselroade, Schaie, and Labouvie, 1972; Fur
by, 1973). Rather than abandon the study of change altogether, as som
researchers have suggested (Cronbach and Furby, 1970), it seems mor
reasonable to search for ways to control or compensate for the effects c
regression to the mean. One way to protect against regression to th
mean is to use highly reliable measures. It is very rare, however, t
obtain perfectly reliable assessments. The problem of statistical regres
sion can be alleviated, in many cases, by including more than two mea
surement occasions in one's design (see Nesselroade, Stigler, and Ba
tes, 1980).

The various factors mentioned above interfere with the interpreta
tion of the results of cross-sectional and longitudinal studies. In som
cases the problems can be addressed through the use of control group:
but in other circumstances the results may be hopelessly confounded. I
such cases design decisions ultimately become a matter of priorities an
trade-offs.

External Validity of Developmental Designs. Thus far we hav
considered threats to the internal validity of developmental researc
designs. In addition to these weaknesses, the conventional develop
mental designs also suffer from limitations in external validity. Extern
validity is concerned with the generalizability of research findings acros
persons, measurement variables, treatments, settings, and time. Ca
the results found be applied to other people in other places at othe
times? In longitudinal studies, the findings for one cohort may not k
applicable to other cohorts who have grown up under a different set
historical conditions. Thus, under conditions of rapid cultural chang
there are restrictions placed on the generalizability of findings fro
single-cohort research. Another external validity problem involves sele
tive attrition. If those who drop out of a study differ from those wl

main, then the results will be limited in generalizability. For example, those who remain in a longitudinal study are better educated, the sults may not be applicable to those with less education. It is recomended, therefore, that statistical tests of differences between the droputs and the longitudinal sample be performed in order to determine the xtent of selective attrition (for examples of methods of testing for differtial dropout, see Nesselroade and Baltes, in preparation; Siegler and otwinick, 1979).

There is, unfortunately, a trade-off between internal and external alidity. If one conducts a highly controlled, internally valid study in the boratory, this is usually done at the expense of external validity conrns. On the other hand, if one tries to maximize external validity by nducting research in real-life settings, the amount of rigor and control ver internal validity invariably will suffer. Traditionally, psychologists ave given primary attention to internal validity at the expense of exteral validity. However, some life-span developmental psychologists ave suggested that at least equal concern should be given to external alidity (Baltes *et al.*, 1977; Bronfenbrenner, 1979; Hultsch and Hickey, 78; Schaie, 1978). The underlying value is that researchers have an oligation to design research that has application and relevance beyond e specific observations made in one study in an artificially contrived tuation.

equential Research Designs

As discussed in the previous section, there are a number of serious eaknesses associated with the conventional cross-sectional and longidinal designs. In the cross-sectional design, age and cohort effects are nfounded, and in the longitudinal design, age and time of measureent are confounded. Moreover, major discrepancies have been found tween the results of cross-sectional and longitudinal studies. In the omains of personality and intelligence, for instance, cross-sectional sults have been indicative of decrements in functioning beginning in idlife. On the other hand, longitudinal findings have revealed few anges and little evidence of declines in functioning throughout adultod (Baltes *et al.*, 1977). It was the widespread occurrence of these ntradictory findings in cross-sectional and longitudinal studies that imulated the development of more sophisticated models and dataithering strategies. These new strategies are referred to as sequential esigns. The major advantage of these designs is that they provide plication of age effects and controls for various sources of invalidity.

Sequential designs have been approached from a variety of different rspectives (e.g., Baltes, 1968; Glenn, 1977; Ryder, 1965; Schaie, 1965).

The approach recommended by Schaie and Baltes (1975) will be present-ed here for illustrative purposes. They have identified two types of sequential strategies: cross-sectional and longitudinal sequences. The major distinction is that in the former, independent samples are tested over time, and in the latter, the same sample is repeatedly tested over time. Cross-sectional sequences involve the replication of a cross-sectional study over the same age range for at least two times of measurement. Longitudinal sequences require repeated measures of at least two cohorts over the age range of interest on at least two occasions. Thus, sequential designs are straightforward extensions of the conventional cross-sectional and longitudinal designs. Through the replication across either cohorts or time, it becomes possible to separate age from cohort or time effects. Thus, it is possible to disentangle the effects that are confounded in cross-sectional and longitudinal designs.

In Table 2 the horizontal segments represent cross-sectional sequences. On three occasions (1940, 1960, 1980) samples ranging in age from 20 to 80 are assessed. With this design, it is possible to examine whether the same developmental pattern holds true for more than one cohort. Since the groups at each occasion are independent (i.e., new representatives of each cohort are selected on each occasion), there can be no retesting effects.

The vertical sections in Table 2 depict longitudinal sequences. Three cohorts (1920, 1940, 1960) are followed over a 60-year period as they age from 20 to 80. Since the same age range is observed across multiple cohorts, it is possible to determine whether age changes are generalizable across cohorts that are developing during different historical periods.

It must be recognized that sequential designs are not the developmental researcher's panacea. In fact, because of their status as quasi-

Table 2. Cross-Sectional and Longitudinal Sequences[a]

Time of measurement	Cohort					
	1960	1940	1920	1900	1880	186
2040	80					
2020	60	80				
2000	40	60	80			
1980	20	40	60	80		
1960		20	40	60	80	
1940			20	40	60	8(

[a]Entries are age levels. Vertical rectangles are longitudinal sequences. Horizontal rectangles are cross-sectional sequences.

xperimental designs, there are still potential threats to the validity of
1ese designs. For example, the problems of testing and selective attri-
ion, which plagued single-cohort longitudinal designs, still can be trou-
1esome in sequential longitudinal designs. Through the use of control
roups, however, it becomes possible to address some of these concerns
5chaie and Hertzog, 1982). For example, the use of cross-sectional se-
uences in combination with longitudinal sequences is one effective way
) control for effects of retesting. The cross-sectional sequences, which
re independent assessments, can serve as a posttest-only control group
)r the longitudinal sequences. Differences between cross-sectional and
)ngitudinal sequences could be attributed to effects of retesting.

As mentioned earlier, there are several approaches to sequential
esigns. The methods presented here represent the position agreed
pon by Schaie and Baltes (1975). Initially, Schaie (1965) and Baltes
.968) disagreed on several points, which have since been resolved. In
1eir discussion, three major issues were raised: (a) the need for two-
1ctor versus three-factor models, (b) the use of sequential designs for
escriptive versus explanatory purposes, and (c) the use of sequential
esigns as data-analytic versus data-collection strategies. Their resolu-
on of these issues is briefly summarized below. (For more extensive
)verage, see Baltes *et al.*, 1979; Schaie and Hertzog, 1982; Schaie and
altes, 1975.) First, it was concluded that only two factors are necessary
)r the sequential methods, since the third factor is always inextricably
nked to the other two, and, therefore, it is represented in the interac-
on of the other two factors. Second, sequential designs can only pro-
ide descriptive information about development. Age and cohort vari-
bles may be indicators of change, but they do not reveal anything about
1e underlying sources of development. Third, sequential strategies are
ata-collection strategies. With cross-sectional or longitudinal se-
uences, it is possible to collect all data necessary to separate the vari-
bles that are confounded in the conventional designs. The recom-
1ended data collection arrangement for developmental psychologists
1terested in intraindividual change and interindividual (cohort) dif-
2rences in change is the age-by-cohort matrix. However, there are other
ossible arrangements (time by cohort or age by time) that are more
ppropriate when designs include only a few occasions of measurement
r a few cohort groups. As for data analysis, there are several appropri-
te techniques that can be applied to the sequential designs. The most
)mmonly applied techniques for data analysis are analysis of variance
Nesselroade and Baltes, in preparation) and multiple regression (Buss,
)79–1980; Mason, Mason, Winsborough, and Poole, 1973). Structural
quation models represent an alternative analytic method (Rogosa,
)79). With newly developed computer programs for structural equation

analysis, it is possible to consider quantitative and qualitative aspects of change simultaneously for multiple cohorts (Jöreskog and Sörbom, in preparation).

In summary, sequential designs may be effective in eliminating the major confounds in the single-occasion cross-sectional and the single cohort longitudinal designs. This is accomplished by replicating age effects across time and cohorts. One major drawback of the sequential designs is that they are time-consuming and costly since they require multiple assessments on multiple groups. To complete the longitudinal sequences depicted in Table 2 would take 100 years! Fortunately, there are some reasonable variations of the sequential designs, such as the "convergence" method (Bell, 1953), which make it possible under certain conditions to approximate long-term age functions with short-term longitudinal data (Wohlwill, 1973).

Alternative Research Designs

Often it is not possible or feasible to employ longitudinal (repeated measurement) methods even though one is interested in how a phenomenon or characteristic has changed over time. One alternative means for studying change is the retrospective method. This usually entails asking subjects to recall what they felt, thought, or did on previous occasions. Of course, such retrospective reports are subject to distortion because of the role of intervening events and problems of memory, and methods for checking accuracy should be adopted (Finney, 1981; Gutek, 1978; Powers, Goudy, and Keith, 1978). The retrospective procedure is often used in studies of adjustment to critical life events. With unexpected events such as widowhood, it is difficult to anticipate the event. In these cases the subjects are usually identified after the event has occurred; therefore, retrospective methods may be the most feasible.

For the study of anticipated events such as the birth of a child, it may be possible to follow subjects longitudinally or to use prospective methods. In prospective accounts, subjects may be asked to make predictions about what they think things will be like in the future.

Another procedure for studying adjustment to events was adopted in the Normative Aging Studies at Duke University, where they selected a sample that was "at risk" for one or more life events such as retirement (Siegler, 1977). Thus, they were able to obtain assessments before and after the occurrence of events, and did not have to rely on retrospective accounts. Moreover, they could make comparisons with those in the sample who did not experience the events.

Prospective and retrospective methods provide subjective rather an objective accounts of development. Within a phenomenological amework, subjective expectations and interpretations take on central eaning. These perceptions of change, from past to present and present future, are more salient than objective indicators of change within a henomenological framework (Ryff and Heincke, 1981; Thomae, 1970).

plicatory Research

The developmental designs that have been discussed thus far are seful for descriptive research. They can be applied to chart the course intraindividual change and interindividual differences in change. The oss-sectional, longitudinal, and sequential designs do not, however, rmit the study of the sources or causes of change. In order to go yond description to the level of explanation, it is necessary to employ her techniques.

AGE SIMULATION. Traditionally, psychologists have applied the ex-rimental paradigm for explanatory research. However, as mentioned rlier, experimental techniques often are difficult to apply in develop-ental studies because many of the independent variables of major terest (e.g., age, history) cannot be subjected to direct manipulation or ndom assignment. Some of the desirable features of the experimental signs may be captured with age-simulation strategies (Baltes and oulet, 1971). Age simulation involves the manipulation of variables pothesized to be associated with age. Through the examination of age treatment interactions, the key developmental parameters that lead existing age differences can be identified.

There are several methods available for age simulation. The most mmon form involves the application of treatment manipulations of riables such as practice, speed, or sensory deprivation, which are pected to be related to age differences. Other types of simulation volve age-hypnotic regression (Baltes et al., 1977) or computer-gener-ed models (Baltes, Nesselroade, and Cornelius, 1978). The major value age simulation strategies is that it permits the analysis of sources of velopment in a shortened period of time. However, because age sim-ation does not involve the monitoring of developmental changes in eir naturalistic form, their major weakness is one of external validity. uestions typically arise as to whether the simulated developmental ocesses would occur in the same way in vivo.

CAUSAL METHODS. Another methodological option for explanatory search is causal modeling (Rogosa, 1979). Causal modeling does not volve the manipulation and isolation of a causal variable, as is true for experimental research. Rather, it involves considering whether a given causal hypothesis is consistent with a particular set of correlational data. Causal modeling involves making explicit statements about the relationships among a set of variables. It is possible to set up competing theoretically based models and to test the adequacy of these models for representing observed data. Earlier versions of causal models such as path analysis and cross-lagged panel models have been greatly improved through the development of computer programs that allow for multiple indicators of latent factors (Jöreskog and Sörbom, 1978). Several techniques are available for the analysis and estimation of causal models. The interested reader should refer to the following sources for an introduction to this area (Jöreskog, 1979; Kenny, 1979; Rogosa, 1979). Although causal models are commonly used in sociology and economics, it is only recently that psychologists have begun to apply them to the study of adult development and aging (e.g., Lachman, 1983). Causal models enable researchers to examine the antecedents of development through the use of naturalistic–correlational data. This combination of explanatory power and emphasis on external validity makes causal models particularly desirable for life-span developmental research.

CONCLUSIONS

The goal of the present chapter has been to apply the conceptual and methodological features of a life-span developmental perspective to the study of women in the middle years. For those readers who already have formulated research questions, this chapter has been intended as a source of methodological suggestions and answers. For those who do not yet have specific questions, it also has been the aim of this chapter to facilitate the formulation of research questions on development during midlife. Although one ideally expects to choose an appropriate method or design for study after determining the questions to be researched, there is in reality a two-way interaction between questions and methods. The questions generated are dependent, in large part, on one's knowledge of research methods. For example, those who do know how to measure change properly will be forced to take a nondevelopmental approach to research. Or, those who are not aware of multivariate techniques will be likely to formulate univariate questions. In alerting the reader to some of the critical issues and pitfalls of developmental methodology and by suggesting some solutions, the present chapter has as part of its overall agenda the stimulation of new types of research questions as part of an effort to enrich and advance the study of women in midlife.

References

Achenbach, T. M. *Research in developmental psychology: Concepts, strategies, methods.* New York: Free Press, 1978.

American Psychological Association. *Standards for educational and psychological tests.* Washington, D.C.: American Psychological Association, 1974.

Anastasi, A. *Psychological testing* (3rd ed.). London: Macmillan, 1968.

Baer, D. M. An age-irrelevant concept of development. *Merrill-Palmer Quarterly,* 1970, *16,* 238–246.

Baltes, P. B. Longitudinal and cross-sectional sequences in the study of age and generation effects. *Human Development,* 1968, *11,* 145–171.

Baltes, P. B. Life-span developmental psychology: Some converging observations on history and theory. In P. B. Baltes and O. G. Brim, Jr. (Eds.), *Life-span development and behavior* (Vol. 2). New York: Academic Press, 1979.

Baltes, P. B., and Baltes, M. M. Plasticity and variability in psychological aging: Methodological and theoretical issues. In G. Gurski (Ed.), *Determining the effects of aging on the central nervous system.* Berlin: Schering, 1980.

Baltes, P. B., Cornelius, S. W., and Nesselroade, J. R. Cohort effects in developmental psychology. In J. R. Nesselroade and P. B. Baltes (Eds.), *Longitudinal research in the study of behavior and development.* New York: Academic Press, 1979.

Baltes, P. B., Cornelius, S. W., Spiro, A., III, Nesselroade, J. R., and Willis, S. L. Integration vs. differentiation of fluid-crystallized intelligence in old age. *Developmental Psychology,* 1980, *16,* 625–635.

Baltes, P. B., and Goulet, L. R. Exploration of developmental variables by set manipulation and simulation of age differences in behavior. *Human Development,* 1971, *14,* 149–170.

Baltes, P. B., and Nesselroade, J. R. The developmental analysis of individual differences on multiple measures. In J. R. Nesselroade and H. W. Reese (Eds.), *Life-span developmental psychology: Methodological issues.* New York: Academic Press, 1973.

Baltes, P. B., and Nesselroade, J. R. History and rationale of longitudinal research. In J. R. Nesselroade and P. B. Baltes (Eds.), *Longitudinal research in the study of behavior and development.* New York: Academic Press, 1979.

Baltes, P. B., Nesselroade, J. R., and Cornelius, S. W. Multivariate antecedents of structural change in development: A simulation of cumulative environmental patterns. *Multivariate Behavioral Research,* 1978, *13,* 127–152.

Baltes, P. B., Nesselroade, J. R., Schaie, K. W., and Labouvie, E. W. On the dilemma of regression effects in examining ability-level related differentials in ontogenetic patterns of intelligence. *Developmental Psychology,* 1972, *6,* 78–84.

Baltes, P. B., Reese, H. W., and Lipsitt, L. P. Life-span developmental psychology. *Annual Review of Psychology,* 1980, *31,* 65–110.

Baltes, P. B., Reese, H. W., and Nesselroade, J. R. *Life-span developmental psychology: Introduction to research methods.* Monterey, Calif.: Brooks/Cole, 1977.

Baltes, P. B., and Willis, S. L. The critical importance of appropriate methodology in the study of aging: The sample case of pyschometric intelligence. In F. Hoffmeister and C. Muller (Eds.), *Brain functions in old age.* Heidelberg: Springer, 1979.

Baruch, G., Barnett, R., and Rivers, C. *Lifeprints: New patterns of love and work for today's women.* New York: McGraw-Hill, 1983.

Bell, R. Q. Convergence: An accelerated longitudinal approach. *Child Development,* 1953, *24,* 145–152.

Bereiter, C. Some persisting dilemmas in the measurement of change: In C. W. Harris (Ed.), *Problems in measuring change.* Madison: University of Wisconsin Press, 1963.

Block, J. Advancing the psychology of personality: Paradigmatic shift or improving the quality of research. In D. Magnusson and N. S. Endler (Eds.), *Personality at the crossroads: Current issues in interactional psychology*. Hillsdale, N.J.: Erlbaum, 1977.

Bornstein, R., and Smircina, M. T. The status of the empirical support for the hypothesis of increased variability in aging populations. *Gerontologist*, 1982, *22*, 258–260.

Brim, O. G., Jr., and Kagan, J. (Eds.). *Constancy and change in human development*. Cambridge, Mass.: Harvard University Press, 1980.

Bronfenbrenner, U. *The ecology of human development: Experiments by nature and design*. Cambridge, Mass.: Harvard University Press, 1979.

Buss, A. R. Methodological issues in life-span developmental psychology from a dialectic perspective. *International Journal of Aging and Human Development*, 1979–1980, *10*, 121–163.

Campbell, D. T., and Stanley, J. C. *Experimental and quasi-experimental designs for research*. Chicago: Rand McNally, 1963.

Carmines, E. G., and Zeller, R. A. *Reliability and validity assessment*. Beverly Hills: Sage, 1979.

Cattell, R. B. *The scientific analysis of personality*. Baltimore: Penguin, 1965.

Cattell, R. B., Eber, H. W., and Tatsuoka, M. M. *Handbook for the Sixteen Personality Factor Questionnaire*. Champaign, Ill.: Institute for Personality and Ability Testing, 1970.

Clayton, V. P., and Birren, J. E. The development of wisdom across the life span: A reexamination of an ancient topic. In P. B. Baltes and O. G. Brim, Jr. (Eds.), *Life-span development and behavior* (Vol. 3). New York: Academic Press, 1980.

Costa, P. T., Jr., and McCrae, R. R. Still stable after all these years: Personality as a key to some issues in adulthood and old age. In P. B. Baltes and O. G. Brim, Jr. (Eds.), *Life span development and behavior* (Vol. 3). New York: Academic Press, 1980.

Cronbach, L. J., and Furby, L. How should we measure "change" — Or should we? *Psychological Bulletin*, 1970, *74*, 68–80.

Danish, S. J., Smyer, M. A., and Nowak, C. A. Developmental intervention: Enhancing life-event processes. In P. B. Baltes and O. G. Brim, Jr. (Eds.), *Life-span development and behavior* (Vol. 3). New York: Academic Press, 1980.

Demming, J. A., and Pressey, S. L. Tests "indigenous" to the adult and older years. *Journal of Counseling Psychology*, 1957, *4*, 144–148.

Denney, N. W. Aging and cognitive changes. In B. B. Wolman (Ed.), *Handbook of developmental psychology*. Englewood Cliffs, N.J.: Prentice-Hall, 1982.

Eichorn, D. H., Clausen, J. A., Haan, N., Honzik, M. P., and Mussen, P. H. *Present and past in middle life*. New York: Academic Press, 1981.

Elder, G. H., Jr. Family history and life course. In T. K. Hareven (Ed.), *Transitions: The family and the life course in historical perspective*. New York: Academic Press, 1978.

Elder, G. H., Jr. Historical change in life patterns and personality. In P. B. Baltes and O. G. Brim, Jr. (Eds.), *Life-span development and behavior* (Vol. 2). New York: Academic Press, 1979.

Elder, G. H., and Liker, J. K. Hard times in women's lives: Historical influences across 40 years. *American Journal of Sociology*, 1982, *88*, 241–269.

Epstein, S. The stability of behavior: I. On predicting most of the people much of the time. *Journal of Personality and Social Psychology*, 1979, *37*, 1097–1126.

Erikson, E. *Childhood and society* (2nd ed.). New York: Norton, 1963.

Eysenck, H. J., and Eysenck, S. B. G. *Eysenck personality inventory*. San Diego: Educational and Industrial Testing Services, 1963.

Finney, H. C. Improving the reliability of retrospective survey measures: Results of a longitudinal field survey. *Evaluation Review*, 1981, *5*, 207–229.

Flavell, J. H. Cognitive changes in adulthood. In L. R. Goulet and P. B. Baltes (Eds.), *Life span developmental psychology: Research and theory*. New York: Academic Press, 1970.

ries, J. F., and Crapo, L. M. *Vitality and aging.* San Francisco: Freeman, 1981.

urby, L. Interpreting regression toward the mean in developmental research. *Developmental Psychology,* 1973, *8,* 172–179.

;hiselli, E. E., Campbell, J. P., and Zedeck, S. *Measurement theory for the behavioral sciences.* San Francisco: Freeman, 1981.

;iele, J. Z. (Ed.). *Women in the middle years: Current knowledge and directions for research and policy.* New York: Wiley, 1982.

;illigan, C. *In a different voice: Psychological theory and women's development.* Cambridge, Mass.: Harvard University Press, 1982.

;lenn, N. D. *Cohort analysis.* Beverly Hills: Sage, 1977.

;ribbin, K., and Schaie, K. W. *The aging of tests: A methodological problem of longitudinal studies.* Paper presented at the 30th Annual Meeting of the Gerontological Society, San Francisco, November 1977.

;utek, B. A. On the accuracy of retrospective attitudinal data. *Public Opinion Quarterly,* 1978, *42,* 390–401.

Iarris, D. P. (Ed.). *The concept of development.* Minneapolis: University of Minnesota Press, 1957.

Iarris, R. J. *A primer of multivariate statistics.* New York: Academic Press, 1975.

Ieise, D. R. Separating reliability and stability in test-retest correlation. *American Sociological Review,* 1969, *34,* 93–101.

Iultsch, D. F., and Hickey, T. External validity in the study of human development: Theoretical and methodological issues. *Human Development,* 1978, *21,* 76–91.

Iultsch, D. F., and Plemons, J. K. Life events and life span development. In P. B. Baltes and O. G. Brim, Jr. (Eds.), *Life-span development and behavior* (Vol. 2). New York: Academic Press, 1979.

;reskog, K. G. Statistical estimation of structural models in longitudinal-developmental investigations. In J. R. Nesselroade and P. B. Baltes (Eds.), *Longitudinal research in the study of behavior and development.* New York: Academic Press, 1979.

;reskog, K. G., and Sörbom, D. *LISREL IV: Estimation of linear structural equation systems by maximum likelihood methods.* Chicago: International Educational Services, 1978.

;reskog, K., and Sörbom, D. Simultaneous analysis of longitudinal data from several cohorts. In H. Winsborough and O. D. Duncan (Eds.), *Analyzing data for age, period, and cohort effects,* in preparation.

.enny, D. A. *Correlation and causality.* New York: Wiley, 1979.

ohlberg, L. Stage and sequence: The cognitive-developmental approach to socialization. In D. A. Goslin (Ed.), *Handbook of socialization theory and research.* Chicago: Rand McNally, 1969.

.rauss, I. K. Between- and within-group comparisons in aging research. In L. W. Poon (Ed.), *Aging in the 1980s: Psychological issues.* Washington D.C.: American Psychological Association, 1980.

abouvie, E. W. Identity versus equivalence of psychological measures and constructs. In L. W. Poon (Ed.), *Aging in the 1980s: Psychological issues.* Washington, D.C.: American Psychological Association, 1980.

abouvie, E. W., Bartsch, T. W., Nesselroade, J. R., and Baltes, P. B. On the internal and external validity of simple longitudinal designs. *Child Development,* 1974, *45,* 282–290.

abouvie-Vief, G. Adult cognitive development: In search of alternative interpretations. *Merrill-Palmer Quarterly,* 1977, *23,* 227–263.

abouvie-Vief, G. Dynamic development and mature autonomy: A theoretical prologue. *Human Development,* 1982, *25,* 161–191.

abouvie-Vief, G., and Chandler, M. J. Cognitive development and life-span developmental theory: Idealistic versus contextual perspectives. In P. B. Baltes (Ed.), *Life-span development and behavior* (Vol. 1). New York: Academic Press, 1978.

Lachman, M. E. Perceptions of intellectual aging: Antecedent or consequence of intellectual functioning? *Developmental Psychology*, 1983, *19*, 482–498.

Lachman, M. E., Baltes, P. B., Nesselroade, J. R., and Willis, S. L. Examination of personality-ability relationships in the elderly: The role of the contextual (interface) assessment mode. *Journal of Research in Personality*, 1982, *16*, 485–501.

Lerner, R. M. *Concepts and theories of human development*. Reading, Mass.: Addison-Wesley, 1976.

Lerner, R. M., and Ryff, C. D. Implementation of the life-span view of human development: The sample case of attachment. In P. B. Baltes (Ed.), *Life-span development and behavior* (Vol. 1). New York: Academic Press, 1978.

Levinson, D. J. *The seasons of a man's life*. New York: Knopf, 1978.

Looft, W. R. Socialization and personality throughout the life span: An examination of contemporary psychological approaches. In P. B. Baltes and K. W. Schaei (Eds.), *Life-span developmental psychology: Personality and socialization*. New York: Academic Press, 1973.

Lord, F. M., and Novick, M. R. *Statistical theories of mental test scores*. Reading, Mass.: Addison-Wesley, 1968.

Lowenthal, M. F., Thurnher, M., and Chiriboga, D. *Four stages of life*. San Francisco: Jossey-Bass, 1975.

Mason, K. O., Mason, W. M., Winsborough, H. H., and Poole, W. K. Some methodological issues in cohort analyses of archival data. *American Sociological Review*, 1973, *38*, 242–258.

McCall, R. B. Challenges to a science of developmental psychology. *Child Development*, 1977, *48*, 333–344.

Morrison, D. F. *Multivariate statistical methods* (2nd ed.). New York: McGraw-Hill, 1976.

Nesselroade, J. R. Issues in studying developmental change in adults from a multivariate perspective. In J. E. Birren and K. W. Schaie (Eds.), *Handbook of the psychology of aging*. New York: Van Nostrand Reinhold, 1977.

Nesselroade, J. R., and Baltes, P. B. Adolescent personality development and historical change: 1970–1972. *Monographs of the Society for Research in Child Development*, 1974, *39*(1, Serial No. 154).

Nesselroade, J. R., and Baltes, P. B. Sequential strategies and the role of cohort effects in behavioral development: Adolescent personality (1970–1972) as a sample case. In S. Mednick and M. Harway (Eds.), *Longitudinal research in the United States*, in preparation.

Nesselroade, J. R., and Bartsch, T. W. Multivariate perspectives on the construct validity of the trait-state distinction. In R. B. Cattell and R. M. Dreger (Eds.), *Handbook of modern personality theory*. Washington, D.C.: Hemisphere, 1977.

Nesselroade, J. R., Stigler, S. M., and Baltes, P. B. Regression toward the mean and the study of change. *Psychological Bulletin*, 1980, *88*, 622–637.

Neugarten, B. L. (Ed.). *Middle age and aging*. Chicago: University of Chicago Press, 1968.

Nunnally, J. C. *Psychometric theory* (2nd ed.). New York: McGraw-Hill, 1978.

Popkin, S. J., Schaie, K. W., and Krauss, I. K. *Age-fair assessment of psychometric intelligence*. Paper presented at the 33rd Annual Scientific Meeting of the Gerontological Society of America, San Diego, November 1980.

Powers, E. A., Goudy, W. J., and Keith, P. M. Congruence between panel and recall data in longitudinal research. *Public Opinion Quarterly*, 1978, *42*, 380–389.

Quayhagen, M., Gonda, J., and Schaie, K. W. *Are familiar tasks always meaningful?* Paper presented at the 32nd Annual Meeting of the Gerontological Society. Washington, D.C., November 1979.

Reese, H. W., and Overton, W. F. Models of development and theories of development. In L. R. Goulet and P. B. Baltes (Eds.), *Life-span developmental psychology: Research and theory.* New York: Academic Press, 1970.

Reinert, G. Comparative factor analytic studies of intelligence throughout the human life-span. In L. R. Goulet and P. B. Baltes (Eds.), *Life-span developmental psychology: Research and theory.* New York: Academic Press, 1970.

Reinert, G. Prolegomena to a history of life-span developmental psychology. In P. B. Baltes and O. G. Brim, Jr. (Eds.), *Life-span development and behavior* (Vol. 2). New York: Academic Press, 1979.

Rogosa, D. Causal models in longitudinal research: Rationale, formulation, and interpretation. In J. R. Nesselroade and P. B. Baltes (Eds.), *Longitudinal research in the study of behavior and development.* New York: Academic Press, 1979.

Rossi, A. S. Life-span theories and women's lives. *Signs: Journal of Women in Culture and Society,* 1980, *6,* 4–32.

Rubin, L. B. *Women of a certain age: The midlife search for self.* New York: Harper & Row, 1979.

Ryder, N. B. The cohort as a concept in the study of social change. *American Sociological Review,* 1965, *30,* 843–861.

Ryff, C. D., and Heincke, S. G. *The subjective organization of personality in adulthood and aging.* Paper presented at the Biennial Meeting of the Society for Research in Child Development, Boston, April 1981.

Schaie, K. W. A general model for the study of developmental problems. *Psychological Bulletin,* 1965, *64,* 92–107.

Schaie, K. W. Quasi-experimental research designs in the psychology of aging. In J. E. Birren and K. W. Schaie (Eds.), *Handbook of the psychology of aging.* New York: Van Nostrand Reinhold, 1977.

Schaie, K. W. Toward a stage theory of adult cognitive development. *International Journal of Aging and Human Development,* 1977–78, *8,* 129–138.

Schaie, K. W. External validity in the assessment of intellectual development in adulthood. *Journal of Gerontology,* 1978, *33,* 695–701.

Schaie, K. W. The primary mental abilities in adulthood: An exploration in the development of psychometric intelligence. In P. B. Baltes and O. G. Brim, Jr. (Eds.), *Life-span development and behavior* (Vol. 2). New York: Academic Press, 1979.

Schaie, K. W., and Baltes, P. B. On sequential strategies in developmental research: Description or explanation. *Human Development,* 1975, *18,* 384–390.

Schaie, K. W., and Hertzog, C. Longitudinal methods. In B. B. Wohlman (Ed.), *Handbook of developmental psychology.* Englewood Cliffs, N.J.: Prentice-Hall, 1982.

Shannon, J., and Kedar, H. S. Phenomenological structuring of the adult lifespan as a function of age and sex. *International Journal of Aging and Human Development,* 1979–80, *10,* 343–357.

Siegler, I. *Stress and adaptation in later life: Description of study population sample, major life events, and resources.* Paper presented at the 30th Annual Scientific Meeting of the Gerontological Society, San Francisco, November 1977.

Siegler, I. C., and Botwinick, J. A long-term longitudinal study of intellectual ability of older adults: The matter of selective subject attrition. *Journal of Gerontology,* 1979, *34,* 242–245.

Stewart, A. J., and Platt, M. B. Studying women in a changing world: An introduction. *Journal of Social Issues,* 1982, *38,* 1–16.

Thomae, H. Theory of aging and cognitive theory of personality. *Human Development,* 1970, *13,* 1–16.

Thurstone, L. L., and Thurstone, T. G. *SRA primary mental abilities: Intermediate ages 11–17.* Chicago: Science Research Associates, 1948.

Thurstone, T. G. *Primary mental abilities for grades 9–12.* Chicago: Science Research Associates, 1962.

Turner, R. R., and Reese, H. W. *Life-span developmental psychology: Intervention.* New York: Academic Press, 1980.

Vaillant, G. E. *Adaptation to life.* Waltham, Mass.: Little, Brown, 1977.

Wheaton, B., Múthen, B., Alwin, D. F., and Summers, G. F. Assessing reliability and stability in panel models. In D. R. Heise (Ed.), *Sociological methodology, 1977.* San Francisco: Jossey-Bass, 1977.

Wohlwill, J. F. The age variable in psychological research. *Psychological Review,* 1970, 77, 49–64.

Wohlwill, J. F. *The study of behavioral development.* New York: Academic Press, 1973.

Chapter 3

Middle-Aged Women in Literature

Carolyn G. Heilbrun

> The upshot of all such reflections is that I have only to let myself *go!* So I have said to myself all my life—so I said to myself in the far-off days of my fermenting and passionate youth. Yet I have never fully done it. The sense of it—of the need of it—rolls over me at times with commanding force: it seems the formula of my salvation, of what remains to me of a future. I am in full possession of accumulated resources—I have only to use them, to insist, to persist, to do something more—to do much more—than I *have* done. The way to do it—to affirm one's self *sur la fin*—is to strike as many notes, deep, full and rapid, as one can. All life is—at my age, with all one's artistic soul the record of it—in one's pocket, as it were. Go on, my boy, and strike hard; have a rich and long St. Martin's summer. Try everything, do everything, render everything—be an artist, be distinguished, to the last. (James, 1947, p. 106)

Henry James was nearly 50 when he wrote those words in his notebook; 10 years later he would begin *The Ambassadors*, the first of his last three great novels. Its hero is a man of 55, a man who has failed to live his life until now—even, perhaps, to recognize that he has not lived it. Henry James and his generation of American men provide all of us with a model for late achievement. Two friends from his youth, Henry Adams and Oliver Wendell Holmes, were, like James, to flower late: Adams did not write *Mont-Saint-Michel and Chartres* until he was 65 and his *Education of Henry Adams* until he was almost 70. Holmes reached his full powers when he was appointed to the Supreme Court at 61 (Matthiessen, 1944, p. 30). Henry's brother, William James, whose youth was a long exercise in indecision, did not produce his first book, the important *Principles of Psychology*, until he was 47.

I speak of men because it is possible, even likely, that the pattern of male lives in the 19th century suggests the pattern of female lives in the

CAROLYN G. HEILBRUN • Department of English, Columbia University; home address: 151 Central Park West, New York, New York 10023.

20th. More than a hundred years ago, for example, young men were troubled by the whole question of "vocation," by the hard task of choosing the path of life that promised the most passion and the most joy Vocation was new for men at that time, and not allowed for women Maggie Tulliver in George Eliot's *The Mill on the Floss* wishes she might have a steady purpose in life, and says to her brother: "You are a man Tom, and have power, and can do something in the world," and Tom replies, "Then if you can do nothing, submit to those who can" (Mintz 1978, pp. 45, 62). Today, young women need no longer submit and, like the men of the 19th century, long to be called to something but are uncertain what that something may be. Similarly, a middle-aged man like Strether in James's *The Ambassadors,* who has always failed to "live," who has swerved from the direct assault of experience, fearing it, "always considering something else; something else, I mean, than th thing of the moment," (1964, p. 26) not only adumbrates the condition of middle-aged women today but, indeed, reflects that condition.

When we move from middle-aged men to women, seeking an im age of middle-aged women in literature, we must look not only at char acters in novels but also at the women who created those characters. S ignored has the middle-aged woman been, so rare a bird is she as protagonist in literature that we must watch first how the idea of middl age struck the women artists themselves, and then explore how she ha been represented in literature.

Inevitably, happily, one begins with Colette. More and more doe she appear to present, in her life, the paradigm of female autonomy, an in her writings the way toward treasured solitude and the vitality of th open life. Colette was born into one destiny and lived, in later years, t achieve another. From an idyllic childhood (though no childhood i idyllic in the sense of being without conflict, without repressed resent ment against even the most loving mother) Colette, dowry-less, wa married off to a man very much older than she, a profligate and pimp c other people's talents. She had never dreamed of being a writer, ha never consciously thought of it: Her recent biographer has been struc by "the exceptional process by which [Colette] was brought to write, and "the time required before she achieved recognition as a writer (Sarde, 1981, p. 16). The exceptional process, of course, was that c being forced by her husband to write books about her girlhood exper ences (the Claudine books), which—incredible though it seems—wer published under *his* name. Colette was just 50 when she first publishe a novel under her own name, the single name she had chosen for her self: Colette. Meanwhile, she had married twice, appeared in musi halls and on the stage, been a journalist and a lover of men and womer When she died, she was the first woman ever accorded a state funeral i France.

With the early process we need not concern ourselves here. It is
ifficient to record that Colette needed to be forced into her profession,
to the practice of what now strikes us as the natural flowering of an
born talent. Indeed, she wrote that she had no early desire to write.
what a blessing that I could experience such an absence of literary
ocation!" (Mallet-Joris, 1981, p. 7). The blessing, of course, is men-
oned in the knowledge of achievement. Yet this, as Mallet-Joris says,
lls us much about the question of "creativity" in women (Mallet-Joris,
81, p. 8). So entrenched is the long cultural constraint against wom-
n having ambitions as opposed to erotic daydreams that some pres-
ure appears necessary to overcome the dire effects of confining women,
s Freud does, to what literary critics now call the erotic plot (Freud,
57, pp. 176–177). In the past decade and more, expectations of and
ncouragement for some commitment to a life not confined to the need
r love and children have been provided women by the culture as a
hole. It is clear, however, that few women, not even a Colette, can be
xpected without great external support or coercion to overcome societal
nctions against nonerotic ambitions.

But it is the middle-aged Colette who must interest us here. Her
me came late, as has the fame of many notable women writers in our
vn time. May Sarton's fame has steadily increased as she grows older,
nd Doris Grumbach became a successful novelist very late. Stevie
nith, the English writer, was to declare: "I am becoming quite famous
 my old age, isn't it funny how things come 'round?" (1981, p. 313). It
 those who achieve great stature long after youth who offer us, like
onne's lovers, a pattern for our lives.

As Colette's biographer said of her at 50: "Man had finally been
orn of his magical and commanding force; he no longer either barred
oors or opened them. For Colette, the days of compromise and sharing
ere over." She entered on a period that Valery has named *Le Bel
ujourd'hui,* the "lovely present" (Sarde, 1980, p. 360). The ambition for
iddle-aged women must be to render the present "lovely," which
eans not that it is calm and without pain—such contentment may be
und in a front porch rocker—but that it offers its own intensity, and is
perienced in non-nostalgic relation to the past. Renunciation must be
rt of it, as with Colette's Lea in *The Last of Cheri,* who, Sarde tells us,
sembles Colette in her "penchant for renunciation for the sake of
eedom, in the abstention Colette praised so highly" (1980, p. 351). And
hat is renounced, abstained from? Love. Not, of course, love of
iends, colleagues, companions, even family if they are capable of be-
oming friends. What is renounced is the erotic dream that can take, in
s most acceptable middle-aged form, the wish for an "escort," for that
knowledgment of personhood that, in the restricted world of feminin-
y, only a man can bestow. Colette herself saw the opportunities of

middle age as a project "when you set out across the undulating barrier" (Sarde, 1980, p. 379). At this time also, Sarde tells us, Colette rejoiced no longer to feel a rival for men, but rather to discover that as a woman she could now enjoy "the highest type of female relationship, without boasting or braggadocio, void of any desire to save face, full of jokes and mutual understanding" (p. 383). This friendship with women is one of the rare prizes of middle age, ironically offered not to those who are refugees from married life but to those who share new experiences in the public sphere. For the ultimate joy of middle age is work.

Many women artists have agreed. Käthe Kollwitz wrote in her diary that she found familial ties growing slacker; "for the last third of life there remains only work. It alone is always stimulating, rejuvenating, exciting, and satisfying" (Kearns, 1976, p. 125). Women, an Isak Dinesen character says, "when they are old enough to have done with the business of being women, and can let loose their strength, must be the most powerful creatures in the world" (1972, p. 119). The feminists among us hope for a time when "the business of being woman" shall not be distinguished from the business of being human, and Dinesen's middle-age change into power will not be so noteworthy. Meanwhile, her phrase is apt.

The messages from and to middle-aged women are all alike in this: that life for such women can indeed be an undiscovered country, but to enter it requires not only amazing courage but the secret knowledge that men have not kept the joys of accomplishment to themselves because these joys are negligible. They claimed them because, among other reasons, they alone can make life, once youth is past, compelling. The hard part is for women to see youth go, and believe something lies beyond. Fromm-Reichmann has put it well: "The shock . . . of middle age is threshold shock. A door is closing behind us and we turn sorrowfully to watch it close and do not discover, until we are wrenched away, the one opening ahead."

Middle-aged women, until very recently, found more encouragement in life than in art. Indeed, middle age itself has had such a bad press that it is startling to find it praised at all, even by men. Samuel Butler, here, as elsewhere, set out to shock, and did: "To me it seems that youth is like spring, an overpraised season. . . . Autumn is the mellower season, and what we lose in flowers we more than gain in fruits. Fontenelle at the age of 90, being asked what was the happiest time of his life, said he did not know that he had ever been much happier than he then was, but that perhaps his best years had been those when he was between fifty-five and seventy-five" (Butler, n.d., p. 38). Women of middle age seldom appeared in novels of the 18th and 19th centuries, unless as someone's mother or surrogate mother, and then only to affect the younger women's erotic plot, her finding a husband

ınd and thus a "destiny." The significant fact about women, in fiction
; in life, is that, after youth and childbearing are past, they have no
lot, there is no story to be told about them. In 1908 Arnold Bennett
ıund it easy enough to startle the world in this regard: "I had always
•volted against the absurd youthfulness, the unfading youthfulness of
ıe average heroine. And as a protest against this fashion, I was already,
ı 1903, planning a novel (*Lenora*) of which the heroine was aged forty,
ıd had daughters old enough to be in love. The reviewers, by the way,
ere staggered by my hardihood in offering a woman of forty as a
ıbject of serious interest to the public" (Bennett, 1928, vi–viii).

Young women and girls do not have individual stories, only varia-
ɔns upon the same story, the waiting for sexual maturity, the selection
ʏ an acceptable man, or not, and the children who will follow. Simone
ɛ Beauvoir put it concisely: "She is twelve years old and already her
ory is written in the heavens. She will discover it day after day without
ʲer making it; she is curious but frightened when she contemplates this
ɛe, every stage of which is foreseen and toward which every day moves
ʳesistibly" (1957, p. 298). For women in literature who avoid, or are
ɛprived of, this erotic-marriage plot, no story remains to be told. Such
omen cannot write their own stories; no narrative will ever be told
ɔout them. So in George Gissing's *The Odd Women*, two of the three
sters do not marry and are thus wholly unworthy of narrative: They
ıve no story. Their youngest sister, Monica, lives out the erotic plot,
hich ends in marriage and death. Gissing's novel, indeed, explores the
ıestion of whether any other narrative *is* possible for women.

The question is answered in certain 20th-century novels, where it
ɔpears that the middle-aged woman may, at her rebirth, hold the secret
˙ a new plot. Virginia Woolf's (1925) Clarissa Dalloway, who has just
oken into her 52nd year, will undergo a profound transformation in
rs. Dalloway. Clarissa Dalloway is to be contrasted with Woolf's more
·pical, and more conventionally appealing, middle-aged woman, also
ʲer 50, Mrs. Ramsay, of *To the Lighthouse*. Mrs. Ramsay has all the
•ductive, overwhelming charm of the beautiful mother but has no story
·her own, and is eventually drained of life by the unremitting de-
ands and needs of others. Her urging of all women to marriage marks
ɛr inability to reconsider the pattern of her own life, or to question the
·omise of the marriages she has encouraged. Lily Briscoe, 44, must
·sist the attractions and advice of Mrs. Ramsay, must release herself
om that feminine source of power if she is to paint her own picture at
·e end of the novel, and have her own vision.

But Mrs. Dalloway, unlike Mrs. Ramsay, will become Clarissa by
·e end of the novel, that is to say, will become herself. The first sen-
nce of the novel is: "Mrs. Dalloway said she would buy the flowers

herself." The last two lines are: " 'It is Clarissa,' he said. For there sh was." *Mrs. Dalloway*, almost infinitely reverberative, most not be sin plified by description as the story of how a middle-aged woman reir vents her self (the novel is careful to separate these two words), but th transformation is at the heart of the novel. Clarissa glances in the mirro seeing herself (one word):

> How many million times she has seen her face, and always with the same imperceptible contraction! She pursed her lips when she looked in the glass. It was to give her face point. That was her self—pointed; dartlike; definite. That was her self when some effort, some call on her to be her self, drew the parts together, she alone knew how different, how incompatible and composed so for the world only into one centre, one diamond, one woman who sat in her drawing-room and made a meeting point, a radiancy. . . . (p. 55)

Many elements figure in the transformation—her past, the return an old lover and present friend, her husband's being invited to lunc without her, "how it is certain we must die" (p. 267). Central to tl story is also the passage into madness and death of a young man, h sanity destroyed by the war. Clarissa and he are, in a sense, double and this identification of a young man, condemned to a monstro "manly" death, and an older woman, restricted to a proper "ladylike" life, is one of the revolutionary themes of the work. It w with this novel that Virginia Woolf, as she said, found her own voice last. She was 44 at the publication of *Mrs. Dalloway*, the same age as Li Briscoe when Lily became certain of what she wished her destiny to b and painted her picture.

Doris Lessing has been, in our own time, the outstanding portray of middle-aged women in the crisis of discovering that they exist only their relationships to others; they are only ancillary. In "To Room 19 Lessing wrote the terrible and terrifying story of a woman who deser her profession, marries, has the "ideal" life, and eventually goes search of her lost self in a lonely London room in a sleazy hotel; sh seeks nothing but solitude. Her husband believes she has a lover; he se detectives to spy on her. Realizing that she is soon to lose the room, sl kills herself. The story is shattering and, in its honesty, incomprehen ble to those women who fear to consider themselves entitled to a destir separate from a family's, or who do not wish to face the anxiety ar dubious rewards of singularity. The rewards are dubious, not becau they are unimportant, or not life-enhancing, but because all birth, b especially birth at middle age, is painful and does not lead (as wome have been taught their lives must lead if they are good and loving) peace, acceptance, and appreciation. Perhaps the hardest task of midd age is to enter upon a new experience that must be, as all adventure i painful and risky.

Lessing's bridge from "To Room 19" to *The Summer Before the Dark*, as Roberta Rubinstein has pointed out, a novella about a 50-year-old an entitled *The Temptation of Jack Orkney* (Rubinstein, 1979, p. 200). The minent death of Orkney's father shocks him into awareness of his piritual drift toward inertia, the temptation of doing nothing. Kate rown of *The Summer Before the Dark* also will discover that she is, in ubinstein's words, "on the verge of a shift in her life's preoccupations id identity" (p. 200). Kate will experiment with sexuality, new as-urances of her attractiveness, but above all she will dream repeatedly of rrying a dying seal toward water, necessary to its survival. The seal is ate's identity, her selfhood, her hope of rejuvenation that will not be sy at her age. Rejuvenation for women is not a replay of youthful iccess—charm, male attentions, serving the needs of children. Rather, ate must enact all the rejections of age—*not* to be found alluring, entic-g—that her society has taught her are the rejections of womanhood id personhood. Even if she can, by dressing a certain way, evoke histles from construction workers, is this reassuring? She must instead scover a strength, or the chance for strength, that does not end with arriage and "they lived happily ever after" but rather begins with the nowledge of old age and death as they come to all, but not with espe-al harshness to women. Bearing the great weight of her own self, she ruggles toward life.

Women who are artists in life rather than in literature have taught s that work is the great redeemer. But women often deny this because tey have been trained to dream, not of opening doors, but of closure, ie safe house whose threshold, symbolically speaking, they have eeded to cross only once. Women's romances, like television commer-als, provide easy resolutions, and a cast of characters who speak as xpected. Do the right thing and they will love you. Those who have ritten of middle age in literature speak less of work, more of the need eschew closure, to choose risk, to know that, as with those feared aralyzed, pain is the sign of life, the hope for recovery.

In 19th-century novels, the most middle-aged women were allowed as another marraige, another manly chest to subside upon. Perhaps e closest we come in a 19th-century novel to a middle-aged woman's vareness of these modern questions is Daniel Deronda's mother. She unique, perhaps, in all literature. She is a woman who did not wish to ve out the erotic plot, who particlarly detested the role of women in wish tradition. The patriarchal tradition has long seen daughters, par-cularly when they are only children, as the means of acquiring a grand-n, a continuation of the paternal line (think of Shakespeare's Juliet). s Daniel Deronda's mother says of her father, "I was to be what he lled 'the Jewish woman' under pain of his curse. I was to feel everything I did not feel, and believe everything I did not believe" (Eliot, 1967, p. 692). She tells her son, "Every woman is supposed to have the same set of motives, or else to be a monster. I am not a monster, I have not felt exactly what other women feel—or say they feel, for fear of being thought unlike others" (p. 691). Her father, Daniel's mother says, "cared more about a grandson to come than he did about me: I counted as nothing" (p. 698). "You are not a woman," she tries to explain to him: "You may try—but you can never imagine what it is to have a man's force of genius in you, and yet to suffer the slavery of being a girl. To have a pattern cut out—'this is the Jewish woman; this is what you must be; this is what you are wanted for'; a woman's heart must be of such a size and no larger, else it must be pressed small, like Chinese feet" (p. 694). Daniel's mother was a great artist, a great singer, and in middle age, what can she do but lament? In the modern novel, she may dare more, if not as a girl, then as an older woman. While George Eliot seems almost to have determined to doom this woman, how differently the voice sounds from that of Miss Havisham in Dickens's *Great Expectations*, who, deserted on her wedding day by her bridegroom, froze into permanent dejection and the unending repetition of that terrible moment. Nor might one answer that, had she married elsewhere, she might have lived. As I have suggested, Katherine Anne Porter shows us in "The Jilting of Granny Weatherall" that finding another man and having your life "like any other woman" does not mean that you have found your destiny, that you have been the author of your own story. Granny Weatherall might have said, with a character in Djuna Barnes's *Nightwood*, "I've not only lived my life for nothing, but I've told it for nothing" (1937, p. 165).

Male writers in the 20th century began also to portray middle-aged women characters in new and provocative ways. We might remember Kate of D. H. Lawrence's *The Plumed Serpent*, who is 40 at the book's opening, and profoundly dissatisfied with her life. While many readers and critics have found much that is troubling in this novel, Lawrence's presentation of a middle-aged woman's sense of meaninglessness in life is perceptive, even though her destiny does, in the end, revolve around a charismatic male leader, male violence, and a regrettable (though prophetic) religion. It is the beginning of the book that arrests us.

Closer to the central problems of middle age is Angus Wilson's *The Middle Age of Mrs. Eliot*, a study of the sudden awakening of a self-satisfied woman after the accidental shooting of her husband. She discovers that all her committees, good works, social acceptance have arisen from her position as "Mrs." Eliot, and not from herself as a person. "She thought, if Bill gave everything to me, what was my life for? It had no meaning except in him. They had set out together to climb

•mewhere; but she had been only a rope, not a guide, for she had
•ver known their destination or asked it, only judged its approach by
s look of certainty, reading his face for portents of success or failure.
•ere was not a single way that she could live for him now; or die for
m" (1960, p. 103). Wilson, unlike Lawrence, sees her through to a new
ceptance of selfhood; he has said that Mrs. Eliot is, of all his charac-
rs, the one closest to himself. The need of men to find an identity
•yond that of their business or corporation or government agency is
•e that renders the female character human for them, rather than
erely female.

In the years following Betty Friedan's *The Feminine Mystique*, many
omen authors have given us heroines who strike out in early middle
•e for themselves, leaving stifling marriages and seeking some degree
autonomy. Many of these might profitably be discussed here, but I
•all conclude with a current author who, now just 70, has long written
the middle-aged woman, and did so before the subject became fash-
nable or even respectable. May Sarton wrote a poem on her 50th
•rthday, which she celebrated in Greece, praising Athene:

> Not she of the olive,
> But she of the owl eyes,
> A spear in her hand. (1965a, p. 47)

She had first met this Athene in youth, and now, 50, knows this is
•t a place for the young: It is right, rather, to meet Athene on one's
•th birthday:

> It was the right year
> To confront
> The smile beyond suffering. (p. 49)

Sarton has written of married women, lonely within "happy" mar-
•ges, but she has also written of middle-aged women loving other
omen, finding in these loves the sources of poetry, of art. In *Mrs.*
evens Hears the Mermaids Singing, she portrays women lovers lost in the
•ppiness of discovering each other, while appearing to those who pass
•em like two dull middle-aged women: "There was a secret joy when
•ey walked down the street together (for at this time they often set out
• long walks) to know that from the outside what people saw was two
•iddle-aged women, but inside they were wild children, wild with joy,
•eling each of them that this (surely last and best) love affair was a great
•esent from life, a source of renewed energy" (1965b, p. 165). Sarton is
•riting of women who find renewed energy and passion in the love of
•her women late in life. But even for those who will not move into
•other and different passionate love, intimacy with women is an unex-
•cted reward of their new freedom to move outside of a constrained

destiny. Although Sarton has only touched upon this, many wome today have noticed how marriages have been preserved because of th wife's discovery of intimacy with other women, the release of hone conversation, the wonder of deep personal trust in friendship. Mar marriages have escaped dissolution because of the safety valve provide by these new friendships.

For women as for men, middle age must avoid the feverish ar fruitless search for fading youthful passions and reassurances; rather must seek a new country, new accomplishment, adventure, and th pain that is the price of adventure. Women have often to find thes adventures in a new world—of work, institutional struggle, ambition the agony of competition and compromise. (Men, already living in th world, may find their middle-aged adventure in personal tasks, and th private acts of nurturance.) Erik Erikson has written of generativity a the mature choice—the working for something beyond oneself, for fi ture generations. In late middle age, furthermore, one can afford to ta risks the young cannot afford: to speak out, to affront convention opinion and demands. Women, having been private people, perhap may now reach out and work in organized numbers, within existin institutions or in their own new groups. E. M. Forster, writing in the ba times between the world wars, regretted the need for the middle-age if they were not to retire from life altogether, to join a movement. I saw the time through which he had lived as a tragedy in three acts. "I the first act the individualist hopes to improve society, in the second, I tries to improve himself, in the third act he finds he's not wanted, ar has either to merge himself in a movement or to retire" (Colmer, 197 pp. 210–211).

Most of us now in late middle age were taught to be, as Forster wa wary of movements. But in the world of today, concerted action required, and required particularly of those, like women, who have live their lives devoted to personal and familial pursuits. Generativity tod may be possible only in a movement, or at least a communal effo whether political, artistic, or ideological. If one might end with a prop ecy, it is that, even for individualistic artists, generativity for women middle age will be found in bonding with other women, for mutu support, in an ambience of productive work and accomplishment.

References

Barnes, D. *Nightwood*. New York: New Directions, 1937.
Bennett, A. *The old wives' tale* (New ed. with preface). New York: Doubleday, Doran, 19.
Butler, S. *The way of all flesh*. New York: Modern Library, n.d.
Colmer, J. *E. M. Forster: The personal voice*. London: Routledge and Kegan Paul, 19
de Beauvoir, S. [*The second sex*] (H. M. Parshley, Ed. and trans.). New York: Knopf, 19.

esen, I. The monkey. In *Seven gothic tales.* New York: Vintage Books, 1972.

t, G. *Daniel Deronda.* New York: Penguin, 1967.

ud, S. The relation of the poet to daydreaming. In *Collected Papers* (Vol. 4). London: Hogarth Press, 1957.

lbrun, C. G. On Katherine Anne Porter . . . . In C. Skaggs (Eds.), *The American short story* (Vol. 2). New York: Dell, 1980.

es, H. *The notebooks of Henry James* (F. O. Matthiessen and K. B. Murdock, Eds.). New York: Oxford University Press, 1947.

es, H. *The ambassadors.* New York: Norton, 1964.

rns, M. *Käthe Kollwitz: Woman and artist.* Old Westbury, N.Y.: Feminist Press, 1976.

llet-Joris, F. A womanly vocation. In E. M. Eisenger and M. McCarty (Eds.), *Colette: The woman, the writer.* University Park: Pennsylvania State University Press, 1981.

tthiessen, F. O. *Henry James: The major phase.* New York: Oxford University Press, 1944.

tz, A. *George Eliot and the novel of vocation.* Cambridge, Mass.: Harvard University Press, 1978.

instein, R. *The novelistic vision of Doris Lessing: Breaking the forms of consciousness.* Urbana: University of Illinois Press, 1979.

de, M. *Colette: Free and fettered* (Richard Millder, Trans.). New York: William Morrow, 1980.

de, M. The first steps in a writer's career. In E. M. Eisenger and M. McCarty (Eds.), *Colette: The woman, the writer.* University Park: Pennsylvania State University Press, 1981.

ton, M. Birthday on the Acropolis. In *A private mythology.* New York: Norton, 1965. (a)

ton, M. *Mrs. Stevens hears the mermaids singing.* New York: Norton, 1965. (b)

ith, S. *Me again: Uncollected writings of Stevie Smith* (J. Barbera and W. McBrien, Eds.). London: Virago, 1981.

son, A. *The middle age of Mrs. Eliot.* New York: Meridian, 1960.

olf, V. *Mrs. Dalloway.* New York: Harcourt Brace, 1925.

olf, V. *To the lighthouse.* New York: Harcourt Brace Jovanovich, 1949.

oles and Relationships

'he Middle Years
hanges and Variations in Social Role ommitments

ELENA Z. LOPATA AND DEBRA BARNEWOLT

ıman beings are involved in many social roles in a lifetime, con-
cutively and within time-bound clusters. One can be a student, work-
, wife, and mother either simultaneously or at different times. At any
e stage of life, however, a person is involved in a cluster of roles, each
th its own cycle of involvement. Each role consists of a set of mutually
terdependent relations with members of a social circle for whom du-
s are performed and from whom rights are received (Lopata, 1971,
73; Lopata, Barnewolt, and Norr, 1980; Znaniecki, 1940, 1965).

The fact that several social roles are carried forth during the same
ne or stage of life and that each role involves many different people
n lead to problems, as sociologists and social psychologists have long
cognized (Biddle and Thomas, 1966; Newcomb, Turner, and Con-
rse, 1965; Ritzer, 1977). These problems have been labeled *role conflict*
d *role strain*. *Role conflict* arises when the demands of one role conflict
th those of another, as when two or more roles must be engaged in
thin too short a time period, or when they require psychologically
compatible sentiments or self-concepts. Even the same role can induce
casions of *role strain*, since it involves relations with several circle
gments (Gouldner, 1957; Merton, 1968; Merton *et al.*, 1957). Mothers
ay be faced with conflicting demands from children and their fathers,
may have each child demand attention at the same time. Role strain
mes from *role overload*, when circle members make too many demands;

ELENA Z. LOPATA AND DEBRA BARNEWOLT • Department of Sociology, Loyola Univer-
y, 6525 N. Sheridan Road, Chicago, Illinois 60626.

intersender strain, when two or more members of the social circle mak
conflicting demands; *intrasender strain,* when the same role partner give
inconsistent messages; and *role–person strain* when the demanded be
havior goes against the person's set of values or self-images (this is
slight modification of Kahn *et al.,* 1964; see also Biddle and Thoma:
1966; Goode, 1960; Gross, Mason, and McEadern, 1958; Ritzer, 1977
We can also look at conflict between roles or strain within a role over th
life-course. This enables us, for example, to examine the problems c
people caught in a social role that they feel interferes with their futu
plans. Many a young man felt such conflict when faced with inductio
into the armed services, which would disrupt preparation for his chose
occupation. Strain over the life-span of a role can occur when a moth
learns one way of relating with her children, only to find that this styl
becomes more and more dysfunctional as the children grow. Finally
problems in role performance may come from the ambiguity with whic
all participants, including the social person, view the role. Mack (195
analyzed the consequences of occupational indeterminateness an
found this to be one of the main problems of the role of housewife. Th
composition of the social circle of that role and the exchange of dutie
and rights within it are open to great variation and misunderstanding
On the other hand, as Coser (1975) points out, the complexity of soci
roles contributes to the complexity and autonomy of personality, and t
the feelings of accomplishment and competence.

The complexity of social circles of just four social roles of a woman
role-cluster at the peak stage of involvement can be partially understoc
from Figure 1. The possibilities of role conflict and role strain, as well a
for feelings of satisfaction, are limitless, not only in terms of duties be
also in the receipt of rights.

Dealing with Role Strain and Role Conflict

Goode (1960) outlines some ways in which a person or an organiz
tion can deal with the inevitable role strain experienced at some time c
another within their lives. The person can compartmentalize relation
with the various circle segments, postponing and sequencing deman
from each. Negotiations can reduce demands or change their timin
Some duties can be ignored or carried out with passive resistance
such ineffectual ways as to push the sender into the job herself or hir
self or into turning to someone else. There are numerous methods b
which workers learn to deal with role overload, intersender or intr
sender strain, or role conflict. Roles can be dropped, assisting segmen
of circles brought in, intermediaries found, and so forth.

Both role strain and role conflict are difficult to avoid and to de *ure 1. Generalized composition of the social circles of four major social roles of American women.*

en there is commitment by the social person to each role and to many ;ments of each social circle. Women committed to the role cluster of 'e/mother/employee/homemaker and the related roles of daughter, ughter-in-law, neighbor, friend, union member, etc., often report role ıflict (Bernard, 1971, 1973, 1974, 1975a, 1975b, 1981; Chapman and tes, 1977; Komarovsky, 1946). Not only do husband and children nand attention at the same time but they require different kinds of

behavior and sentiments. Being a perfect housekeeper is often perceive
in terms of the product—a spotless and neat home—a difficult accom
plishment in the presence of offspring and a not-very- "housebroken
husband (Lopata, 1971). The role of employee requires absence from th
home even at times when the roles of wife and mother require presence

One way in which people deal with role strain is by arrangin
duties in the different segments of the circle hierarchically, both in tern
of the importance assigned to the segment and in terms of the impo
tance assigned to specific duties toward each segment. A woman ma
feel, for example, that the duties to her children are more important tha
duties toward the grandparents concerning these children. She ma
further evaluate time spent companionately with the children as mo
important than focusing on their physical appearance (even when th
grandparents want them "looking pretty"). Role conflict can be partial
decreased through a hierarchical arrangement of the roles in the cluste
giving priority to the duties and rights of the roles by order of the
assigned importance (Lopata, 1971). Such ranking of roles can be situ
tional, time-bound, or considered as permanent. Problems arise,
course, if members of the different segments of one circle or of differe
social circles do not agree with the rank order an individual assigns
their segment or role—which is apt to happen if they are more involve
in one of the circles than in another. A man may resent having a woma
assign the role of wife, when he is the husband, to a second place
importance to the role of mother, even if he is the father of the childr
(Dyer, 1963; Hobbs, 1965; LeMasters, 1957; Rossi, 1968).

Each society and the smaller social units within it appear to recc
nize the problems of role conflict and role strain and encourage, or ev
enforce, hierarchies among different kinds of roles or for different kin
of members. American society has developed strong expectations th
men emphasize their occupational role and that circle members of th
other roles adjust their demands to those made by that role (Fowlk
1980; Pleck, 1975; Whyte, 1956) Wives and children, parents and frien
are expected, according to the American success ethic, to reduce th
demands upon the male worker, especially the career-minded prof
sional and business executive, if they interfere with the demands of t
job (Mortimer, Hall, and Hill, 1978). Although Pleck (1983) claims,
the basis of much research, that the American male has decreased
prior emphasis on his occupational role, others find it still dominant a
spreading to other societies. Evans and Bartolome (1980) studied Eu
pean middle managers who have adopted the American values of sι
cess, and concluded that the man's strong commitment to his occu
tion resulted in a great deal of spillover and strain to family life, w
which wives must deal.

The American woman, on the other hand, has experienced several anges in the expected composition and hierarchical arrangement of r social roles over the past century or so. Numerous historians and cial scientists have documented the shift in the role structure of mar-d women from kin, community, and occupational involvement to most exclusive focus upon home roles between the early 1800s and the 50s (Bernard, 1974, 1981; Easton, 1976; Lerner, 1971; Rothman, 1978; herman, 1975). As the society turned from agricultural to industrial d business life, with its focus on growth and technological change, ork became organized into jobs within large complex organizations vay from homes, to be performed mainly by full-time, continuously ployed men. These men, in turn, were expected to economically pport their wives, whose basic roles were homemaker, wife, and other.

The duties of these roles included the physical and emotional care the husband and children, home maintenance, and the conversion of jects for home use as one of the stages of production. Women's in-vement in economic life away from home was encouraged only prior marriage, or in cases of dire necessity, and women accepted this finition of the world, or had little power to change it. In any event, by turn into the 20th century and for many years after, only about one-h of the American women worked outside of the home in paid jobs. e figures vary by race and ethnicity, or at least immigrant status, inly because of necessity, but the ideal remained for married women stay home and not be involved in paid employment.

Role conflict within the family institution has resulted from the mpetition between two focal roles of women and the shift in the portance assigned to them at different times in American history. The sening of authority and power of the patrilineal line accompanying gration, democratization, mass education, and the creation of jobs shed obligations to in-laws and kin into a position of secondary im-rtance. "Family duties," generalized without specifying the main neficiary in traditional families, usually consisted of housekeeping ks, whether performed by the woman directly or through the work of ers (Lopata, 1966, 1971). Gradually, however, the romanticization of role of wife separated it from the general family maintenance and ded numerous personal duties. At the same time, the role of mother ned in complexity, with the addition of health maintenance duties ompanying the "germ theory" of illness and child developmental ties thanks to new theories of psychology (Ehrenreich and English, 9; Rothman, 1978). Thus, the roles of both wife and mother increased specialized importance, separating from the role of homemaker.

Although the "two-person career"—as sociologists have renamed

the situation in which the man takes on the public aspects of a profes
sional or business career while the wife forms the backup support
providing him with needed resources—continues to be idealized iⁱ
managerial, medical, religious, and even academic worlds, wives ar
seeking out careers of their own in increasing numbers (Fowlkes, 198(
Mortimer et al., 1978; Vandervelde, 1979). Social scientists have studie
ways in which professional and managerial men have been affected bⁱ
the career demands of their wives, the effects on family life and powe
distribution of dual-career marriages, and the consequences of caree
decisions of husbands on the careers of wives (Nadelson and Nadelsor
1980; Poloma, 1972; Poloma and Garland, 1971; Rapoport and Rapopor
1971, 1976). These studies have been accompanied by research on thⁱ
role conflict expected to be facing women as they leave the traditiona
and supposedly compatibly combined, cluster of housewife/wife/mothe
and add the role of worker (see Bird, 1979; Lopata and Pleck (1983). ,
few authors, such as Pleck (1975, 1979, 1983) point to the role conflic
experienced by men because of demands in the roles of worker, hu
band, father, and home-maintainer. Concern over the alleged role coⁱ
flict of women arises out of the historically dominant emphasis that the
carry the main, even total, responsibility for the maintenance and deve
opment—physical, social, and emotional—of the child. Although moⁱ
American women have small children at home for only a limited numbⁱ
of years of their nearly 80-year-life span, and although only very smⁱ
children are home during the whole day, the women are expected
keep themselves in a holding pattern in their preparation for adult rolⁱ
and throughout life in order to be able to stay home during these fe
years. The emphasis on the ideology defining women as primariⁱ
mothers who should be home constantly during the years when the
children are young is evident in three ways: first, the failure of tⁱ
society to provide alternate child care resources; second, the tendency
women to drop out of paid employment after childbirth; and third, tⁱ
constriction of most discussion about women's employment to thoⁱ
years (Lopata, Barnewolt, and Miller, in press; Lopata, et al., 198
Lopata and Norr, 1979, 1980).

Awareness of the possibility of role conflict in the lives of Americⁱ
women and of the culturally prescribed, though not consistent, hiⁱ
archical arrangement allegedly decreasing this conflict leads to maⁱ
sociologically interesting questions. Which of the currently discuss
roles of women—wife, mother, employee, or homemaker—are chos
as the most important by different types of women? What factors, suⁱ
as involvement in a role, the composition of the core role-cluster, baⁱ
ground, age of children, family income, or own earnings, most contr
ute to the probability that a woman will select one of these roles as tⁱ

ost important to her at the present time? What are the cohort dif-
rences in the role selected as the most important? How do women
xpect their role focus to change over time? What changes in life circum-
ances, experienced or projected, influence the hierarchical consistency
r flexibility during the middle years of life? We now turn to an examina-
on of the roles women in the middle years of life consider the most
nportant, emphasizing both the similarities and the differences among
em.

METHODS AND SAMPLES

The first study of women's role hierarchies conducted by the senior
uthor utilized questions from several waves of interviews. A 1956 sam-
e consisted of 300 suburban homeowners who were married and had
least one pre-high school child in the home (Lopata, 1966, 1971). Most
ere white but they varied in social class, with lower-class women
owing a definite variation in role orientation from their middle-class
unterparts in that they were less oriented to roles outside of the home
d to the role of wife. Second- and third-wave interviews used the
me schedule, or a more formalized variation, and reached full-time
memakers and employees in older suburbs and in the central city. A
tal of 571 interviews, including the 300 original ones, were selected out
a total of over 1000 for analysis (Lopata, 1971). Although a subset of
e sample responded to a structured question by ranking 12 roles from
set list, most of the respondents were asked an open-ended question:
What are the most important roles of a women (in order of impor-
nce)?" The research yielded a sevenfold classification of women:

1. The husband-oriented woman sees her basic role as that of wife,
   grouping other sets of relations around it; husband-oriented
   wives have successful husbands.
2. The child-oriented woman believes that the basic unit of the
   family consists of herself and her children.
3. The house-oriented woman establishes her major area of interest
   in her home and its maintenance. She often feels that people
   impinge upon this relation, upsetting her equilibrium by disar-
   ranging the house.
4. The life cycle woman decreases her concentration on the role of
   wife after the children are born but returns to it in later years,
   either as her children mature or when the retirement, work dis-
   engagement, or "phasing-out" stages are reached by her husband.
5. The family-oriented woman blends all roles related to the home,

those of wife, mother, and housewife, into a single "family care package.

6. The self-directed woman refuses to focus upon any of these role as basic to her. She is more concerned with herself as a tota individual and with satisfying what she defines as her need than with any role.

7. The woman oriented toward roles outside of her home tend toward such activities as that of worker, community membe: volunteer, friend, neighbor, member of a religious organizatio (Lopata, 1971, pp. 64–66).

The most recent study of American urban women, with interview in 1978, focused on their construction of reality and included a prob bility sample of 966 metropolitan Chicago respondents aged 25 to 5 Oversampling of currently nonmarried women resulted in a weighte total of 1,877.[1] The construction of reality theoretical framework aims the interpretation people have of the world around them and of the place in it. It is concerned with the definition of the situation with whic people approach all of the aspects of their lives and their self-images The role-order question came first in the interview in order to prevei bias arising from the focus of the interview itself and read as follows

Please tell me which of these roles is the most important one to you now?
Which role is second in importance.
Which role is third in importance?
Which role is fourth in importance to you now?
Here is a list of social roles which women can perform at different stages in their lives:

daughter
student
worker
friend
active/involved citizen
mother

[1]Research on the changing commitments of women to work and family roles is the basis this study and was funded by the Social Security Administration (Contract No. SSA600-: 0190, 1975–1979). Dr. Henry P. Brehm was the SSA project officer, Dr. Helena Lopata w principal investigator, and Dr. Kathleen Norr was deputy director. Interviews were cc ducted in 1977–1978 by the staff of the Survey Research Laboratory of the University Illinois, Circle Campus. Our thanks go to Kathy Norr, Cheryl Miller, Suzanne Meyerir Marlene Simon, and Jennifer Ettling of the Center for the Comparative Study of Soc Roles, Loyola University of Chicago, for their contributions to various stages of research.
[2]The interview, whose theoretical foundation aimed at the construction of reality of t respondents, contained 31 areas of "competence" and "characteristics" items, whi factored into six clusters. These are summarized into leadership, competence, successf ness/intelligence, emotionality, social interaction, and creativity factors.

career woman
homemaker
volunteer worker
wife
member of a church, synagogue, or other religious group
grandmother

The same set of questions was asked for "thinking about when you
ere 24" and "looking ahead, which of these roles do you think will be
e most important one when you are 55?" In the course of this chapter,
e will look at the roles the women chose as the most important ones at
e present time and through their adult years.

The recent study (1978; see Lopata and Norr, 1979, 1980) involved
omen who are representative of those who live in the Chicago area,
cept for the fact that they are more highly educated, due to their
lative youth. Thirty-nine percent are Catholic, 48% are Protestant, 4%
e Jewish, and the remainder are either without religious identity or
attered among other groups; 73% are white and the majority of the
nwhites are black. The ethnic background of this part of America is
flected in the fact that 46% of the women grew up in families that are
osely identified with a national or ethnic group. The women are diver-
ied educationally; 58% have no more than a high school degree, while
% graduated from college, some of them obtaining more advanced
hooling. Most of the women (74%) are married and have children in
e home (77%); only 8% live alone. Although almost a third of the
ungest women aged 25 to 34 have no children, the percentage drops
6 for the oldest age cohort. Ten percent of the respondents have never
arried. As for employment characteristics of the sample, 58% of the
omen are currently holding a job outside of the home in addition to
memaking activities. The employees are mainly in occupations tradi-
nally held by women. The professional women are mainly in the
miprofessions such as teaching or nursing. The other white-collar
orkers are concentrated in clerical jobs, and the blue-collar workers are
edominantly operatives or service employees.

IE MOST IMPORTANT ROLE OF WOMEN

Table 1 summarizes the role the women consider most important in
eir lives at the present time. Few women consider a role in which they
e currently not involved as the most important, so we have organized
e respondents by such involvement in the major roles of American
omen: employee, wife, mother, homemaker, member of society and
 groups, and kin member. Such a small number of the respondents
e involved in the role of wife alone, without combining it with em-

Table 1. The Most Important Role by Role Involvement of Chicago Area Women (Percentage Distribution)

Role involvement	Role preference						
	Employee	Wife	Mother	Homemaker	Societal member	Kin member	Total (N)
Employee only	78	0	1	1	14	6	(16
Employee and wife	17	63	8	7	5	0	(11
Employee and mother	24	1	63	2	7	4	(17
Employee, wife, and mother	7	33	48	7	4	0	(61
Wife and mother	1	34	52	10	2	1	(65
Mother only	6	0	70	9	11	5	(10
Total	14	27	45	7	5	2	(183

ployment or the role of mother, that they have been removed from thi analysis. There are 168 women in the sample who are employees but nc wives or mothers, 104 who are mothers but not wives or employees, 11 who combine the role of wife and employee, and 174 involved in bot mothering and working outside of the home. By far the largest numbe of women (651) are wives and mothers but not employees, or combin the home involvements of wife and mother with employment (617 Interestingly enough, there are more women who have not ever entere marriage than who have never been employed for at least 6 month:

Employees who are not also wives and mothers are much more a to rank the role of worker or career woman as the top role than ar women involved in family roles. They are also the most frequent liste of societal roles such as church member, friend, student, citizen, (volunteer, in that order of frequency. Only two women list volunteer a their most important role at the present time, and the number increase to only 24 for the future time period of when they are age 55. Th addition of the role of wife immediately moves a woman's role emphas away from employment, making her husband-oriented, and the add tion of the role of mother also dramatically alters the importance a signed the role of worker. The combination of the roles of wife ar mother decreases the importance of the employee role, so that only 7 of the respondents involved in all three roles assign first place in order importance to a role external to the family. Married workers withou children are most heavily concentrated on the role of wife, largely due

ıe fact that the addition of motherhood splits commitment between
ıese two roles. Whether or not a woman is employed does not notice-
bly influence her tendency to select wife or mother as the most impor-
ınt role, since few choose employee over the role of wife or mother.
Vomen lacking either the role of wife or the combination of wife and
mployee are the most committed to motherhood. Concentration on the
ɔle of mother by nonmarried homemakers is only slighly relieved by
ıe importance of the role of homemaker or member of a set of relations
ıtside of the home. The role of homemaker does not receive "most
ıportant" ranking for the most part, but full-time homemakers who
re also mothers, whether married or not, are the most likely to rank
omemaker as the most important role. The downplaying of this role
ifferentiates the 1978 women from those studied in the 1950s and
ᴐ60s, since women in that era were twice as likely as women in 1978 to
ıve it first place in the order of importance. All in all, the role of mother
ır outweighs any other role, including that of wife, as most important
ɔr Chicago area women. We shall now examine the characteristics of
ᵒomen who stress the different roles as important to them now, focus-
ıg only on the roles of employee, wife, and mother.

ᴴE WORK- OR CAREER-ORIENTED WOMAN

Although only 14% of the Chicago area women list worker or career
ᵒoman as the most important role at the present time, distributions
ıry, depending on several factors. As mentioned before, the work-
ᵣiented women do not face competition from the other two roles
ᵉemed important for their sex in American society because they are less
ᵪely to be married and to have children. Interestingly enough, and
ɔntrary to expectations, it is the blue-collar woman, rather than her
ʰite-collar counterpart, who is most apt to list the role of employee
ᵣst in the absence of the roles of wife and mother (see Table 2).

In addition, the blue-collar worker who is married continues to
ᵉlect the role of worker, while the other workers drop their emphasis
ı the job when marriage is added, with a sizable exception in the case
ᶠ professional and managerial women. Duncan socioeconomic scores of
ıe respondents' jobs are not, however, significantly related to their role
ᵣientation, as far as the employee role is concerned. Educational
ᵪhievement is not as important an influence on role choice as was
ıticipated, although it has more impact on women who went to college
ıan on those who ended their education before reaching that level.
ımily background is also not significantly connected with the place-
ent of the employee role in first order of importance, whether it be
ᵈexed by the father's education or occupation, the mother's education

Table 2. The Most Important Role by Role Involvement and Last or Current Occupational Category of Chicago Area Women

Role involvement	Employee role			Wife role			Mother role		
	Professional	White-collar	Blue-collar	Professional	White-collar	Blue-collar	Professional	White-collar	Blue-collar
	(%)	(%)	(%)	(%)	(%)	(%)	(%)	(%)	(%)
Employee only	82	67	88	0	0	0	1	0	0
Employee and wife	26	6	67	62	70	0	0	12	33
Employee and mother	26	28	18	0	0	1	53	61	68
Employee, wife, and mother	9	6	8	44	40	17	37	42	61
Wife and mother	2	1	1	36	34	28	53	51	50
Mother only	0	4	8	0	0	0	100	77	67

r experience in paid employment when the daughter was growing up,
r the general socioeconomic status of the home. Also insignificant in
ifluencing the woman's tendency to list the role of worker first are the
usband's characteristics, such as his education, occupational category,
r Duncan score. The work-oriented women tend to see themselves as
taders and successful people, and they are less likely to see themselves
s emotional than are women who give first importance to other roles. It
, the age of the children, rather than the age of the respondent, that is
te crucial variable. The presence of small children, at least one of whom
, under age six, dramatically decreases the choice of employee as the
tost important role. The work-oriented women tend to live alone, or
/ith someone other than a husband and children. The only other impor-
int factors, out of many hypothesized about the women's past or pre-
ent situation, are the respondent's earnings and her dependence upon
tese in the absence of other sources of income. This circumstance is
sually due to the absence of a husband and thus competition from the
ile of wife.

HE HUSBAND-ORIENTED WOMAN

Twenty-eight percent of the women in our sample list the role of
/ife as the most important one at the present time. These respondents
:nd to be wives who are currently employed but without children.
hey tend to have entered that role between the ages of 22 and 24 and to
ave been married a high proportion of time since age 18. The woman's
ackground characteristics appear not to influence her willingness to list
te role of wife first. The "strongest" relation exists between the fre-
uency with which the wives list that role and the characteristics of the
usband's job and earnings. The more education the husband has, the
igher the Duncan score of his occupation, the more often he is in
rofessional or managerial positions, and the more he earns, the more
ot is the woman to place the role of wife first in order of importance.
/omen whose husbands earn little in low-status jobs are definitely not
usband-oriented; instead, the focus of their attention is on the mother
ile. For example, only 25% of the women whose husbands did not
nish high school list the role of wife first, but 45% of those with college-
lucated husbands do so. The distribution is practically duplicated
hen Duncan socioeconomic status scores are considered (these figures
'e in the "Now" column of the role of wife in Table 4). If the family
.come without the respondent's earnings is under $10,000, the wife is
ot apt to list that role first, with only 4% doing so. However, 39% of the
ives living on incomes of over $25,000 (in addition to their own earn-
igs, if any) are husband-oriented. These are similar to findings of the

1956–1965 studies of women living in the same metropolitan area (Lopata, 1971).

THE CHILD-ORIENTED WOMAN

Women oriented toward the role of mother are most often characterized by having a child under the age of 3 at home. Interestingly enough, increase in the number of children tends to decrease orientation toward the role of mother. Women who had their first child at age 27 or later are more apt to list the role of mother first than are women who entered the role at the early age of 19 or less (61 to 43%). The most apt to be oriented toward this role are women who either live alone with their children or share the household with someone else, but not a husband. Child-oriented women tend to be of a lower socioeconomic background and current standing than are the others, mainly because they experience less competition from the role of wife. When compared to women of other role orientations, child-oriented women are not as apt to be employed, thus decreasing the likelihood of role conflict. Both they and their husbands, if any, reached minimal educational levels. Finally, these women are not apt to see themselves as successful leaders, although the factor of emotionality is not related to the frequency of listing the role of mother first. Of course, the self-images are related to socioeconomic background and status, as is the tendency to list the role of mother first, rather than being directly related to that variable.

MULTIPLE CLASSIFICATION ANALYSIS OF ROLE IMPORTANCE

The use of multiple classification analysis enables us to assess the individual and collective impact of nominal and ordinal variables on a woman's likelihood of describing a role as "most important" at the time of the interview. In addition, multiple classification analysis is especially useful because it calculates the impact of each variable controlling for the other variables in the equation. Because not all of the relationships analyzed here are strictly linear in character, the amount of explained variance remains low, but observing the deviation from the mean gives us added insight into the role hierarchies of the women in our study. This enables us to construct a profile of women who are very likely to select role as important and a correspondent profile of women who are most unlikely to choose that role.

Involvement in the employee role, combined with the exclusion of familial roles, is the most important factor in the choice of worker or career woman as a woman's most important role. In addition, women who have been employed in professional occupations more than 60% of the time since they were 18 years old and who have a high family income are most likely to choose employee as their most important role. Surprisingly, when controlling for the above variables, women with relatively low educational levels of less than high school are also most apt to choose employee as their most important role. Respondents with high levels of education (college completion) are least likely to choose the role of worker or career woman as important when factors of involvement are controlled. Contrary to initial assumptions, older women choose employee as the most important role more often than do young women, probably because of the lesser significance assigned to the role of mother. Deviations from the mean in the opposite direction are not as strong, possibly because the mean proportion of women who choose employee as the most important role is relatively low. The least likely to choose employee are women who are wives and mothers but are not in paid work, who have worked less than 30% of the time since they were 18 years of age, and who did so in blue-collar occupations. Thus, commitment to the employee role is largely dependent on the lack of involvement in competing familial roles, coupled with long duration of involvement in employment, particularly in professional occupations.

Involvement in the role of wife is the single most important factor in determining whether or not a woman will choose that role as most important, but other characteristics of her involvement in that role have additional impact. The woman most likely to choose the role of wife is married and working outside of the home, but is not a mother. In addition, women aged 45 to 54 who were married at age 18 or younger, whose marriage did not end in divorce or death of the spouse, and whose husbands have graduated from college and have high status and high income jobs are most apt to list the role of wife as of greatest importance to them. Those least likely to so rank the role of wife are employees and mothers now aged 25 to 34 who are not currently married and who were between the ages of 22 and 24 when married the first time. From this information we can see that women highly committed to the role of wife have been in that role continuously and with the same man. In addition, their husbands are likely to be occupationally successful men, a finding that shows little change in the last 20 years.

Actual involvement in the role of mother is the main variable when assessing influences on the importance of that role to women. In addition, the other roles in which a woman is involved in tandem with that of mother strongly affect her choice of that role as the most important. Women who are mothers only—that is, who are not wives or employees at the same time—are the most likely to choose mother as the most important role. Those who are both mothers and wives but not employees are the least likely of the women with children to list the role of mother as most important. A variety of factors that reflect the extent of involvement in the role of mother have added impact on the likelihood of choosing that role. Women currently aged 25 to 34, those who entered the role of mother at a relatively late age of 27 or older, those currently with a child less than 3 years old in the home, and those with either an only child or with five or more children were most likely to choose mother as their most important role at the time of the interview. Older women (aged 45–54) who became mothers while still teenagers and had two children who are already grown are least likely to choose mother as the most important role in their lives at this time. It becomes apparent that *active* involvement in mothering young children is statistically the *most significant* indicator of the likelihood of choosing mother as one's most important role.

CHANGES IN COMMITMENTS TO BASIC ROLES IN THE MIDDLE YEARS

The Chicago area women aged 25 to 54 report some very interesting beliefs as to shifts in their focal role within their middle years of life (see Table 3). Of course, the role hierarchies are affected not only by age and stage in the life-course of the woman but also by historical cohort effects. Women in their early 50s in 1978, when they were interviewed, were born between 1923 and 1928. They experienced the depression when very young but were entering marriage and motherhood during the post-World War II baby boom years in which the roles of mother and wife were accentuated in the extreme in American society (Elder, 1974; Friedan, 1963; Lopata, 1971). Women now in their 20s are apt to have been influenced, on the other hand, by feminism and the push of women to paid employment. The differences are somewhat visible in Table 3 in that more of the youngest cohort of women than of the oldest place the role of worker or career woman in first place in order of importance now, when they were age 24, and when they will be age 55. Still, the differences are not large and could be accounted for by the absence of children, indicating the possibility that this much-publicized shift to the world of work might be exaggerated as far as commitment rather than simple involvement is concerned.

Commitment to the role of wife shows interesting variation, by age and in the life-course overview. The youngest women think that they will be much more oriented toward this role when they reach age 55 than are women now approaching age 55. The older women do not see themselves as having gone through a dramatic swing in their commitment to the role of wife, while all the other women see themselves as having major life or family-cycle shifts. The differences between what the young women think will be important to them at age 55 and what

Table 3. Perceived Life-Course Changes in Focal Role by Current Age of Chicago Area Women

Most important role at age	Current age						All
	24–29	30–34	35–39	40–44	45–49	50–54	
	(%)	(%)	(%)	(%)	(%)	(%)	(%)
Employee							
24	25	20	19	14	13	16	19
Now	21	12	9	11	6	15	14
55	18	16	16	15	9	10	15
Wife							
24	35	31	38	36	33	37	34
Now	26	20	28	29	35	31	28
55	47	49	51	49	48	38	47
Mother							
24	24	34	34	31	36	32	31
Now	39	58	51	46	33	31	44
55	14	7	7	13	10	22	12
Homemaker							
24	5	4	2	4	7	1	4
Now	4	6	6	7	12	12	7
55	3	5	4	2	5	5	4
Other							
24	11	11	7	15	11	14	12
Now	10	4	6	7	14	11	7
55	18	23	22	21	28	25	22
Total (N)[a]	500	346	320	251	237	222	1876

[a] 100% is obtained by adding percentages in cells of roles at each time period.

women who are now approaching that age think is also evident, though a less extreme, when we look at the role of mother. Women in their 30s, who are the most likely of any cohort to list the role of mother as very important now, expect it to fade into lesser importance when they get older, while women now in the 50-to-54 age range still consider it important much more frequently. The difference in the percentage of women aged 25 to 29 and those 50 to 54 listing the role of mother as important to them at age 24 is probably due to the fact that the youngest women have delayed motherhood until a later age than the older women.

Whether it is a matter of historical cohort differences or stages in the life-course, the older women in our sample are much more apt than are the youngest respondents to list the role of homemaker as the most important to them now, although it is difficult to explain their antici-pated drop in importance of this role within the next few years. It is quite possible that they anticipate a reduction in the size of the house-hold as a source of decreasing the complexity of that role (Lopata, 1966). Finally, we find that all women expect an increase in the importance they will assign to social roles outside of the basic four of wife, mother, homemaker, and employee when they reach age 55. Women in the middle years of life are especially apt to ignore roles outside of this cluster, such as friend, member of a religious group, or citizen. They, as well as women who are now aged 45 to 54, expect to turn to these roles in the future. Only 10% of this increase in the number of respondents expecting such a shift is accounted for by an expansion of the role of grandmother; other roles each contribute a few women. There is surpris-ingly little variation among the different age cohorts in their view of life-course changes in commitments, except for the women in their 30s who are so heavily involved in the role of mother at the present time.

Looking now at the three roles most apt to be listed as of importance at the top level—those of employee, wife, and mother—by actual in-volvement we find further corroboration of some of the previous state-ments. The role of employee is considered the most important "now" by many more employed women who are not also wives or mothers than at "age 24" or "age 55." This is very interesting and supports theories of midlife phasing out of interest in one's occupation first developed by Brim and Wheeler (1966) and Neugarten (1973); see also Ritzer (1977). An alternative explanation is that the younger women expect to enter the roles wife and mother and thus to decrease the importance of the role of career woman or worker in the future. This appears to be true of respondents who are now combining the role of employee and wife and who report that they gave the first of these roles greater importance when they were age 24 than they do now.

Life-course variation in commitment is very evident when we look at the roles of wife and mother (see Table 4). Many of the women who are combining marriage and employment, but not motherhood, at the present time may be anticipating having children, since they drop of the commitment to the role of wife at age 55. Full-time homemakers who are wives and mothers anticipate a definite drop of orientation toward the children when they reach age 55. The same is true of women who combine wife, mother, and employee roles. Interestingly enough, few expect to increase the importance assigned the role of worker and few obviously expect to become widowed.

Although most of the associations are not statistically significant

able 4. Perceived Life-Course Changes in the Focal Social Role by Role Involvement
Chicago Area Women (Mean Proportion Selecting Role as Most Important)

ole	Employee role			Wife role			Mother role		
volvement	24[a]	Now[b]	55[c]	24	Now	55	24	Now	55
mployee only	.56	.78	.45	07	.00	.27	.01	.01	.03
mployee and wife	.24	.17	.17	.54	.63	.56	.02	.08	.20
mployee and mother	.14	.24	.26	.31	.01	.05	.42	.63	.24
mployee, wife, and mother	.12	.07	.10	.35	.33	.54	.39	.47	.08
ife and mother	.18	.01	.07	.40	.33	.64	.32	.51	.10
other only	.10	.06	.15	.21	.00	.04	.49	.70	.29
ll	.19	.14	.15	.34	.28	.47	.31	.44	.12

t age 24 (respondents were all between age 25 and 54 at time of interview).
t the time of the interview.
nticipated at age 55.

ome of the variations within the "most important role" assignment
elated to such variables as the respondent's education, her earnings,
amily income, and the family income minus her earnings are worth
xamining (see Table 5). Although education increases interest in the
ole of employee, it does not influence life-course attachments. The
woman most apt to focus on the role of employee, with a peak at the
resent time, is one who is totally financially dependent upon her earn-
ngs and who does very well in bringing home the money. The drop she
xpects in focusing on the role of employee is probably due to antici-
ated marriage, or remarriage, since more women give the role of wife
s the most important role of age 55 than do so now, if they are currently
ngle breadwinners. The respondents whose family income is pro-
uced mainly by someone other than themselves and is high tend to be
usband-oriented, as mentioned before, and a dramatic 71% of all wom-
n living on a high income not earned directly by themselves expect to
e husband-oriented at age 55. Thus, the pattern is clear: The husband's
arnings influence the emphasis by the wife on her relation with him, in
he past, present, and future, more than any other variable.

Looking at the life-course commitment to the role of wife by the
haracteristics of the husband, which proved so important in the "now"
eriod, we find an especially strong trend by wives of highly educated
en in prestigious jobs to anticipate a strong orientation toward those

Table 5. Perceived Life-Course Changes in the Importance of the Roles of Employee, Wife, and Mother by the Respondent's Education and Earnings, Combined Family Income, and Family Income without Respondent's Earnings of Chicago Area Women (Mean Proportion Selecting Role as Most Important)

Education, Earnings, Income	Employee role			Wife role			Mother role		
	24[a]	Now[b]	55[c]	24	Now	55	24	Now	55
Respondent's education									
Less than high school	.13	.10	.11	.23	.16	.23	.46	.53	.21
High school graduate	.15	.09	.11	.36	.31	.52	.36	.46	.09
Some college	.21	.18	.16	.40	.30	.56	.30	.41	.08
College graduate	.30	.21	.23	.37	.29	.51	.10	.35	.11
Respondent's earnings									
$1,000–$5,999	.17	.06	.10	.38	.34	.52	.26	.43	.08
$6,000–$9,999	.16	.16	.11	.34	.26	.46	.38	.43	.13
$10,000–$14,999	.24	.33	.23	.31	.23	.40	.25	.32	.10
$15,000+	.35	.46	.40	.25	.21	.30	.21	.26	.09
Family income									
Less than $10,000	.18	.16	.17	.20	.06	.15	.40	.53	.23
$10,000–$14,999	.23	.28	.19	.26	.11	.28	.27	.37	.11
$15,000–$19,999	.20	.05	.10	.38	.32	.60	.34	.52	.09
$20,000–$24,999	.16	.10	.13	.47	.41	.64	.25	.36	.07
Income without respondent's earnings									
0	.35	.54	.35	.16	.04	.18	.21	.29	.15
Low	.17	.11	.14	.26	.19	.29	.39	.48	.18
Medium	.16	.07	.12	.39	.35	.56	.33	.47	.10
High	.17	.04	.09	.47	.39	.71	.25	.43	.06

[a] At age 24 (respondents were all between age 25 and 54 at time of interview).

Table 6. Perceived Life-Course Changes in the Importance of the Role of Wife by Husband's Education, Occupational Category, and Duncan Socioeconomic Score for Chicago Area Women (Mean Proportion Selecting Wife as Most Important Role)

Husband's characteristics	Wife role		
	24	Now	55
Husband's education			
Less than high school	.27	.25	.33
High school graduate	.36	.35	.55
Some college	.35	.31	.67
College graduate	.52	.45	.69
Husband's occupation			
Blue-collar	.30	.30	.46
White-collar	.33	.42	.67
Professional	.48	.40	.67
Husband's Duncan score			
0–19	.25	.21	.36
20–39	.36	.35	.47
40–59	.31	.37	.60
60–69	.43	.41	.66
70+	.56	.42	.70

nen in the anticipated future (see Table 6). The overall pattern is strong, lthough the measures of significance are lowered by the lack of consistency. Women whose husbands are in low-prestige jobs certainly never anticipate becoming oriented toward them above all other sets of elations.

The lower the education of the woman, on the other hand, the more pt she is to list the role of mother as the most important role to her now nd at the age of 24. And although this emphasis is expected to decrease t age 55 for such women, the stress on motherhood continues more requently than is true of the women at other educational levels. The igher the earnings of the respondent, the less apt she is to list the role f mother as the most important; such women stress the employee role nd are apt not to have children. Total family income has an uneven ssociation with emphasis on the role of mother, except that the women vith the least amount of funds tend to be more child-oriented in memoies of age 24, at the present time, and in the future.

Finally, a look at Table 7 shows interesting trends in the importance ssigned to the role of mother. Respondents for whom the role of moth-

Table 7. Perceived Life-Course Changes in the Importance of the Role of Mother by Age of Respondent at the Birth of the First Child, Age of Youngest Child, and the Number of Children for Chicago Area Women (Mean Proportion Selecting Mother as Most Important Role)

Mothering characteristics	Mother role		
	24	Now	55
Age at birth of first child			
19 or younger	.56	.43	.1?
20–22	.58	.52	.1(
23–26	.30	.49	.1(
27 or older	.15	.61	.1(
Age of youngest child			
Less than 3 years old	.25	.75	.0*
3 to 5 years old	.45	.64	.1!
6 to 17 years old	.38	.51	.1
No child less than 18 years old	.18	.12	.0*
Number of children			
0	.01	.03	.1*
1	.24	.64	.1.
2	.33	.51	.0?
3–4	.39	.50	.1
5 or more	.55	.49	.1?

er was of primary importance in the remembered age of 24 becam mothers at age 22 or younger, but even those who were not yet mother at that time were oriented toward children in 15% of the cases. On th other hand, mothers who entered that role at a later date, as state before, really focus on it now and even tend to anticipate a similar focu at age 55 more often than do the other women. The age of the younge* child is an important variable; respondents listing the role of mother a the most important to them now typically have small children. Th association is very strong, compared to other associations. On the oth hand, the connection between the number of children and the perceive importance of the role of mother is uneven. As mentioned before, it the mother of one child, rather than the one with multiple offspring who most often concentrates on this role for now. As the number c children goes up, however, the probability of the mother finding th role important at age 24 and carrying over this importance into old years increases, only the mother of one child expects continued cor centration on the role of mother as often as does the parent of five c more children. The one-child mother is likely to have that offspring a bit later in life and to have it by choice. She is also more educated than are the mothers of two or three children, and thus more conscious of the importance of the mother for developing the child.

SUMMARY AND CONCLUSIONS

The series of studies of metropolitan women just described indicates how they organize their roles within the role-cluster and over time, assigning hierarchical rank to those in which they are actually involved. The role of employee takes primary focus mainly when the roles of wife and mother are absent from a woman's current life, and only 14% of women aged 25 to 54 in the most recent study assign it first place. Thus, the mass media image of the "new American woman," committed to occupation above family, is simply not reflected in reality, at least among Chicago area women, a finding consistent with those reported in *The Inner American* (Veroff, Douvan, and Kulka, 1981). Even the professionals do not rank it first if they are wives or mothers, and especially if they are both. Husband-oriented women tend not to have children and/or are married to men with a high educational background who are in high-paying and high-prestige jobs. One assumes that such marriages are more demanding of the role of wife and that the woman is more conscious of the contribution made to the home by the husband than are women whose spouse brings home relatively little money from a low-prestige job. Child-oriented women tend to have only one child or to have very young children and to have entered this role relatively late in life. They often lack the role of wife and even employee. The home-oriented woman is almost absent from this sample, although twice the proportion of such Chicagoans existed in the 1956–1965 data (14 to 7%; see Lopata, 1971). Societal and kin roles outside of the family of procreation did not fare well in this study, except among employees who are not married or mothers.

The women in the recent study tend to see their involvement in social roles in life-course terms, expecting a shift from the role of mother to that of wife if they are involved now in child-rearing. Women close to the age of 55, which was used for projections of role importance in the future, tend to see themselves as having shifted emphasis much less often than do the younger women. Those nearing age 55 do not anticipate major changes in the near future, except for an increase of involvement in roles outside of the basic complex of wife and mother. There is no strong projected shift by any women toward the role of employee in the future, in spite of the probability of divorce or widowhood by the time they reach age 55. Roles outside of the home, such as those of friend, member of a religious group, citizen, or neighbor, are expected to increase in importance in their future on the part of women of all ages in 1978, although the respondents now between age 50 and 54 are not as yet so involved. Over twice as many expect roles outside of the family to be of primary importance at age 55 than are so involved at ages 50 to 54.

The strong emphasis on the role of mother, especially by women who have young children and who themselves tend to be in their 30s, as well as the anticipated shift to the role of wife as children become less dependent, reflects American culture and the reality of life. Women's projections into the future show strong differences between what younger women think they will value most when they become age 55 and what women close to that age regard as important at the present time. The younger women think the role of mother will recede in importance much more often than is true of the older women. The younger women are also much more apt to expect the wife role to become very important in the future than older women find it to be. Of course, we do not know if this is a historical or an age phenomenon.

The Chicago area women whom we have studied over the years tend to be relatively traditional. Their stress on the role of mother reflects the value system of American culture. A major difference between the 1956 and the 1978 respondents is the devaluation of the role of housewife, which is not surprising in view of the modern trends in the society. Role conflict is alleviated through the process of assigning hierarchical placement to roles in which the women are actually involved and that demand most from them according to the value system: motherhood when the children are small, wifehood if the husband is in a demanding and rewarding occupation, and employment if those two roles are absent from the role-cluster.

REFERENCES

Bernard, J. *Women and the public interest.* Chicago: Aldine, 1971.

Bernard, J. *The future of marriage.* New York: Bantam, 1973.

Bernard, J. The housewife: Between two worlds. In P. L. Stewart and M. G. Cantor (Eds.) *Varieties of work experience.* New York: Wiley, 1974.

Bernard, J. *Women, wives, mothers: Values and options.* Chicago: Aldine, 1975. (a)

Bernard, J. *The future of motherhood.* New York: Penguin, 1975. (b)

Bernard, J. *The female world.* New York: Free Press, 1981.

Biddle, B. J., and Thomas, E. J. (Eds.). *Role theory.* New York: Wiley, 1966.

Bird, C. *The two-paycheck marriage.* New York: Rawson Wade, 1979.

Brim, O., and Wheeler, S. *Socialization after childhood.* New York: Wiley, 1966.

Chapman, J. R., and Gates, M. (Eds.). *Women into wives: The legal and economic impact of marriage.* Beverly Hills: Sage, 1977.

Coser, R. L. The complexity of roles as a seedbed of individual autonomy. In L. A. Coser

(Ed.), *The idea of social structure: Papers in honor of Robert K. Merton*. New York: Harcourt Brace Jovanovich, 1975, Pp. 237–263.

Dyer, E. D. Parenthood as crisis: A restudy. *Marriage and Family Living*, 1963, *25*, 196–201.

Easton, B. L. Industrialization and femininity: A case study of 19th century New England. *Social Problems*, 1976, *23*, 389–401.

Ehrenreich, B., and English, D. *For her own good: 150 years of the experts' advice to women*. Garden City, N.Y.: Anchor Books, 1979.

Elder, G. H. *Children of the Great Depression: Social change in life experience*. Chicago: University of Chicago Press, 1974.

Evans, P. A. L., and Bartolome, F. The relationship between professional life and private life. In C. B. Derr (Ed.), *Work, family and the career*. New York: Praeger, 1980. Pp. 281–317.

Fowlkes, M. *Behind every successful man: Wives of medicine and academe*. New York: Columbia University Press, 1980.

Friedan, B. *The feminine mystique*. New York: Norton, 1963.

Goode, W. A theory of role strain. *American Sociological Review*, 1960, *25*, 483–496.

Gouldner, A. W. Cosmopolitan and locals. *Administrative Science Quarterly*, 1957, December, 281–306.

Gross, N., Mason, W., and McEadern, A. *Explorations in role analysis: Studies of school superintendency role:* New York: Wiley, 1958.

Hobbs, D. F., Jr. Parenthood as crisis: A third study. *Journal of Marriage and the Family*, 1965, *17*, 367–372.

Kahn, R. L., Wolf, D. M., Quinn, R. P., Snoeck, J. D. and Rosenthal, R. A. *Organizational stress: Studies in role conflict and ambiguity*. New York: Wiley, 1964.

Komarovsky, M. Cultural contradictions and sex roles. *American Journal of Sociology*, 1946, *52*, 182–189.

Laws, J. L. *The second X: Sex role and social role*. New York: Elsevier, 1979.

LeMasters, E. E. Parenthood as crisis: *Marriage and Family Living*, 1957, *19*, 252–355.

Lerner, G. *The woman in American history*. Menlo Park, Calif.: Addison-Wesley. 1971.

Lopata, H. Z. The life cycle of the social role of housewife. *Sociology and Social Research*, 1966, *41*, 5–22.

Lopata, H. Z. *Occupation: Housewife*. New York: Oxford University Press, 1971.

Lopata, H. Z. *Widowhood in an American city*. Cambridge, Mass.: Schenkman, General Learning Press, 1973.

Lopata, H. Z. *Women as widows: Support systems*. New York: Elsevier/North Holland, 1975.

Lopata, H. Z., Barnewolt, D., and Miller, C. A. *City women: Work, jobs, occupations, careers*. New York: Praeger, in press.

Lopata, H. Z., Barnewolt, D., and Norr, K. Spouses' contribution to each other's roles. In F. Pepitone-Rockwell (Ed.), *Dual career couples*. Beverly Hills: Sage, 1980. Pp. 111–142.

Lopata, H. Z., and Norr, K. *Changing commitments of American women to work and family roles and their future consequences for social security*. Final report to the Social Security Administration, 1979.

Lopata, H. Z., and Norr, K. Changing commitments of American women to work and family roles. *Social Security Bulletin*, 1980, *43*, 3–14.

Lopata, H. Z., and Pleck, J. H. (Eds.). *Research in the interweave of social roles: Jobs and families*. Greenwich, Conn.: JAI Press, 1983.

Mack, R. W. Occupational determinateness: A problem and hypothesis in role theory. *Social Forces*, 1956, *35*, 20–25.

Merton, R. The role set. *British Journal of Sociology*, 1957, *8*, 106–120.

Merton, R. *Social theory and social structure*. Glencoe, Ill.: Free Press, 1968.

Merton, R. K., Reader, G. G., and Kendall, P. L., eds. *The student-physician*. Cambridge
    Mass.: Harvard University Press, 1957.
Mortimer, J., Hall, R., and Hill, R. Husbands' occupational attributes as constraints on
    wives' employment. *Sociology of Work and Occupations*, 1978, 5, 285–314.
Nadelson, C. C., and Nadelson, T. Dual-career marriages: Benefits and costs. In F
    Pepitone-Rockwell (Ed.), *Dual career couples*. Beverly Hills: Sage, 1980. Pp. 91–110
Neugarten, B. L. *Middle age and aging*. Chicago: University of Chicago Press, 1973.
Newcomb, T. M., Turner, R. H., and Converse, P. E. *Sociol psychology: The study of huma*
    interaction. New York: Holt, Rinehart & Winston, 1965.
Pleck, J. H. *Work and family roles: From sex-patterned segregation to integration*. Paper present
    ed at the annual meeting of the American Sociological Association, 1975.
Pleck, J. H. Men's family work: Three perspectives and some new data. *Family Coordinator*
    1979, October, 481–488.
Pleck, J. H. Husband's paid work and family roles: Current research issues. In H. Z'
    Lopata and J. H. Pleck (Eds.), *Research in the interweave of social roles: Jobs and families*
    Greenwich, Conn.: JAI Press, 1983: 251–333.
Poloma, M. M. Role conflict and the married professional woman: In C. Safilios-Rothschil
    (Ed.), *Toward a sociology of women*. Lexington, Mass.: Xerox College Publishing, 1972
    Pp. 187–198.
Poloma, M. M., and Garland, T. The married professional woman: A study of tolerance (
    domestication. *Journal of Marriage and the Family*, 1971, 33, 531–540.
Rapoport, R., and Rapoport, R. N. *Dual career families*. Harmondsworth, England: Per
    guin, 1971.
Rapoport, R., and Rapoport, R. N. *Dual career families re-examined*. New York: Harpe
    Colophon, 1976.
Ritzer, G. *Working: Conflict and change*. Englewood Cliffs, N.J.: Prentice-Hall, 1977.
Rossi, A. Transition to parenthood, *Journal of Marriage and the Family*, 1968, 30, 26–3'
Rothman, S. M. *Women's proper place: A history of changing ideals and practices*. New Yor
    Basic Books, 1978.
Sicherman, B. Review essay: American history. *Signs*, 1975, 1(Winter), 461–485.
Vandervelde, M. *The changing Life of the corporate wife*. New York: Mecox, 1979.
Veroff, J., Douvan, E., and Kulka, R. *The inner American*. New York: Basic Books, 198
Whyte, W. H., Jr. *The organization man*. New York: Simon & Schuster, 1956.
Znaniecki, F. W. *The social role of the man of knowledge*. New York: Columbia Universi'
    Press, 1940.
Znaniecki, F. W. *Social relations and social roles*. San Francisco: Chandler. 1965.

Chapter 5

Multiple Roles of Midlife Women

A Case for New Directions in Theory, Research, and Policy

JUDY LONG AND KAREN L. PORTER

INTRODUCTION

The flexible boundaries of the midlife period are sometimes said to include persons from ages 35 to 64. Midlife is a heterogeneous category, subsuming decisively different life courses. What "midlife" entails is a function, at least in part, of experiences and transitions in earlier periods. Women who currently fall into this category include the first of the baby boom, the veterans of the Feminine Mystique and the Great Depression eras and more than a few flappers. Different birth cohorts among today's midlife women experienced predictable life transitions in different historical times. In addition, individuals within birth cohorts differ in the timing, sequencing, spacing, and duration of such life transitions as completing schooling, starting a family, and establishing careers.

Schooling, working, and family life can be thought of as multiple careers, developing at different rates within the individual's life-span. Midlife represents a period in the unrolling of the multiple careers that stems from the multiple roles enacted by women. The midlife period brings a series of life transitions that may include changes or disruptions in family life, changes in labor force participation, and alterations in emphasis or priority among women's multiple roles.

JUDY LONG • Department of Sociology, Syracuse University, Syracuse, New York 13210. KAREN L. PORTER • Maxwell School, Health Studies Program, 712 Ostrom Avenue, Syracuse, New York 13210.

Our particular interest in this chapter is with how women's role affect their economic viability at midlife and after. Occupational an marital careers, in particular, are major determinants of a woman's ecc nomic situation both at midlife and in old age. Many women who ar now in midlife will face poverty in old age, given their current em ployment and marital history and the existing public programs availabl to aid them. There is clearly a role for public policy in ensuring th future well-being of today's midlife women. Public programs must b responsive to the diverse needs of distinct subpopulations within th midlife category. Innovations and modifications in public policy are ir dicated on the basis of analysis of the needs of current midlife womer

Existing public programs appear to be informed by faulty socia science. Distortions in social science theorizing and research on olde women are reflected in the provisions and rationales of programs o which many women will depend in old age. The shortcomings of cui rent social science perspectives on older women must also be corrected they are to be the basis of a rational and equitable social policy.

The latter half of the female life cycle has been too little studiec Perhaps as a consequence, midlife has more often been treated as terminus than as a transition. An overemphasis on women's family role has led to characterizations of midlife as a time of loss and diminishmer for women. Current research contests the pervasive images of midlif women as losers and has-beens. The focus on women's family roles ha led to a neglect of economic outcomes for women. When employment c women who are in midlife today is analyzed, it is usually in terms c "jobs" rather than "careers." Many questions concerning women's ex perience in the labor market have not been investigated. Among th most critical are the questions of long-run economic outcomes for en ployed women.

At present, of a total female population of 116 million, slightly mor than 36 million (or 31%) are between the ages of 35 and 64 (U.S. Burea of the Census, 1981). Midlife women, as a share of the population, ca be expected to increase in the future as a result of both the size of th younger birth cohorts and gains in life expectancy. The life expectancie at birth for women born in 1920, 1930, and 1940 are 55, 62, and 65 year respectively (U.S. Bureau of the Census, 1976). Women aged 45 in 197 can now expect to live to age 80 (U.S. Bureau of the Census, 1981 According to the most conservative census projections, by the year 200 the number of midlife women between the ages of 35 and 64 will hav increased to slightly more than 50 million, approximately 42% of th entire female population (U.S. Bureau of the Census, 1978).

Each birth cohort ages in a unique way, as it lives through a distin history. Nevertheless, women who are now in midlife shared certai

:periences that distinguish their life trajectories from those of women
)w in their 20s or early 30s. Available options in life-styles, as well as
e timing, spacing, sequence, and duration of major life transitions, are
ajor factors determining the situation of women at midlife.

Most of the women now in midlife married. When they reached
ibility at or after the Second World War, the marriage rate reached a
cord high. Between 1945 and 1947, an average of 143 first marriages
ere taking place for every 1000 single women aged 14 to 44. Since 1947,
e marriage rate has declined steadily and the divorce rate, declining
ıtil the 1963–65 period, has risen steadily since. Between 1970 and
'78, the number of never-married women between the ages of 25 and
: increased by 111%, the number of divorced women of the same ages
ho had not remarried rose by 170%, while the number of married
omen climbed only 17% (U.S. Bureau of the Census, 1978). The result
an increase in the number of single older women in the 1980s.

Most of today's midlife women remain married, however. In 1980,
all women aged 35 to 64, 77% were married either in a first and only
arriage or by remarriage after widowhood or divorce. Another 9%
ere divorced, 5% single, and 9% widowed (U.S. Bureau of the Census,
•81).

Most of today's midlife women bore children. Women now in their
ırly 40s to early 50s married at earlier ages, gave birth to more children,
•gan childbearing sooner, and completed childbearing in a span of just
'er 7 years, on the average, compared to their mothers and older
ısters (Norton, 1980). The diminution of family responsibilities has im-
ıcations for women's availability for labor force participation in mid-
•e. The contraction of the child-intensive phase of family life, in the
•ntext of ever-increasing life expectancy, has implications for a wom-
ı's work expectancy at midlife, whatever her work history in previous
:riods.

Though normative disapproval of working mothers was strong dur-
g the years when today's midlife women had young children, the
atistics show that labor-force participation of this group has never been
egligible. At midcentury, the labor force participation rates for women
;ed 2O to 24 and 25 to 34 were among the highest of all groups of
omen (46 and 34%, respectively; U.S. Bureau of the Census, 1976).
'oreover, the greatest increases in labor force participation since World
'ar II have been among mothers with school-age children. Currently,
•% of the women aged 35 to 44, 60% of the women aged 45 to 54, and
:% of the women aged 55 to 64 are employed in the civilian labor force
J.S. Bureau of the Census, 1981). Estimates of work-life expectancy
dicate that the labor force attachment of women at midlife and after
ceeds that of men (Laws, 1979). Though midlife women are the fast-

est-growing segment in the female labor force, the poverty rates f(
women at midlife (aged 35 to 44—11%; 45 to 54—9%; 55 to 59—11%; an
60 to 64—13%) are rather high compared with the rates for men of th
same ages (8%, 7%, 6%, and 8%, respectively; U.S. Bureau of the Cer
sus, 1982). A wage differential between the sexes persists. Women wh
exhibit labor-force participation patterns different from those of me
receive penalties in the form of lower wages for comparable jobs. Di
ferences in labor force histories among midlife women place them i
different positions with respect to economic viability in later life.

A study by Neugarten and Brown-Rezanka (1978) illustrates th
heterogeneity of the midlife population. The authors compare demo
graphic features and life outcomes of three adjacent cohorts of womer
The cohort exiting midlife contains a disproportionate number of wom
en who remained single until age 30 or older, and many married wome
who delayed childbearing until their late 20s or remained childless a
together. The cohort entering midlife married earlier and had more chi
dren, on the average, than the preceding cohort. The cohort that was t
enter midlife by the end of the 1980s exhibited lower fertility expect;
tions and higher educational rates than either previous cohort.

Today it makes sense to ask what the latter half of life holds f(
women, in terms of work rewards, success, satisfaction, and econom
security. It is revealing and significant that these questions have on.
rarely been asked. Though social scientists have, in recent years, take
cognizance of women's work roles, discussion has for the most pa
assumed that women have jobs, and men careers. Consequently, su
cess, level of rewards, and commitment are rarely the focus of researc
on women's employment. Conversely, women in the first half of li
have been discussed primarily in terms of family roles. Only recent
has the second half of the female life-span been examined in detail. Y
current work has made it clear that many aspects of women's lives
midlife are problematic. Among the most notable features of midlife
an economic vulnerability that derives directly from the combination
work and family history.

With changing marital status and childbearing patterns, more an
more women are finding themselves alone in midlife. Changes in fami
roles and the timing and spacing of births have resulted in longer pe;
ods of time after the youngest child leaves home and before retiremer
age: It tends to be assumed that income is accumulating during th
time. For the married woman, midlife may be a period of income a
cumulation. But for the woman who has lost her spouse, the risk
poverty is great.

The ideal of economic self-sufficiency among women was not pa
of the sex-role script when today's midlife women were being socialize
for their adult roles. More to the point, the sex-role prescriptions for th

arital relationship required the husband to support his wife, and often
deal with all financial matters. The sexual division of labor minimized
omen's financial responsibilities. One consequence is that most wom-
n are poorly prepared to support themselves, and to compete in the job
arket when separated from their husband's income. Women at midlife
ho are widowed, separated, or divorced are at risk of poverty.

As we seek to assess the condition of women at midlife, and to
redict their future well-being, three strands of social science theory and
search have contributions to make: the literature on occupations and
reers, the work on "dual roles," and the tradition of the study of the
e-course. In each of these are to be found omissions and distortions
at limit their applicability to the situation of midlife women today.
ew orientations and new research are required in order to realize the
tential benefits of these three perspectives.

Research on occupational roles and the research on the articulation
work and family roles have a common basis in role theory. Research
careers and the life-course share a common focus on transitions
nong statuses over time. Nevertheless, these traditions, which have
tentially so much to contribute to each other, have developed in paral-
l, with very little intercommunication or complementarity. In part, this
tcome can be traced to the different subject populations studied under
ch focus. Ideally, theories of roles, careers, or the life-course should be
neric in form, capable of explaining variations in terms of the same
neral principles. In fact, however, most of the research on careers has
cused on men. Research on "dual roles" has until recently dealt ex-
usively with women. Much of the life-course research has focused on
ansitions among what used to be called "stages of the family life cy-
e," which were widely assumed to have their primary impact on wom-
. Role theory is generic in form but rests upon research in which
en's work experience predominates. Thus, theory and research that
ar on midlife women are substantially sex-segregated, thereby impos-
g regrettable limits on social science contributions to date.

In this chapter, we will attempt to integrate the contributions from
e literature on occupations and careers, role theory, and the life-course
rspective. We will indicate directions for future research to carry for-
ard the understanding of midlife women. In addition, a rational social
licy relates to the economic vulnerability of midlife women based on
eir roles will be provided.

CCUPATIONS AND CAREERS: "GENERIC THEORY"

The world of work, and social science portraits of it, is dominated
imagery, vocabulary, normative judgments, and timetables that are
asculine in culture and framed to the experience of males (Derr, 1980).

Each of these elements carries a freight of evaluation (which is generall
not subjected to analysis), so that vocabulary, imagery, and timetable
that describe men are considered dominant and normal, and those tha
characterize women are considered deviant.[1] Such judgments, uncor
scious though they are, constitute a normative climate in which th
occupational efforts of midlife women are received. Public policy an
social science theory appear to be colored with the same normativ
slant, and do injustice to midlife women in similar ways.

Theories of vocational development set the tone for the normativ
manner of participation in the labor force. A good deal of convergence i
apparent in commonly cited models of career choice and career commi
ment. They picture a world in which the young person moves upwar
in an educational structure that contains information about possible o
cupational options. Social and familial networks contain role model
sponsors, and advisors. Opportunities for role rehearsal, for summer c
part-time work may be made available. Education, its content and dire
tion, is assumed to be instrumental for future occupational attainmen
Adults' ambitions are often projected onto the young person; they fe
involved and have a stake in future success that will reflect upon them
A unified atmosphere of expectation, support, and benevolent anxiet
about future occupational success hovers throughout the school years,
not before. Occupational choices themselves reflect success or failur
before occupational role enactment—the occupational career *per se*–
begins.

The normative timetable for careers assumes entry into the wor
force and the establishment of a career as a task of early adulthood. Fc
men, it is the primary task, and violation of the timetable tends to b
seen as a reflection on the individual and a threat to ultimate caree
success. Occupational success is assumed to follow a parabola of ir
creasing rank and reward throughout early and middle adulthood, pe
king and then reaching a plateau that may be maintained through lat
adulthood to retirement. The presumed isomorphism of this occupa
tional script and the human life-span has been attacked by Saraso
(1977).[2]

---

[1]The usage of the terms *dominant* and *deviant* is taken from Laws (1975).

[2]Nevertheless, the unconscious sexism of this normative model continues to be perpet
ated in current work on careers. For Karp and Yoels (1981), the chronological life a
work life are virtually coterminus, illustrating the essence of "career" as an order
progression of ages or stages. Their unexamined assumptions about the nature of t
occupational career include the following: that it involves an individual for the enti
period from approximately age 18 to age 65; that it requires an early start; and that it
always "regular," i.e., upwardly mobile in a steady, predictable fashion. When it is n
regular, it is deviant. The discussion of why women were excluded from their analysis
relegated to a single *footnote*.

It has now become commonplace to criticize these theories for their
ck of applicability to women. The critique has been instrumental in
imulating inquiry into the processes by which young women develop
'cupational intentions (Laws, 1979) and choose adult life-styles (see
ngrist and Almquist, 1975). Undoubtedly, the critique has under-
rded the great increase in detailed studies of women's occupational
'es that have appeared in the last decade.

The availability of such a body of data permits comparisons be-
'een the occupational experiences of women and men. These, in turn,
ied new light on the theories and allow us to identify more clearly the
ibstructure of male cultural experience on which the theories are con-
ructed. Among the dimensions that enhance the fit of theories of oc-
ipational careers and male experience are the following: (1) It is clear
at the theories assume continuity between childhood and adulthood,
tween school life and work life. (2) The career and the demands of the
cupational role take clear priority over other roles and commitments.
) The peers who monitor and the superiors who reward occupational
rformance are men. Careers that follow this script are normal, and
ese features of a career are assumed to be requisite for success.

These elements seem to be part of the structure of careers, and of
reer success. In the occupational world, for example, the most pres-
tious and best-paid occupations are those in which the concentration
males is very high, especially in the upper ranks. It is understood that
ectacular careers require sacrifices, particularly in the early years. For
e professions, this means extended schooling. For business and the
ofessions, it means that the time demands of the job may be double
e standard work week. Compartmentalization of work and personal
e may be impossible. In addition to long hours, career commitment
quires open-ended and flexible availability to the demands of the work
' the employer. Lower priority plans such as recreation, or activities
ntered on self or family, may be canceled when duty calls. Through-
ıt the world of work, the highly significant distinction between exempt
ıd nonexempt employees is understood to mean that the former do not
't paid for overtime. When we are speaking of careers (as contrasted
ith jobs), it is understood that *any* organization or employer possesses
e characteristics of the "greedy institutions" analyzed by Coser (1974).

These dimensions of the career script operate not only in the expec-
tions of recruits and those who supervise and reward them but in
stitutional arrangements as well. Researchers have written about the
ıpact on women of entering and trying to function in work settings
at are predominately and traditionally male (Bayes and Newton, 1978;
rnard, 1964; Harragan, 1977; Kanter, 1977a, 1977b; Laws, 1975; Laws
ıd Tangri, 1979; Lorber, 1975; Wolman and Frank, 1972).

For the most part, these writers have neglected the role of pric socialization—sex-role socialization, in essence—in rendering such er vironments intelligible and conquerable. Yet for each of the dimensior of the career script discussed above, evidence is available that shows th link to sex-role socialization. The experiences of females and males d verge long before high school students seek vocational counseling, an long before individuals encounter the first day on the job.

Both girls and boys acquire detailed cognitive maps of the se> segregated labor market early, and can render them for the social re searcher by the time they are in the second grade; not only do boys an girls project different future occupations, but girls project marriage an family life, while boys do not even mention them (Looft, 1971). A di ference in expectations regarding occupational planning is apparent i even second-graders. Females envision their future lives in terms of du, roles. Familial roles enter their calculations even when they are explicit being queried about future occupational roles. Marital and familial rol(do not loom so large in the future planning of school-age boys. Eviden(that young girls expect to give priority to family obligations can be foun very early. Later, even when occupational aspirations are being artic lated, there is some awareness that the exigencies of marriage may inte fere with occupational intentions (Davis, 1964; Mahajah, 1966).[3] R search demonstrating that it does so is plentiful (Mulvey, 1963; Tangr 1972; Harmon, 1969; Levitt, 1971).

Even in the absence of awareness, discontinuities occur in th female life-span. Research on sex-role socialization indicates that boy are more rigorously sanctioned for sex-role conformity than are girls, preschool and schoolage. Until puberty, girls enjoy greater license fe androgyny than boys. At puberty, however, new restrictions are place on girls. For college-going youth, the student role may offer a mo atorium on adult sex roles. For the female student, this may mean su port for serious academic commitment and career preparation. Howe er, at some point the sex-role norm according priority to family roles applied, and the student, dismayed, finds that parents are no long(interested in what she is learning and achieving, but only in her soci life (Komarovsky, 1946).

The expectation of marriage brings with it the expectation of disco tinuity in labor force participation. Although current data show a cle, trend for women's labor-force attachment to converge with that of me

---

[3]Data collected in 1980 from kindergarten and fourth-grade boys and girls by Grace Baru and Rosalind Barnett indicated that with respect to occupational aspirations, boys ma more traditionally sex-typed and more prestigious choices than did girls, and these (ferences were more pronounced among the older group (fourth-graders).

Creps and Clark, 1975), it is still considered normal for women to remain home with young children, perhaps reentering the labor force when the children are in school full time. For women now at midlife, the force of this norm was even stronger than it is at present. (For a compilation of public-opinion data on employment of mothers during the years when midlife women were in their childbearing years, see Oppenheimer, 1970, 45 ff.)

Intermittent labor force participation, as both norm and behavior, illustrates the priority that family responsibilities are supposed to have for women. This priority, the converse of that which is normative for men, is imputed *even where it does not apply*. Women in the labor force are treated *as though* they are mothers with unremitting and overriding responsibility for children who have not yet achieved basic competence. Suwhill (1973) has demonstrated that sex differentials in earnings, often attributed to women's intermittent labor force participation, persist in lifetime earnings curves *even of women with no intermittency*. Studies of male managers' attitudes toward women in management show that they believe women would refuse transfers, increased responsibilities, and extra time demands—elements consistent with the male career script. In these studies, the attitudes are not connected with the respondents' experience with females in management (Rosen and Jerdee, 1974a). Lorber (1975) has pointed out that male colleagues and superiors feel a concern for women's loyalty as organization members that is linked to their putative status as mothers. That is to say, the norm of dual role enactment and priority of family responsibilities suffices to create in men the *expectation* that women colleagues are of a different motivational type than themselves.

The difference between women and men in expectations for the share of responsibility they will take for their home and children appears to be established early in the process of sex-role socialization. As we have seen, dual role expectations are in evidence very early in girls. Boys, on the other hand, are sanctioned for exhibiting any "contrasex" attributes or interests, among which nurturing ranks high. Interestingly, it is men who sanction sex-role behavior, particularly in boys. A strong negative connection is established between the self and anything that is sex-typed as feminine. A reaction of "not me" in response to "feminine" spheres affects males' occupational choices and, indeed, their orientation toward spouse and family roles in relation to their work role in adulthood. As a result of sex-role socialization, it seems likely that males grow up with stronger boundaries dividing them from girls than the girls experience, and greater psychological distance from females than females feel toward males. This discrepancy will affect women's occupational mobility at any age. Although their own expectations are

likely to correspond to the male career script, their bosses will have grea
difficulty in applying the male career model to women (Laws, 197£
Nieva and Gutek, 1980).

The analysis of sex-role socialization suggests dimensions that ur
derlie and affect the interactions of women and men in mutually cor
tingent work roles in their adult years. Even where work roles are syn
metrical or complementary, women and men are likely to have differer
expectations of each other, as a function of sex-role socialization. Avai
able literature suggests that sex-role scripts may be more definitive i
men's treatment of their female colleagues than the reverse. In man
work organizations, both women and men confront a situation in whic
the normal incumbent of their occupational role is male and a femal
incumbent is anomalous. The impact of this situation on female an
male is likely to be quite different.

Part of this difference results from sex differences in earlier socia
ization, for immersion in male work groups and peer groups, headed b
male authority figures, is a component of male sex-role socializatior
Harragan (1977), in describing the corporate work environment, empha
sizes the importance of team sports and the armed forces as models f(
work life and as training grounds for participation in a world of wor
organized along similar principles. Team sports, in particular, provic
another source of continuity from school to work for many men who ar
now adults and for very few women of the same birth cohorts. F(
women who are now at midlife, compulsory and desultory gym clas
was their only involvement in athletics during the school years, ar
provided little in the way of models for adult work life. Bernard (197
has commented on how different the organizational environment is f(
female and male, where the latter is secure in being backed up by h
peers and the former becomes increasingly aware that she is in alit
territory. Laws (1975) holds that individuals who are in the structur
niche of the "token woman" do not initially perceive much differen
between themselves and male peers, and assume that gender is irrel
vant for the latter, too. They are concentrating on the task; they defir
themselves, in the work context, in terms of their skills and credential
The irony is that both the token woman and her majority peer a
focusing on what is unusual about her: For the woman, it is her achiev
ments and abilities, and for the man, it is her gender. The differe
contexts in which they have grown up account for a difference in p(
ception that is unlikely ever to be discussed or analyzed.

The literature on careers, then, is of limited relevance for midli
women—or midlife men (see Sarason, 1977; Brim, 1975; Weick, 1976)
in its present form. Both theory and research need to be developed
the direction of incorporating the multiple roles of workers and tl

varying trajectories of work and other roles over the life-span. It will be of primary importance, if outcomes for midlife women are to be understood, to study the sex structuring of work roles and the world of work.

"DUAL ROLES" AND ROLE CONFLICT

Sociology, as the study of the doings of men, reflects an emphasis in "public" life and public deeds as more important, more challenging, and altogether more worthy than the study of private life. The relative prestige of the study of social stratification and the study of marriage and the family, or the sociology of science versus the sociology of sex roles, tells that story.

It is in this context that we must understand the characteristics of the sociology of occupations and careers. Two characteristics of particular relevance to the study of women at midlife are the neglect of family roles and the normative status of a *single role* vision of work and success. As the preceding section made clear, workers (particularly in the professions, from which models of work and careers appear to be drawn) are viewed as though they occupy only one role or (what is normatively the same) as though only one role matters. This "myth of monism" (Laws, 1976) means that one role is normal and "dual roles" are deviant. When we examine the literature on dual roles for its contributions to the study of women at midlife, we must bear this in mind.

On no other basis can we understand the fact that the term dual roles, with the tradition of analysis peculiar to it, is used with reference only to women, even though a superficial recognition of men's roles is to be found in the literature. This recognition does not enter into discussion of men's occupational role enactment and careers, however. Men's dual roles do not officially exist. In contrast, women do not officially exist in discussions of careers except in the context of dual roles.

The study of role conflict has been an enduring concern of role theory in its generic form. However, research attempting to study the causes of and defenses against role conflict as set forth in theory has focused on men (Ritt, 1971; Ritzer, 1969; Rizzo et al., 1970). Research on role conflict in women, on the other hand, has an *ad hoc* quality and ordinarily tests no systematic theory. Thus, the work on men neglects their multiple roles, while the work on women remains outside the mainstream of role theory.

Role Conflict in the World of Work: Generic Theory

A strong theme in the study of people at work has been the problem of role conflict. A number of different forms or aspects of role conflict have been discussed over the years, although not all have received

empirical confirmation. Role conflict may arise from incompatible expec
tations associated with two different roles occupied by an individual, o
from contradictory expectations that are part of the same role, or fron
lack of congruence between the role and the person (or role incumbent)
Role ambiguity and role overload are also discussed as sources of role
strain, the former referring to problems arising in knowing how to be
have, due to inadequate specification of role expectations, and the latte
to an excess of demands over time available for role enactment, althougl
the demands themselves are not incompatible. Role diversity, or the
number of different role relationships in which a person is involved, i
also mentioned as a source of strain (Snoek, 1966). A distinction is some
times made between objective role conflict and subjective role conflict
The term *role strain* is often used in the sense of subjective role strain
Indications are that the distinction between objective role conflict (the
existence of the conditions listed above) and subjective role conflict (
psychological phenomenon) is one that should be observed more fre
quently in the study of role conflict.

Goode (1960) holds that role strain, or felt difficulty in fulfilling role
obligations, is a normal condition and not a crisis or a disaster. It is
direct consequence of two related facts. Multiple role occupancy ensure
that there will be contradictory demands on the person—that is, inter
role conflict—at least some of the time. A second factor probably in
creases the occurrence of role conflict: By implication, role partners rusl
in to fill this vacuum, and the role pressures they generate are the direc
source of conflict for the focal person. *The importance of role partners as
source of role conflict has been consistently underestimated in theory and re
search.* Yet, as we shall see, role partners are particularly critical in wom
en's experience in the world of work.

As role strain is normal, so are the maneuvers by which role incum
bents lessen, neutralize, or redefine the role expectations that, mediate
by role partners, induce role strain. Mechanisms of role articulatio
include (1) compartmentalization of roles, (2) delegation of role perfor
mances, (3) elimination of roles, and (4) role accumulation (Goode
1960). It is possible that various styles in enacting roles also constitut
strategies for reducing role conflict—as, for example, Goffman's (1961
notion of role distancing.

The use of strategies of role articulation (Coser and Rokoff, 1971) i
taken for granted, and evidence of their utilitization has been found i
studies of men in industry (Pugh, 1966; Ritzer, 1969) and stockbroker
among others (Evan and Levin, 1966). Indeed, adeptness in role articula
tion appears to be one of the skills required by the work role. Strategie
for reducing role strain are discussed in the vocabulary of games as rule
governed exchanges in which players can appreciate skillful move

ven when these do not advance their own side (cf. Spreitzer, Snyder, nd Larson, 1979). Goode (1960) and others who followed employ an laborate economic metaphor in discussing the active negotiation of the ole incumbent in seeking to establish a "role bargain" with his role artners. Given the fundamental reality of role strain resulting from ultiple role incumbency, the individual cannot satisfy all role expecta- ons and hence bargains for the best deal he can make (Goode, 1960). In rms of the dimensions later developed by Sieber (1974), the individual ies to gain the maximum role rights in combination with the minimum ole obligations. One of the most important issues as yet unaddressed in e role theory corpus is the bargaining positions of women and men *qua* omen and men, and their bargaining positions vis-à-vis each other.

Although there is consensus on the range of strategies available to e individual suffering from role stress, there is little research as yet at sheds light on the factors that determine which strategy the indi- idual selects. It seems likely that situational and personal characteris- cs have some influence. In addition, the source of role pressures— hether time pressure, simultaneous competing demands, or role part- ers—might indicate what response is most likely to be selected. Ritzer 969) found that male personnel managers selected different strategies or reducing role conflict, depending on the relative power of them- elves and their role partners. Independent, unilateral action was the ost preferred response, but compromise or conformity was the choice the role partner was more powerful than the focal person. Among en, withdrawal was the least favored response. The issue of relative ower of women and men has become a ubiquitous issue in research on omen and men in business and the professions (cf. Laws and Tangri, 979) and will surely need to be addressed in research and policy bear- g on careers of women at midlife and after.

Another issue that deserves the attention of researchers is the ques- on of differential outcomes resulting from strategies for reduction of ole conflict. Hall (1972) found that of three fundamental strategies for onflict reduction—structural role redefinition, personal role redefini- on, and reaction role behavior—the first resulted in substantially great- r satisfaction in a study of female college graduates. Findings of this tudy also indicated that various strategies may be differentially avail- ble to women who are situated differently in life.

Reduction of Role Conflict in Employed Women

The applicability of the generic theory and findings concerning role onflict to the situation and experience of midlife women must be care- ully assessed. Though in principle a general theory is capable of sub-

suming the special cases of female and male, in practice, in social sci
ence, it is more common for the theory to be based on the normal cas
(male) and to require modification for the analysis of "deviant cases,"
that is, of women. Assumptions that do not apply to females cause the
theory to fit this case poorly. In the literature on role conflict, these
assumptions deal with power and parity. Substantial differences in
power and peer status that have their roots in sex roles make the man
agement of role conflict in the workplace more problematic for women
than for men. This can easily be seen for the basic strategies enumerated
by Goode (1960).

COMPARTMENTALIZATION OF ROLES. The effectiveness of compart
mentalization as a means of reducing role conflict relies on a prior condi
tion that Goode takes for granted: the existence of specified times and
locales for role enactment. For most men, the work day is "off limits" to
family demands, permitting compartmentalization. In addition, a princi
ple of priority also separates the sets of role demands as well as the
locales reserved for role enactment. A professor may work at home if his
or her study is off limits and work time is uninterruptible. One limitation
on the efficacy or availability of compartmentalization as a means to
stress reduction is the specificity versus diffuseness of the role involved
A "master status" such as gender transcends specific locales and ac
tivities and elicits role demands transsituationally. These role demands
may well disrupt enactment of occupational roles, in spite of the best
efforts of women workers to employ the mechanism of compartmental
ization to reduce role stress. Many women have reported that others
treat their work as interruptible without qualification—a carry-over from
the way the role of mother is defined in our culture.

DELEGATION OF ROLE RESPONSIBILITIES. Goode suggests that at
tributes or performances that are central to the role in question may not
be delegated, but others may be. When we look at employed women in
their dual roles, there seems almost a qualitative difference between the
way familial roles and work roles are regarded by society at large. Tradi
tional sex-role expectations for women have a sacred quality that con
trasts greatly with the robustly secular tone of discussions of work roles
Wife, mother, and housewife roles do not seem to lend themselves to
analysis of central and peripheral expectations. Expectations are diffuse
as may be seen in the instance above, in which the mothering figure is
expected to be always there and always available. A certain amount of
bias may be detected when social scientists seek to analyze housework
as a job (Oakley, 1974) or when employed mothers assert that what is
important is quality, not quantity of time with their children.

Public opinion research has tracked attitudes toward women's ex
trafamilial role enactment (evidently a problematic reality) for better

ꓺan 30 years. The tone of censure that pervades laypersons' attitudes ꓺas not been absent from social scientists' discussions of "working ꓺives," "latchkey children," and "broken homes." The persistence of ꓺe "maternal deprivation" shibboleth in both lay and professional cir- ꓺes is testimony to the normative status of full-time involvement of ꓺomen in family roles. This normative climate severely limits employed ꓺomen's ability to delegate role responsibilities as a means of reducing ꓺle conflict.

ELIMINATION OF ROLES. In the traditional sex-role script, work roles ꓺe expendable for women, but family roles are not. A woman who ꓺooses work to the exclusion of family roles is still treated as a de- ꓺatured female. At present, the climate of opinion in the United States ꓺems punitive toward women who choose marriage-only as a life-style ꓺption. Marriage-cum-*some* employment (but not a career in the sense ꓺscussed earlier) is the expected pattern today (Pleck, 1977). Yet where ꓺimination of roles is used to reduce role conflict in women, it seems ꓺore likely to lead to abandoning or reducing commitment to work roles ꓺther than family roles. Epstein (1970) has suggested that women are ꓺwarded for resolving any work–family conflict in this direction. The ꓺistence of this cultural pattern has implications for the careers of mid- ꓺfe women. They are likely to have intermittent labor-force participation ꓺ a feature of their work history before midlife, and they may be vul- ꓺerable to pressures to eliminate newly acquired work roles if family ꓺressures are still strong.

ROLE ACCUMULATION. Goode suggested that taking on additional ꓺle obligations (accumulating roles) has the advantage for the focal ꓺerson that role partners will adjust (reduce) their expectations in the ꓺght of the focal person's new obligations. In this way, role accumula- ꓺon results in reduction of role strain.

Sieber (1974) has extended this analysis, challenging the perspective ꓺat has become conventional, that multiple role occupancy inevitably ꓺxposes the individual to role strain, which in turn results in decrements ꓺ role performance and in personal adjustment. Sieber, to the contrary, ꓺrgues that role accumulation, rather like capital accumulation, presents ꓺ net gain rather than a penalty: The individual acquires privileges, ꓺghts, or resources by taking on new roles that may, within limits, be ꓺsed to profit the individual as well as the role incumbent. The new ꓺcquisitions may be used to facilitate goals of the person. Sieber dis- ꓺsses four sorts of gains the individual may realize through role ac- ꓺmulation: role privileges, enhanced status security, resources for sta- ꓺs enhancement, and gratification of ego and personality.

Sieber assumes that role accumulation leads to an ever-increasing ꓺrplus of role privileges over role obligations, since he makes the prior assumption that individuals strike role bargains having this feature. He dismisses in one parenthetical phrase the "exploitive" role relationships where obligations exceed privileges. He does not question who the role partners may be who accept an excess of obligations over privileges complementary with the generic "he" of Sieber's analysis.

Role privileges include those aspects of the role that ordinarily act as inducements for the individual to enact it—e.g., legitimate authority. In addition, role incumbents gain "liberties" that do not involve the role partner. Some of the "liberties" one can gain via role accumulation seem more accessible to men than to women. The reduction of visibility has already been discussed; theoretical consensus seems to be that it is more difficult for a woman than for a man to escape surveillance in the occupational world, where she is viewed as a deviant by virtue of her "master status." The extension of authority without formal authorization is another such liberty. Research indicating the difficulties women have in exercising their legitimate authority suggests that extension may be an unlikely payoff for women at present (Bayes and Newton, 1978 Sterling and Owen, 1982).

Sieber suggests that role accumulation is a means to "status security," in the sense of offering compensatory success in one area in case of difficulties in another. There is, indeed, some evidence that work serves this function for women who are less than perfectly happy in their marriages (Spreitzer *et al.*, 1979; Rapoport and Rapoport, 1969). However, the interchangeability of successes must surely be conditioned by the priority the individual gives them, and this, in turn, by the normative forces that operate so powerfully to give preference to women's family roles.

Role accumulation also provides gains in the form of status enhancement of the role incumbent. Sieber uses the example of useful introductions and use of equipment and other resources of the employer, or the accumulation of status resources that can translate into power across different spheres. Insofar as status enhancement rests upon the facilitative operation of male networks, this payoff for role accumulation may be unavailable to women (Hoferek and Sarnowski 1981; Albrecht, 1976). A number of writers have noted the difficulty women have in gaining access to or making use of such networks in business and the professions (Epstein, 1970; Laws and Tangri, 1979 Laws, 1980; Lorber, 1975). Female networks are not usually available in these work sites, because of the sex ratios that obtain in management ranks and in the professions. In addition, a woman's transferral of resources across institutional spheres is less likely if her access to those spheres is problematic in itself. To the extent that spheres of "public"

ctivity remain socially masculine, women are unlikely to parlay re-
ources acquired via the work role into, for example, the political scene.

Sieber also notes personal growth and ego gratification payoffs to be
ained from multiple role occupancy: e.g., gains in sophistication, ap-
reciation for one's own competence. A good deal of research evidence
omparing housewives with employed women suggests that the latter
eport gratification through work and higher self-esteem (Birnbaum,
971; Baruch, Chapter 6, this volume). However, there is no reason to
ttribute these effects to multiple role occupancy; indeed, these studies
o not measure the extent of role accumulation in the two groups. These
tudies straightforwardly reflect the rewards available from working in
he public world of paid employment. Women who do not occupy fami-
′ roles report, without distortion, even greater levels of reward or satis-
action in many such studies (Birnbaum, 1971).

Although researchers commonly refer to "dual roles" in such com-
arisons, the effect of role accumulation remains a hypothesis for future
esearch. The facile interpretation in terms of dual roles results from a
amiliar bias that is operating here: Women who occupy both work and
amily roles are assumed to have engaged in role accumulation, since a
ngle role—housewifery—remains the unacknowledged norm in think-
ng about women. It is the position of the present authors that the
everse is the case: Housewife-only is an impoverished life-style, and
ultiple role occupancy is normal. The observed differences between
mployed women and housebound wives are better accounted for by
his formulation than by the more conventional one.

Sieber's (1974) formulation of the benefits of role accumulation has
een much quoted but, as yet, little researched. A number of limitations
re apparent when we seek to apply Sieber's formulation to the situation
f midlife women. First, there is a circularity in Sieber's argument, for all
s appeal: He assumes that gains outweigh strains in role accumulation
terms of the excess of gratifications over strains. Another blind spot in
ieber's formulation is that it refers (and presumably applies) only to
les in formal organizations. Thus, the role privileges he lists as profits
be realized by role accumulation (due process, collective bargaining,
nd protection from physical abuse or arbitrary firing) are not available
those in wife and mother roles.

There are many reasons for doubting the applicability of Sieber's
eneric theory to women, not the least of them his failure to try out the
nalysis on any instances involving women. In discussing roles and role
ettings, however, Sieber clearly has the parameters of male experience
mind. When he discusses gratifications in excess of performance re-
ards, for example, will the proposition hold for members of a category

that is subject to wage discrimination? The level of performance rewards assumed "normal" by this analysis is a far-off goal, not baseline, for the female role incumbent in most occupations. The value of Sieber's notion of role accumulation for understanding midlife women's prospects, therefore, remains to be demonstrated by future research. Given the reformulations made necessary by taking into account women's experiences in the work role, appropriate modifications of Sieber's predictions would be necessary. Nevertheless, when appropriately "grounded" in women's experience, the idea of role accumulation still has a contribution to make to a generic role theory.

To date, only the most elemental prediction from role accumulation has received empirical test. Spreitzer et al., (1979) tested the central proposition of Sieber's formulation with data from a national probability sample. They examined the relationship of multiple roles to a global sense of personal well-being. The analysis involved adults of preretirement age showing different configurations of the following roles: spouse, parent, worker, friend, and church member. Results showed a moderate absolute relationship between number of roles enacted and global well-being. This was moderated by satisfaction with the distinct role spheres: When only women who expressed satisfaction with their roles were included in the analysis, they showed a higher degree of global satisfaction than the comparable group of men.

The Spreitzer et al. data demonstrate another positive consequence of role accumulation: Satisfaction associated with one sphere may compensate psychologically for dissatisfaction in another. Spreitzer et al. did not analyze all possible comparisons, but they reported cross-tabulations of satisfaction/dissatisfaction with other roles when the respondent was satisfied or dissatisfied in the marital role. In this analysis, the picture is far more optimistic for men, in the sense that the compensation or compartmentalization mechanism seemed to work much better for men than for women. When overall happiness was compared for men with unsatisfactory marital roles, in all comparisons men satisfied in the other role (parent, work, friend, church) showed higher global satisfaction than men unsatisfied in the other role. For women, however, the mechanism broke down notably for the parent role, though the pattern appeared for the other roles. Either the spouse and parent roles are not so readily separable for women in this sample as for men, or spouse and parent roles mean different things and operate under different constraints for women and men. Research from other sources offer support for both these possibilities.

When satisfaction in the work role is the pivot for the analysis, both women and men show a regular compensation/compartmentalization effect in all comparisons (Spreitzer et al., 1979). It is surprising, given the mplications of the normative priority of marriage over work for women, the degree to which satisfaction with the job appears to improve one's marriage. In this sample, the power of the "dual roles" to affect global life satisfaction appears stronger for women than for men: 48% of women experiencing satisfaction in both work and marriage roles express high overall happiness in life, as compared with only 40% of men.

ROLE DISTANCE. Goffman's (1961) notion of "role distance" may figure as a coping mechanism differentially employed by women in a dual role situation that is in fact a double bind. Goffman's dramaturgical concept refers to a posture that conveys "disdainful detachment" of the performer from his role. Specifically, the role incumbent acts in such a way as to deny a virtual self implied in the role. It is evident that the self expected in many occupational roles is a male person, possessed of many masculine attributes. Women role incumbents may engage in behaviors that symbolically deny the culturally masculine dimensions of their occupational roles. Or they may behave in ways that attempt to negate or neutralize their femaleness in the occupational role setting.

Women may engage in role distancing as a way of warding off social control maneuvers by role partners. One strategy may be to enact symbolically some aspect of "femininity," denying thereby any contradiction between the feminine self and the "masculine" role. Another may be to disclaim the priority that the role connotes in the life of the male role incumbent by self-limiting commitment through part-time work or modest ambitions. "Cognitive feminization" of occupations traditionally associated with cultural maleness can be accomplished, for example, by emphasizing healing, rather than authority or income, if the woman is a physician. However, role distancing in women has been little studied to date.

Coser's (1966) thinking about role distancing emphasizes the normative dimension. Role distancing is a behavior that occurs when there is a question as to the legitimacy of the role incumbency (or where the incumbency is transitory). It is a defensive strategy, an attempt to ward off a challenge to the legitimacy of role incumbency, or the driving of a wedge between self and role. Stebbins (1967) adds to the analysis in stressing the importance of significant others (role partners, in our terms) in providing support and validation for a challenged role. The other side of this analysis, of course, is the role partners as a source of invalidation and a stimulus requiring defensive coping. The issue of legitimacy, and the evaluation of the role incumbent as communicated through role pressures, is a crucial strand in understanding women's dual role enactment. In communicating role pressures and hence creating role conflict for women, role partners play a decisive and heretofore neglected part.

Role Conflict and Coping in Women's Dual Roles

The third resource for thinking about multiple role enactment by women is the curious literature on *women's dual roles*. The term is restricted to women who "add on" roles in paid employment, the fundamental (and "normal") roles being wife/mother/housewife. Men's work role is not added on; hence, men do not have *dual roles*, with all the freight of normative reaction that term entails. The lack of symmetry in vocabulary and analysis is a signal that the work on role conflict in women is not a subset of the generic role theory or a complement to the empirical tradition of work on role conflict in the work settings of men. Rather, the work on women's dual roles is a ghettoized literature, replete with the limitations and dangers of such intellectual segregation. Connections with popular stereotypes of women—though unacknowledged—appear closer than those with the propositions of generic role theory or with the comparable literature on men in work roles. What marks the research on this topic is the assumption that "dual roles" are unmanageable, leading inevitably to disabling role conflict. Thus, negative outcomes are assumed when women work outside the home. Explicitly, they and their role partners are expected to suffer from this unnatural state of affairs. This appears to be a normative judgment rather than a scientific one, and research on role conflict in women exhibits little attempt to discover or explain variation in the occurrence or severity of role conflict. With rare exceptions, the well-known mechanisms of management of role conflict are not investigated in the research. The woman who is enacting "multiple roles" appears cut off from support, 'tricks of the trade', and mechanisms of role articulation on which her male peers matter-of-factly rely. Another peculiarity of this research is that the "dual role" woman is assumed to suffer an internalized, psychological form of role conflict (guilt?) that is different from that experienced by ordinary multiple role occupants in the ordinary role conflict with which they routinely cope.

In several studies of working wives and mothers (Nevill and Damico, 1972; Hall and Gordon, 1973; Gordon and Hall, 1974; Lashuk and Kurian, 1977; Holahan and Gilbert, 1979), the authors assumed difficulties for a woman attempting to manage both a family and employment. Walberg (1968) looked for person–role conflict in practice teachers. Ziebarth (1972) sought evidence for three distinct types of "feminine role conflict." In general, in such studies, concern is with predicting not the occurrence of conflict but rather its frequency and/or intensity, contingent upon such independent variables as hours worked per week, quality of the work experience, education, marital status, and spousal support. The hypotheses offered by Lashuk and Kurian (1977) and Holahan and Gilbert (1979) exemplify the "internal" nature of conflict assumed to afflict women. Lashuk and Kurian expected employed wives and mothers to experience greater "negative internal effects" such as anxiety, tension, and feelings of inadequacy about the wife–mother role than their full-time housewife counterparts. Holahan and Gilbert expected that employed wives and mothers who perceived their employment as a "career" would suffer more role conflict than those who perceived their employment as "only a job." But in both studies, contrary to the authors' expectations, the hypotheses were disconfirmed. The female respondents, in fact, reported less or no conflict, the more roles they assumed.

Other studies indicate that housewives report more role conflict than women employed outside the home (Baruch, Segal, and Hendrick, 1968). It is possible that conflict between self and role is felt more by women who have not dared to seek expression of some of their talents and skills outside the home. Certainly, there is evidence that women who choose "housewife-only" as a career are women who cannot face the conflict they have been told exists between career and family (Watley and Kaplan, 1971; Birnbaum, 1971). Certainly, many of the compensations that ease role conflict are not available to women who do not work outside the home (Epstein, 1970; Spreitzer et al., 1979; Rapoport and Rapoport, 1969; Gannon and Hendrickson, 1973).

The empirical existence of a distinctively feminine response to role conflict remains to be established. It does not appear when it "ought to," given the underlying assumptions of the dual role conflict literature. More extensive comparisons among women and between women and men are needed in order to ascertain whether there are specifiable conditions under which role conflict has psychological sequelae. At present, we are in danger of calling any role conflict experienced by a female person "psychological." This sort of prejudgment resembles the "motivational deficit" theories that once prevailed about the achievement of black Americans. In careless science like this, it is possible to find discussions of phenomena whose existence remains unsubstantiated. A "blame the victim" tone accompanies the neglect of structural and historical influences on the phenomenon of interest. A description of the *status quo* may be achieved but fall short of causal explanation. Unfortunately, such formulations, whether verified or not, can find their way into popular media and parlance and become self-fulfilling prophecies.

Many of the shortcomings of the research on role conflict in women can be seen in an influential article by Coser and Rokoff (1971). While focusing on women, these authors neglect the implied comparison with men. Indeed, they seem to assume that women are qualitatively different from men. The assumed differences resemble the normative script for women's priorities: Home responsibilities take precedence over work responsibilities. Coser and Rokoff seem to assume an invariant relationship between family and work responsibilities in women; they neither seek variance in this relationship nor seek to explain variance. Coser and Rokoff assert baldly that mechanisms of role articulation available to men—mechanisms that are part of the equipment, standard issue for persons in occupational roles—cannot be employed by women. Disappointingly, Coser and Rokoff fail to analyze the dynamics of gender as they affect the enactment of family and work roles by women and men, and the gender-related assumptions of work and family contexts that affect the definition of work and family roles. They hint that women are prevented from enacting their occupational roles in the normal way, and are confined to a deviant style that is, by definition, ineffective. However, Coser and Rokoff do not develop this allusion to the normative context of dual role enactment. Their failure to analyze the institutional context of occupational role enactment leads them to two errors. In not specifying what structural variables determine individual outcomes, they cut themselves (and their hapless subjects) off from the appropriate analyses of variation and links to generic role theory. They then retreat to a psychological formulation—always uncomfortable, and usually untenable, for sociologists. By default, it seems, Coser and Rokoff locate the problem in the individual woman and reach conclusions that are both static and pessimistic.

The work of Coser and Rokoff has been influential in shaping research on "role conflict" in employed women. Regrettably, the conclusions of this theoretical work have carried so much conviction for some researchers that they have insisted on seeing "intrapsychic role conflict" where their respondents report none (See, for example, Hall and Gordon, 1973). So influential a theoretical paper might very well have the effect of inhibiting research on role bargaining, coping, and innovation among women occupying multiple roles. It may contribute to a posture of pessimism in the literature on women's dual roles, and may create a static image of an eminently dynamic process.

Findings from research on dual careers that reveals the effective use of compartmentalization, and from the family time use studies that show both elimination and delegation of some role functions, apparently result from inadequate socialization of researchers. Researchers who did not know their role theory were able to discover important phenomena that, according to theory, did not exist. Certainly, much more remains to be learned. The existence of multiple roles in an ongoing time stream points toward commitments, rates of development, and priorities that change over time, rather than remaining fixed.

Role Partners and Role Conflict in Women

The existence of sex-role scripts that contain negative evaluations of women's extrafamilial roles is not sufficient, in itself, to produce role conflict in employed women. Indeed, the findings of Gordon and Hall (1974) suggest that even conscious awareness of traditional sex-role scripts does not induce role conflict in working women in and of itself. Pressures for sex-role conformity, like all role pressures, must be directly mediated in a relationship. Role pressures that induce role conflict in multiple-role women can be brought to bear by female relatives, authority figures, peers, or the proverbial mother-in-law. However, although research to date has dealt little with this process, there is evidence that such role pressures are exerted by husbands and by male co-workers. Examined closely, the data indicate that subjective role conflict, with or without disruption of role performance, can be instigated in women by role partners who challenge the legitimacy of dual role enactment or the adequacy of role performance. One can attack a woman's femininity or her competence; one can assert that one who is feminine cannot be competent, or that the female achiever is deficient as a female. One can portray the achieving woman as a ruthless individual whose pathetic family pays the price for her monstrous ambition.

Husbands are particularly efficacious in inducing role conflict in employed women or in neutralizing it (Rapoport and Rapoport, 1971; Weil, 1961; Feldman, 1973; Mahajah, 1966). "Dual career" wives commonly express gratitude that their husbands approve of their careers. However, the emotional support derived from approval may not be accompanied by help with the burdens of dual role responsibilities, and indeed, wives with professional careers report role overload (Rapoport and Rapoport, 1969), In one sample of college-educated women, professional women report more symptoms than a comparable group of wives without dual roles (Powell and Reznikoff, 1976).

Evidence exists, then, for two seemingly contradictory effects of multiple roles. Some studies show the negative effects of role stress and some the positive effects of enrichment or role accumulation. Clearly, more work needs to be done in order to clarify conditions under which multiple roles lead to positive and to negative outcomes for the role incumbents. Barnett and Baruch (1981) have found evidence for both positive and negative effects of women's multiple role occupancy. They found, in a study of 238 women aged 35 to 55, that feelings of role strain were related to the number of roles a woman occupied. Employed women did not report significantly more role strain than did women who worked only in the home. When the roles of wife, mother, and paid worker were examined for their relationship to role strain, only the mother was found to bear a significant relationship. Barnett and Baruch also found the number of roles a woman occupied significantly related to two aspects of personal well-being: mastery and pleasure.

Research on women's life-style planning indicates that they are aware of a potential conflict between the ambitions toward which their abilities lead them and the destination for which the culture intends them (Davis, 1964; Feldman, 1973). There is substantial evidence that boyfriends and, indeed, all potential husbands, have a power over younger women's choices and plans with regard to dual role life-styles that parallels the influence of husbands over wives. Typical data show that an overwhelming majority of college women prefer a dual role life-style, show high career commitment, intend little or no interruption of labor force activity with the advent of children—and would abandon it all, if a future husband disapproved of a working wife.

Current studies of college men (the presumptive future role partners of college women) indicate some support for dual roles in women (Komarovsky, 1973) and increased interest in family roles for men (Rossi, 1980). However, there is no empirical evidence at the present writing for a change in behaviors corresponding to such attitudes. Indeed, Komarovsky's (1973) data show men's attitudes to be much more conservative than those reported by college women in other studies. This corresponds to earlier findings by Siegel and Haas (1963) that men disapproved of employment of mothers to a greater extent than did women. Nelson and Goldman (1969) found that although public attitudes toward employment of women have become liberalized over time, men reject employment as an option for their *own* wives.

Interestingly, it is the sex role *attitudes* of women and men that permit the latter to go on the offensive and the former to become defensive, rather than the objective conditions of multiple role occupancy. Sense of time pressure and role overload are part of the objective role stress (Rapoport and Rapoport, 1969), which remains "external" until a finger of blame is pointed. We may speculate that most women are quite accustomed to dealing with too many things to do and too little time, but few are skilled at rejecting blame. It is the cultural script, specifying domestic concerns as the "one role" appropriate for women (Bernard, 1972b), that permits women to be blamed for enacting multiple roles. This script, coexisting with other cultural themes such as equal opportunity and individualistic achievement, constitutes an ever-present potentiality for conflict. Existing research suggests that both women and men are aware of the existence of the achievement versus femininity formulation (cf. Monahan, Kuhn, and Shaver, 1974). The consequences of the knowledge are different for women and men. However, only women can be impaled and disrupted by the conflict. Possessing the

.nowledge that most women are vulnerable to this latent conflict be-
ween achievement and femininity gives men a weapon to use against
vomen who are invading new occupational turf.

From research on women entering traditionally "masculine" oc-
upations (e.g., the construction trades, steel production, business man-
gement), it is increasingly clear that induced conflict between sex-role
xpectations and work goals may be used as a form of social control of
vomen. Ridicule, sexual challenge, isolation, and seduction are a few of
ne means documented in research to date (Wolman and Frank, 1972;
1ayes, 1976). Out-and-out harassment has been reported in many situa-
ons where women are entering traditionally male-dominated occupa-
ons. Sexual harassment and sexual hazing are frequently used to intim-
late women recruits and throw them off balance (Laws and Tangri,
979). This research makes it clear that some form of sexual harassment
r hazing is part of the working conditions of many, if not most, women
urrently in paid employment. This factor clearly constitutes a job stress
nd can be expected to have effects on women's outcomes in the job
narket. Kahn, Wolfe, Quinn, and Snoek (1964) found that high role
onflict was related to reduced job satisfaction and increased job-related
2nsion. Being subjected to conflicting role expectations reduces career
atisfaction and happiness for women (Hall and Gordon, 1973).

This material on occupational stress of women needs to be incorpo-
ated into the tradition of research on occupational stress, which, regret-
bly, has understudied women (Kahn et al., 1964; Haynes, Levine, and
cotch, 1978). Haynes and Feinleib (1980) make a start with an analysis
f the incidence and antecedents of coronary heart disease in women,
omparing employed women and housewives. Their data show a rela-
onship between role overload and heart disease in women: Number of
1ildren and marital status, as well as employment, contributed to ele-
ated rates of coronary disease in their sample. Single women had the
west rate of coronary disease. Among women, marriage and family
2sponsibilities predicted to coronary disease, although employment per
' did not.

Interestingly, it was not the "demanding" professional jobs that
1rried most job stress but rather the clerical occupations, in which
vomen, locked in by necessity, suffered lack of occupational mobility
1d lack of support from their bosses, and suppressed their anger.
Vhen heavy family responsibilities are added, the risk of heart disease
nong women in clerical occupations is considerably increased.

The Haynes and Feinleib data suggest that relationships with two
nportant role partners—husbands and bosses—are a factor in occupa-
onal stress leading to coronary disease in women. These authors do not,
owever, systematically assess role relationships as a factor in occupa-

tional stress of women. The connection between role partners' behavior and role conflict in employed women needs to be thoroughly researched. The corpus of research on occupational stress is in need of updating to include and reflect the research on women's experience in the world of work.

Sex Structuring of Roles

The sex structuring of work roles is a question that is only now recieving attention from researchers. Past research on "women's occupations" has pointed out continuities between women's work in the home and women's work in the labor market. Underlying this analysis can be discerned a rudimentary sketch of the feminine sex-role script, with a focus on the activities that correspond in the two work environments. The analysis can be extended, however, to show correspondences in *ways of performing work activities,* even where the activities may be different from those found in women's home tasks. In terms of roles and role expectations, we can say work roles and working relationships become colored by characteristics expected of women *qua* women. Of course, men's work roles and working sytles can be analyzed in the same way, as we have suggested at several points in this chapter.[4]

An aspect of sex structuring that has not been investigated to date is the way in which role expectations are adjusted for females and males in the same occupational roles. A fundamental asymmetry in role definitions of women and men in the "same" job are embedded in role expectations and role relationships that are decisively different.

On the basis of research in sex roles, it appears that women and men in the same jobs experience differences with respect to power relations, peer relations, and benefits to self and others. Much of this difference can be summarized, in terms of Sieber's (1974) analysis, by the propositions that (1) men's roles and role relationships are structured in terms of an excess of role privileges over obligations, and (2) women' roles and role relationships are structured in terms of an excess of role obligations over role privileges. The "complementarity" implied by these formulations has very different consequences for women and men in their work roles.

A number of researchers have observed that women in predominately male work settings are responded to by others in terms of a very restricted set of roles strongly marked by sex-role expectations (cf. Kanter, 1977b). Of these, the dominant one is Mother. When women are dealt with as Mother, they are characterized (and treated) as givin

---

[4]The fact that this is rarely done is due more to the psychology of the dominant and deviant than to any inherent difficulty in the analysis. (cf. Laws, 1975).

ithout counting the cost, as ever-available. Their diffuse willingness to cilitate and support others, and the goal attainment of others, is con-asted with a contractual mentality. Self-interest and personal ambition o not feature in Mother's makeup. A willingness to expend time and nergy on others' personal problems is expected of Mother. This kind of vestment is ordinarily not reciprocated: Mother does not receive nur-rance. Mother can be relied on to take care of any (and many) details. he "office wife" is one who performs many small personal services that re beneath the attention of the boss but contribute to smooth mainte-ance and smooth achievement sequences. Although the secretary most ften functions as the "office wife," most women with professional redentials have had the experience of being expected or asked to per-rm Motherly functions in the office.

The casting of female colleagues into stereotypical feminine sex les not only influences the relationships between pairs of women and en in the workplace but also prejudices the woman's chances of being cluded in peer relations. Observational studies of interacting work roups show that normal processes of competition, coalition formation, nd cooperation exclude women (Wolman and Frank, 1972; Mayes, 976). The sole or token woman is isolated, and her contributions are istorted (Laws, 1975; Kanter, 1977b; Taylor and Fiske, 1976). Emphasiz-g sex roles has the effect of polarizing women and men, and of further olating women, in situations where the sex ratios are heavily skewed Grimm and Stern, 1974). Women's access to peer networks and to onsorship that facilitates career success is further compromised by is often unrecognized factor.

Masculine sex roles, too, can be discerned in the work setting. The terature on role expectations for those in management positions is articularly rich in characterizations of masculinity: Men in their organi-tional roles are expected to exhibit decisiveness, authoritativeness, xpertise, or the posture of knowledgeability: firmness. They receive eference. They delegate work. They evaluate. They chew out their ubordinates. They make their subordinates shape up.

Power and the exercise of power are major dimensions underlying e sex structuring of occupational roles. The research on women in anagement shows that men perceive a contradiction between the at-ibutes of women and those required for success in management (Bass, rusell, and Alexander, 1971; Rosen and Jerdee, 1974a). Although stud-s have repeatedly shown that women and men recruits to management ave the same characteristics (Day and Stogdill, 1972; Terborg, 1977), the erception that women cannot command—and in particular, cannot ommand men—persists (Bartol and Butterfield, 1976). The power di-ension clearly enters into consideration of the use of persuasion and negotiation, as in the discussion of role bargains (Merton, 1968; Sieber 1974). If women cannot credibly exercise power, their bargaining position is diminished and the ratio of role privileges to role obligations that the can wring from role partners is accordingly reduced.

The frank pursuit of self-interest is consonant with male sex-rol scripts, in the occupational sphere as in others; it is dissonant with images of femininity. Bluffing and bargaining are skills that prevail and pay off in male games, including occupational games (Harragan, 1977) In light of the cultural penalties for the exercise of power by women women may indeed have difficulty playing these games with the agility and verve that is called for.

The sentimental image of the home as haven from the stresses c the occupational world has a misplaced focus. It is not the home but the homebody to whom the expectations attach. As women have moved into the labor market in increasing number, we find that the asymmetr of spousal roles in the home moves with them.

Midlife women are workers, wives, mothers, daughters, and do mestic workers. In each sphere, they are surrounded by role partner whose roles are complementary to their own. In each sphere, it can b seen that the role expectations for the female role incumbent are frame to an excess of obligations over privileges. This becomes clearer as w examine specific role partnerships.

Female and male partners in marriage can be referred to by the identical term, but their privileges and obligations are asymmetrical b law and custom. In some localities, law and custom are at variance; fc example, custom holds that a husband should support his wife an minor children, but laws currently hold that each spouse is responsible for the other's debts. Husbands have rights of sexual access to thei wives, but the law does not recognize a similar right of wives or a obligation of husbands.

Ironically, research indicates that women and men seek the sam benefits in marriage—nurturance, intimacy, emotional support—an thrive when they encounter them (Kotlar, 1962). However, men expee these attributes in a spouse, as a function of sex roles (or feminir nature), but women are aware that these attributes contradict the mas culinity their spouses are supposed to embody.

Male and female parents, similarly, can be designated by the sam term, but research makes it evident that virtually all the parenting in th United States is done by mothers. The enormous child-care burden i assumed by mothers, and only a trivial amount of it is shared wit spouse, relatives, or paid help. There is some evidence that father when they share in child care at all, by and large limit their contributio to routine custodial activities or "playing with" their children (Laml

)76). Guidance, the inculcation of values, coaching, nursing, and :aching are among the parental responsibilities that seem to follow an on-call" kind of schedule rather than occurring conveniently, say, on unday afternoons. The asymmetrical role demands on parents extend to late life rather than being limited to the period when children are gally dependent. The same asymmetry can be found in other kin rela- ons maintained by the marital pair, as with the care of aged parents by aughters (and daughters-in-law) rather than sons. Many women find ie role obligations of the daughter increasing in midlife as aged parents ome to require care.

The asymmetry in household work is well documented at present .aws, 1979; Robinson and Converse, 1966). Detailed studies of family me budgets make it clear that a rising standard of living has imposed icreased burdens on housewives. Husbands and children bear only a ivial share of the work generated by their joint households, and do not ike a significantly larger share as the children grow older or the moth- -'s total work week is increased by paid work (Walker, 1970).

Dual Roles"/Multiple Roles

As individual roles are structured differently for women and men,) too are their "dual roles" and the multiple role system that is the ontext of all adults in our society. We have pointed out the way in hich sex-role scripts prescribe a different normative weighting of work id family roles for women and men. Women's "dual roles" often mean iding the inflated demands of a male-style (single-role) career to those f a wife's domestic duties, which in themselves frequently add up to a ork week twice as long as the paid work week. When Baird (1967) lentified structural sources of role stress for individuals beginning raduate school, he found that extra-academic roles, and particularly iarital and family responsibilities, exacerbated role stress. Family roles, f course, make far heavier demands on women than on men. Feldman 973), too, found that graduate women's productivity (publications) as impeded by marriage, while men's was enhanced.

If the general principle of sex structuring of roles holds, role ac- imulation—such as may be involved in kin bonds, office in profes- onal associations, committee work, and the like—may well mean in- easing the total role obligations enormously, and increasing the lative excess of obligations over role privileges still more. Role over- ad would be the predicted result. Continuing and chronic stress from verwork might be expected to result in substantial increases in occupa- onal health problems for employed women.

Sex differences found by Spreitzer et al. (1979) reflect the facts of

women's multiple role incumbency as contrasted with that of men.
When women reporting marriage/work combinations were compared
with women reporting marriage/work/family, the percentage reporting
a high degree of happiness was substantially lower (38% as compared
with 44% with an additional role). For men, the difference was only 2
percentage points (37% as compared with 35%). The addition of friend
and church roles did not detract in a comparable way from global happiness, suggesting that these roles are less demanding than work and
family roles. The Spreitzer *et al.* data confirm the problem of role over
load in women documented in the time-use studies.

Data showing husbands' (increasing) leisure relative to their work
week, and wives' (vanishing) leisure relative to their double work day
succinctly tell the story of asymmetry in dual roles of women and men
(Kreps and Clark, 1975). In the light of these trends, it is not surprising
that the wives—and only the wives—in Rapoport and Rapoport's (1969
study of dual career families complained of role overload. The inescapa-
ble conclusion is that "dual roles" and multiple roles make greater demands on women than on men. Beyond the regular "marriage tax" o
heavy home obligations, however, women pay an additional penalty. It
consequences are felt at midlife and later, in the form of economic vulnerability. The period of the life-course when family demands are great
est often coincides with the high investments required by the establish
ment of a career. The "dual roles" of men are engineered to enhance
career investment, while the role expectations for women are designed
to enhance their partners' and not their own career success. It is to be
expected that many midlife women's careers reflect this rather typical
prior experience. At this point in their lives, they have already suffered
the penalties of having chosen the approved life-course for their gender
Very few women have built up the equity in the work world and th
contingent social benefits that their male peers enjoy.

When women seek to compensate for their earlier work history b
retraining or reentering at midlife, however, they feel the sting of th
normative judgments of the world they seek to enter. As students, a
apprentices, or as colleagues, they meet a subtle prejudice to the effec
that if they had possessed the requisite talent and motivation, they
would, of course, have followed different (and incidentally, male) pr:
orities in their 20s and 30s. Teachers and fellow apprentices make it clea
that little contribution can be expected from such "late bloomers" c
"late starters."

[5]Speitzer *et al.* did not attempt to study the lack of symmetry between women's and men
work and marital roles (or other roles). However, the authors note the importance
differential commitment to roles—or priorities, as discussed here—and suggest a focus c
this issue in future research.

Midlife women find it difficult to make a "new" start even when they must or want to do so. Others will not let them; they carry their life histories with them. In order to understand their situation, it is not enough to know what roles they occupy or aspire to in the present moment. Rather, the life they have lived, with its transitions and changes, colors their present and their future. The situation of midlife women calls for a life-course perspective.

WOMEN AND THE LIFE-COURSE

Life-course research has consistently included women, and a great deal of it has focused on transitions in the family life-cycle that are widely assumed to affect women disproportionately. One of the earliest traditions in life-course research subsumes the so-called family life-cycle studies. In this tradition, the family as the unit of analysis is assumed to mature over its life-span with the accomplishment of successive "developmental tasks" (Duvall, 1957). These developmental tasks define the normative requirements for the family throughout the life cycle. Developmental tasks may be individually or socially prompted and include such sets of activities as reproduction, socialization, status attainment, and physical maintenance (Hill and Mattessich, 1979). The family life cycle comprises an orderly progression of life events such as establishment of the family by marriage, birth of the first child, entrance of the first child into school, departure of the last child from the parental home, retirement, and widowhood.

The conceptual thrust of the life-cycle perspective lies in its treatment of the family as a semiclosed system of interrelated positions (i.e., wife/mother, husband/father, sister/daughter) that evolves over time. Each position is occupied by a family member who performs multiple roles. As a result of the inclusion of a time dimension, the family is not perceived as a static entity, but rather a dynamic one with a past, present, and future conceptualized as sequential stages of development. New stages are initiated with change in the system of positions or in the content of any role(s).

Despite the advantages of a life-course perspective (primarily its way of viewing family development longitudinally), there are certain deficiencies, particularly in older work (see Hill and Mattessich, 1979, for an extensive review). Several assumptions made in connection with the way family is defined render this perspective inadequate for studying individuals or any family configuration other than the nuclear one. To begin with, family life-cycle theorists assumed that a family will follow a "predictable natural history" (Hill and Hansen, 1960). Deviations from this normal life cycle were sometimes categorized not only as atypical, random, and disruptive, but also as ultimately unnatural (Rodgers, 1973). Thus, for example, the female-headed family, by virtue of its failure to fulfill the cultural mandate that a family have a male and a female head, was thought weak and incapable of accomplishing further developmental tasks in the family life cycle.

Because the unit of analysis is the family and the family members are expected to perform their roles normatively, individual development tends to be glossed over in the life-cycle perspective. Development occurs in the family only because of individual maturation, yet personality development and individual growth are underrepresented in the family life-cycle vocabulary.[6] Rather, we find that the members growing and working in unison are seen to produce family outcomes, not individual outcomes. The household or family is reified in order to be viewed processually or developmentally (Elder, 1980/1981). The heterogeneity in the population of midlife women and their households is particularly ill-served by the unitary model of family development.

As Elder (1977) has pointed out, the life-cycle model does not offer a precise definition of change or development over time—but merely records a plus or a minus in the configuration of the family. It does not make use of all possible information on the economic careers and work lives of adult family members. The family development stages are not capable of charting the life-course of an individual, or her career path, or the career paths of several adult family members simultaneously. The model usually offered delineates stages in relation to compositional change in the family only, as when a baby is born or a member leaves the household.

To a certain extent, the family was understood as a group capable of development in and of itself. Yet family members develop in spheres other than the family. Women, especially, have been underestimated in the family development literature because of this familial determinism. From this perspective, it appears that women's "developmental tasks" have required that they promote the growth and well-being of others at the expense of their own development. Although a woman may have enacted only her family roles to the exclusion of all others in early adulthood, at midlife as family demands slack off, she is capable of launching a delayed career in spheres other than the family. At this point in her life-course, a woman may complete an education or begin one, train for a new job or seek a promotion, join a volunteer association or found one. A midlife woman is much more than her familial roles.

---

[6]Hill and Mattessich (1979) recognize the need for convergence between family development theory and life-span developmental psychology in remedying this problem and suggest ways in which the convergence might occur.

ore than "just a wife" or "just a mother." The multiple roles of a
idlife woman constitute her biography, each role contributing to her
evelopment.

Another area of life-course research focuses on differences between
rth cohorts in the incidence, timing, sequence, spacing, and duration
major life events, such as school-leaving or the birth of a first child.
ne question for such inquiries concerns the impact and consequences
normative expectations on the timing of life transitions. A second
uestion concerns the impact and consequences of social change on the
ariation and timing of traditional life-cycle events across successive
rth cohorts (Glick, 1957; Uhlenberg, 1974). The social concept of "onne" transitions and the pressure on the individual to follow the social
hedule for life transitions have intrigued researchers in this tradition
f. Modell, Furstenberg, and Herschberg, 1976). One further question
als with the impact of nonnormative events on traditional life-cycle
tterns. Norton (1980) studied the relationship of divorce to standard
e-cycle measures such as age at first marriage, birth of first child, birth
last child, and end of child-rearing for successive birth cohorts of
men who had ever borne children.

Current work in the life-course perspective is open-ended, non-
dgmental, and better equipped to question the effects of certain se-
ences and timing of life events beyond the familial ones on the eco-
mic well-being of women in their middle and later years (Elder, 1977,
81; Riley, 1971, 1979; Brim, 1980; Brim and Ryff, 1980; Featherman,
81). Principles of current life-course theory include the following:

1. The life-course is structured by major life events—events such as
mpletion of training, entry into the labor market, marriage, divorce,
dowhood, birth of a child, departure of the last child from the home,
ntry into employment, retirement—which require role transitions re-
lting in permanent changes in the individual's life. Brim (1980) de-
ibes these as "triggers for personal change and development." At
ch of these transitions, a new period in an individual's life is initiated.
 single period may be adequately understood apart from antecedent
consequent periods.

2. Cohort membership locates an individual within the life-course.
birth cohort refers to a group of people born at approximately the
ne time. They share either birth year or birth period. As Riley (1979)
rns, the term cohort should not be confused with generation, used to
scribe individuals of similar ages within a kinship context. An indi-
ual's age supplies approximate knowledge about one's biological,
ychological, and social experiences.

3. The stages of development implied in the life-course process are
ther fixed nor immutable. Successive birth cohorts do not experience

the same life patterns due to social change and environmental variation
As history unfolds, it influences and shapes the life-course of entire
cohorts of individuals differently because each cohort lives through it in
unique ways.

4. An individual's social roles undergo changes several times over
the life-course and are said to follow careers. An individual's life-course
may be conceptualized as a convergence of career lines or trajectories
that follow a series of age- and sex-differentiated roles across several
spheres—educational, familial, occupational.

5. The life-course covers the entire life-span. As an individual ages
there is an interactive effect involving the biological, psychological, and
social processes of life.

An individual's life-course is made up of interlocking strands of
careers rooted in multiple roles. Multiple role occupancy is not associated with a particular stage in the life-course but continues throughout
the life-span. The various combinations of marriage, parenthood, and
employment across time suggest the diverse trajectories possible for
women at midlife. By paying attention to multiple roles and careers
through time, the life-course perspective offers an understanding of the
individual not only in a familial context but also in the contexts of marriage, fertility, and employment. Too often one context has been singled
out at the neglect of others. For midlife women, the impact of the "empty nest," losing a spouse, entering the labor market, or finishing a college degree is not isolated from other spheres and other careers. In this
chapter, we are most concerned with the impact of changes in multiple
roles at midlife (occupational, marital, parental, and domestic) on wom-
en's economic well-being in later years.

The normative order and timing of life events judges individuals
"on time" if their role behavior accords with the cultural prescription
for their age/sex category and "off time" if their role behavior does not.
The consequences of the nonnormative incidence, sequence, spacing,
timing, and duration of life events are yet to be widely researched (Norton, 1980). Although we know that conformity to traditional timetables
is eroding, women now in midlife were subjected to those traditional
timetables and lived lives "on time" for the most part. Ironically, for a
midlife woman, a lifetime of "on-time" events such as marriage and
childbearing early in adulthood means being vulnerable to economic
declines throughout the latter half of the life-span. Being "off time," for
women, as in completing a college degree, entering an occupation early
in the work life, and postponing marriage and childbearing so as to
advance in the career, usually predicts to economic security in later
years.

Women who are now at midlife may well have chosen their adult
life-styles at a period when women's options were more restricted than

any other time in this century. In their mothers' and grandmothers' nerations, there were more never-married women and more women ho never bore children. The variability in educational attainment was eater, and substantially higher educational levels were attained by omen who did not marry. The characteristics of midlife women's four ajor careers—occupational, marital, parental, and domestic—are portant for determining the needs of future research and policy on omen in their later years.

ie Marital Career at Midlife

Simone de Beauvoir (1974) has argued that most women marry, ve married, or suffer from not marrying. The cultural mandate holds at marriage is of the utmost importance for the well-being of women. midlife, however, a wife's chances of being divorced, separated, or dowed are high and climbing higher. At any given time, divorced omen outnumber divorced men of all ages due to the higher remar-ge rate among the latter. Younger divorced people are more likely to marry than older ones; hence, those who stay divorced tend to be ler and female. Women outlive men more often, and more widowers narry than widows; hence, those who remain widowed are pre-minately older and female. The premature death of a spouse or the ssolution of a marriage may leave a middle-aged wife in dire social and onomic straits, not because she has "lost" the role of wife, as the erature would word it, but because, in a more fundamental sense, the ltural stipulation of female dependence in marriage leaves her finan-lly hard-pressed, occupationally inexperienced, and ill-equipped for lependence.

The literature supplies some evidence to contradict the assumption at well-being for women requires an intact marriage (Bart, 1971; Ber-rd, 1972a; Brown, Feldberg, Fox, and Kohen, 1976). Bart (1971), in a idy of depression of middle-aged women being treated in mental spitals, concluded that if a woman's sense of worth derives from her /n accomplishments, as in initiating or expanding an occupational e, she is less vulnerable to breakdown when other salient roles con-ct or disappear—for example, when a husband dies or children leave me.

For those who remain married throughout midlife, the changes perienced in the wife role appear potentially liberating. Brim (1975) cnowledges that at midlife, wives may be moving toward a genuine owth in self-esteem and self-actualization. Other studies have shown at women at midlife tend to be more eager to strike out on their own in perhaps in their earlier years of marriage (cf. Rubin, 1979). It is at s time in the life-course that the opportunities for involvement with

extrafamilial activities increase for many women. Well-being seems to b
a function of having multiple roles and multiple options rather tha
being "just a wife."

The Parental Career at Midlife

Occupying the role of mother produces lasting effects over the lif
course that influence many aspects of a woman's life. Using retr
spective data collected from a nationally representative sample of mi‹
life women, Borker, Loughlin, and Rudolph (1979) found that the age
which a woman became a mother for the first time determined, to
considerable extent, her socioeconomic status in later life. The autho
found that women who became mothers early suffered lower earnin‚
at midlife relative to those who did not, primarily as a result of the
lower educational levels. Studies of teenage mothers and the rate act
ally completing high school or its equivalent corroborate these findin‚
(Moore, Hofferth, Caldwell, and Waite, 1979).

A life-course perspective defines midlife for mothers, not pri
cipally by chronological age but by the experience of a major life ever
the launching of the last child into the adult world (Neugarten, 196¶
This event initiates the so-called "empty nest" stage, a stage durin
which the mother, married or not, experiences an attenuation of chil
rearing obligations. The menopause and the "empty nest" are typical
associated with the female at midlife as crises. The view that marria‚
and children are essential ingredients for a full and healthy life for
woman is based on a biological determinism that links mind and bo‹
more closely for women than for men (Barnett and Baruch, 197¶
Against this view, Troll and Turner (1978) argue that the majority
midlife women, having identified themselves with other interests, ‹
not experience severe trauma upon the departure of the last child fro
the home. Most midlife mothers, they claim, positively anticipate t
freedom from child-rearing responsibilities and the opportunities to pu
sue their own interests and to spend more time with peers. Mothe
who view mothering as an episode rather than a lifelong occupation,
appears, are better able to facilitate their own as well as their childrer
development. However, mothers who have dedicated their entire liv
to mothering were found in one study to be plagued by adjustme
problems when their children left home (Bart, 1971). The effects of t
emptying nest, of course, depend in part on the degree of independen
achieved by maturing offspring. Present trends indicate that many mi
life women take on substantial responsibility for care of grandchildre
Current economic factors mean that many young adults who have l
home return for longer or shorter periods to live under the parental ro
There is an image of the postparental woman in our society as

ormer achiever" (Mayer, 1969). This image is based on a definition of
ᴐman as "just a mother" and a definition of female achievement as
production of the species. When the duties associated with mother-
od are no longer required, as when a midlife woman watches her last
ᴉld depart the parental home, that certain social recognition she re-
ᴉved as reproducer of the species changes emphasis: An "active"
ᴐther becomes a "former" mother. Retiring from active motherhood
n potentially detract from a woman's economic well-being as well: Her
gibility for public assistance such as Aid to Families with Dependent
ᴉildren or survivor's benefits (if she is widowed with dependent chil-
en) ceases when her children reach age 18. At this time, a woman's
ᴣportunities to receive job training and career placement are in short
pply. Her experiences and skills, accrued while mothering and home-
ᴉking, are unrecognized or underestimated. In general, mothers who
sh to enter or return to the public world as active participants find the
ᴉng difficult and few places or persons willing to offer assistance such
training, career placement, or support.

e Domestic Career at Midlife

Upon reaching midlife, women do not find too many drastic changes
the content of their domestic role. Perhaps with children gone, the
ᴣrk load decreases, but it never disappears altogether. Indeed, some-
ᴉes the middle-aged housewife's work load is increased by the pres-
ᴣe in her home of elderly parents who can no longer care for them-
ves. No matter what her age, the housewife is still expected to meet the
ᴣds of the remaining household members and to perform the domestic
ks until she is no longer capable. She continues to have multiple role
ᴣponsibilities.

e Occupational Career at Midlife

Of all women currently in the labor force, the 35- to 64-year-olds
ᴠe consumed the highest doses of a segregated sexual division of
or in the home and the labor force. Their labor force histories reflect
s exposure to the cultural prescriptions for womanhood. Essentially
ᴉr patterns are distinguishable for midlife women's labor force histo-
s, these being rank-ordered from most to least prevalent (Parnes,
ᴣnius, Blau, Nestel, Shortlidge, and Sandell, 1975; Howe, 1982):

1. Long intermissions between times in the labor force: Usually a
   job is held until marriage or the birth of the first child, followed
   by a protracted absence during the child-rearing years and reentry after children are launched.

2. Short intermissions between times in the labor force, usually t have a child or meet a family exigency.
3. No labor force experience as an adult whatsoever: Usually ma riage and motherhood occupy the woman full time.
4. Continuous labor force employment, until recently an optio exercised mainly by never-married women.

Is outside employment beneficial for a midlife woman's well-being We have reviewed evidence indicating that employment enhances woman's well-being by providing wages with which to maintain a stai dard of living, social status as an incentive to upward mobility, and sense of personal competence that contributes to self-esteem. Howeve it is well documented that female employment is paid less and carri lower social status than most male occupations. Employment tends afford some self-esteem for women, usually more than is accrued in housewife-only existence, but its rewards are less when the job is dea end, tedious, or otherwise demeaning.

Nonetheless, in light of present trends, the role of labor force pa ticipant is an extremely important one for women of every age. A sk rocketing cost of living is encouraging replacement of the husband-a provider with the dual-earner marriage. In addition, a growing segme of highly educated, professional career women in dual-career famili are exhibiting new patterns of family living. Divorce and widowhoc force many women to head their households single-handedly. Midli women, in particular, are entering or returning to the labor force f financial reasons, personal aspirations, or some combination of bot Whereas the midlife male is thought to experience a "time squeeze," realization that time is running out on his career ambitions, the midl female is thought to be experiencing a "time gap," a realization that s has many years left before retirement age with perhaps no husband, children at home, and no means of supporting herself socially and/ economically (Cohen, 1979).

It appears that employment will loom large in the futures of mc midlife women, whatever has been their life-course to this point. F most, the life-course they have lived has not been sufficient to assu them of economic self-sufficiency in later life. There will be an urge need for social programs to meet some of their needs. These progran in turn, must be grounded in an adequate social theory.

FUTURE DIRECTIONS FOR THEORY AND RESEARCH

Recognition of the fundamental reality of multiple roles could sti ulate an enormously fruitful reorientation in role theory and could ge

ate research that will provide for more adequate bases for policy
rmulation. New research in role theory needs to incorporate a time
mension, such as inheres in the life-course perspective, and give par-
ular attention to the dynamic character of role demands, role bar-
ins, and role enactment as multiple careers unfold over the life-span.

A greater variety of life transitions—and their timing, spacing, and
quencing—are now "expected" than was the case in past generations.
future, we can expect more research on the unexpected transitions:
reer change, downward mobility in occupations, remarriages, reen-
es, and exits. We can expect more research on nonunitary career lines,
d a more acute analysis of continuities and discontinuities in the indi-
dual's multiple careers. The time dimension will be taken for granted,
d we will see research not solely on occupational planning but on
anning for multiple roles over the life span. The payoffs of various
ategies—including alternative sequencing and timing of education,
ployment, and family formation—need to be calculated. It is clear
m the situation at present that planners and legislators are unaware
the negative consequences of certain prevalent patterns of educa-
n/marriage/employment. "Social accounting" needs to be informed,
a greater degree than is the case at present, of the outcomes of the
rious paths women take to midlife. It is to be hoped that in the future,
a result of research that demonstrates these causal paths, women will
enabled to make choices that do not doom them to penury in midlife.

A focus on the economic situation of women at midlife and beyond
derscores the need for studies of outcomes. It is essential that the
ths to various midlife outcomes be charted. These paths must further
related to choices that women make, and to choices that women
rceive. Some authors have pointed out that "economic rationality"
sed on differential earning power of spouses dictates that it be the
fe's career that is interrupted by family moves, or her job options that
limited by where the household is located. From other studies we
rn of the effects of family responsibilities on women's occupational
hievements. Studies of "dual career" marriages tell us that wives con-
ously subordinate their careers to those of their husbands. This strat-
y may have different outcomes in the short run—particularly where
rital harmony is given priority—and the long run, where a woman's
nomic viability is at stake should the marriage terminate. A major
ortcoming of the "dual role" research is that it seems to assume a
gle and lifelong marriage. Very few studies contain a time dimension
ended enough to permit the assessment of long-term economic out-
nes of different strategies. Yet this is the kind of research that is most
eded.

Current research has underestimated the importance of employment and employment history for women's future. Indeed, research c "dual roles" evidences a genteel neglect of the economic dimensio New research on women's multiple roles needs to focus more on th salable and transferable skills and experience women gain from er ployment, and less on their husbands' marital satisfaction. Above a there needs to be considerably more work on developing predicti models that chart women's paths to the economic outcomes of midlif

Unacknowledged normative perspectives have distorted existin research on women's multiple roles and options. "Regular" career composed of "on-time" life transitions, have been viewed as more r spectable. "Off-time" transitions are viewed as deviant, giving rise imputations of personal irresponsibility or immaturity. However, a emphasis on outcomes of differing pathways should produce rath different judgments. Some "off-time" transitions may be detrimental women's economic self-sufficiency in later life (for example, very ear childbearing), while others, equally "deviant," may enhance later ec nomic status (for example, "late" marriage contigent upon education and career goals).

In specifying future directions for research, we are stressing th need for sustained study of women's multiple roles, with an emphas on outcomes over longer periods of time. A major thrust must be i creased study of women in their work roles. In the course of our review we have raised many issues that call for comparisons of women ar men in the work world.

Many pressing questions involve the outcomes of multiple role e actment for women and men. Under what conditions does one enjoy th benefits of role accumulation? Under what conditions does role confl occur? Specifically, what elements in the organization, setting, or sta ing of employment facilitate coping strategies of what types? Are the ranks, occupations, or employers that facilitate the acquisition or exe cise of methods of status articulation? And for the range of organizati variables to which our attention is directed, we can ask: How are wom and men distributed over these opportunities?

The study of women's role partners in the world of work deserv much more attention than it has received to date. One focus for need research is the question of women's peers in the workplace, and t related, crucial factor of sex composition of the work group. Past search has shown positive effects of both peers and superiors on t career success of men, but the picture will be more complex for wom When women in sex-typical occupations are studied, the role of pe tends to be overlooked competely. Research on women in sex-atypi occupations suggests negative influences of male peers on wome career progress. The picture will be equally complex with respect 'omen's superiors in the workplace. Researchers have raised issues ɔncerning mentoring and role modeling for long-term occupational ıccess of women, stressing the importance of support and coaching by ıperiors in the organizational structure. Most accounts note the paucity f women at higher ranks as an impediment to career facilitation for ʼomen, but have not systematically examined the role of male superi- ʼs. When researchers document negative attitudes toward female ca- ʼers in men at high organizational ranks, they do not analyze the im- lications in terms of role relationships and face-to-face interaction.

Co-workers, particularly men, are not inert elements of industrial ɘsign in women's work contexts. Rather, they engage women actively ıd, as we have seen, actively impede women's role enactment and ʼreer advancement in some instances. The importance of role partners deliberately inducing role conflict surfaced first in accounts of wom- 1's experiences on the job. By this means, a new and significant type of le conflict was brought to the attention of the social science fraternity. ıe effects of this factor, previously overlooked by researchers in- rested in occupational mental health, are important for the study of job ʼess, in both the short run and the long run. More research is needed 1 the ways in which women's performance in the work role is impeded ıd on the ways long-term outcomes, such as labor force attachment, e affected.

It appears that in her role as worker, a wife has an invisible role ırtner, in addition to peers and superiors on the job. Although re- arch has documented the importance of husband's attitude in a wom- ı's initial decision to embrace employment, his continuing influence is rely taken into account. Systematic research on the interactions of ɔligations and privileges associated with work and family roles for omen and men is called for.

One critical variable that appears in both work and family role rela- ɔnships is power. Current evidence seems consistent with the proposi- ɔn that the acquisition of role privileges in the work organization is ɔilitated by possessing and wielding credible power. Being perceived ıd reacted to as credible wielders of power appears to be problematic ʼ women. Yet the effective use of power contributes to career advance- ent in many ways. As only one example, when one has the power to ımmand desired outcomes for subordinates, their loyalty is strength- ɘd, and the individual's power position is enhanced as grateful for- ɘr subordinates move up in the organizational hierarchy. Lack of ca- ɘr mobility, as much as intermittent labor force participation, produces ʼor economic outcomes for women in midlife.

Another focus for researchers is the connection between role stress women workers and aspects of the organizational context that are susceptible to change. Both the stressors and the need for change have been neglected topics during decades when the norm was the male breadwinner–full-time housewife household. Current interest in the economic status of the midlife woman has led us to reevaluate that path, whose effects are disastrous in the event of marital dissolution. Similarly suspect are the script and associated employment career that define wives' employment as incidental and episodic. When women (and their wages) are viewed as dispensable, public concern about their conditions of employment is minimal. As a result of past definitions of the situation, substantial gaps in both policy and research are evident.

Today it is apparent that continuous labor force participation enhances women's midlife economic outcomes. Women's experiences in the labor market are given increasing importance, and researchers are increasingly drawn to the study of factors that drive women from employment or compromise their productivity. There has been too little research on job satisfaction among women, and its long-term effects on productivity, mobility, and labor force attachment. When we make the linkages between low labor force participation and economic trouble in midlife, we are forced to examine fundamental questions about what paid work offers women of any age. Program policy and planning must also attack these basic issues.

FUTURE DIRECTIONS FOR POLICY

Midlife women are a heterogeneous group, exhibiting varying degrees of economic viability and vulnerability. Although they represent wide range in educational attainment, labor force experience, occupational prestige, marital and family status, and health, they share the need to achieve economic security. For most women, economic security in the latter half of the life-span is often uncertain. Older women are joining the ranks of the poverty-stricken faster than any other group in this country: The poverty rate for women over age 65 is almost twice the rate for men of the same ages (U.S. Bureau of the Census, 1982). A sound economic future can be obtained through a well-paying job with ample benefits and a pension plan, a husband with the same, or both. At midlife, the proportion of women holding well-paying jobs that provide benefits is small, while the chance that they may experience the loss of a husband is large. Employed women, married or not, have better chances for economic survival at midlife and later than women who are unemployed. Women without their own earnings *and* without husband fare the worst.

Social security entitlement programs such as the Old Age, Survivor's, Disability, and Health Insurance (OASDHI) program are sup

ɔsed to provide benefits to persons in need of income and to provide
ɪsurance against economic disruptions resulting from disability, retire-
ent, or the death of an income-producing spouse. Midlife women
ithout incomes or with meager incomes have only these programs to
ɪrn to at midlife and in later years. Some 60% of older single women
ɔllect their major source of income from social security (Miller, 1982).

The system of entitlement programs known simply as "social se-
ɪrity" was created with one role in mind for women, homemaker, and
ɪe for men, breadwinner. While Social Security has tried to keep pace
ith inflation, it has done relatively little to accommodate the changes in
mily roles and life-styles occurring since Social Security was estab-
ɪhed. The once-common pattern of lifelong marriage between a career
ɔmemaker and her breadwinning husband has been replaced by a
owing diversity of marital, familial, and occupational roles of women
ɪd men over the life-course (U.S. Dept. of H.E.W., 1979; National
ɔmmission on Social Security, 1981; Cahn, 1978).

Despite the changing roles of women and men, the objectives of the
ɔcial Security entitlement programs remain much the same as they
ere at the programs' inception in the 1930s: Women are provided for
ainly in their roles as workers' wives and mothers of workers' chil-
ʻen. According to eligibility criteria and benefit formulae, women who
ɔ not have long and continuous labor force histories are entitled to
nefits by virtue of their relationships to men and children. For exam-
e, under Social Security, men "earn" disability benefits and retire-
ents benefits (if and when they need them) by paying taxes on their
rnings. In most cases, women also "earn" disability and retirement
nefits, not because they may be paying taxes on their own earnings
ɪd require such benefits but because they are related to disabled or
tired men and qualify for benefits as "dependents" rather than "work-
s." Social Security pays a widow with dependent children a care-
ʻer's allowance, but only until her children reach age 16. Social Se-
rity then does not supplement the widow's income again until she
ɪches age 60 (age 50 if she becomes disabled). (For a thorough descrip-
ɪn of federal programs and their treatment of women, see Griffiths,
76; Kinsley, 1977; Gordon, 1979; Miller, 1982; Mudrick, 1983.)

The midlife woman who has never been employed is usually a
ɪeer wife and homemaker. Her husband's pension and future retire-
ɪnt benefits will support the couple in their later years. Their monthly
cial Security check will amount to the husband's full benefit plus an
ditional half for his wife. However, if the husband should die or the
ɪrriage dissolve before retirement age, financial security for the widow
divorcee is severely diminished. Private pensions and life insurance
ntribute to the widow's economic well-being in only a small percent-

age of cases. Survivor's Insurance provides relief in this situation, bu
only to midlife widows who are disabled or have dependent children
Employment remains the sole option for formerly married women with
out dependents before retirement age, yet the government provide
little in the way of job placement and training to upgrade educationa
credentials or teach profitable skills for these women.

The midlife woman who has been continuously employed through
out adulthood is least likely to experience poverty at midlife or later. Sh
is, however, treated unfairly in public program definitions. Continu
ously employed married women receive no return on *their own* contribu
tions to the Social Security system unless their entitlement (on accour
of their own earnings record) is larger than half their husbands' fu
benefit. The same applies to divorced women whose marriages lasted a
least 10 years and who have not remarried. As a result of these stipula
tions, married and divorced midlife women whose lifetime earnings ar
less than their husbands' or ex-husbands' (of 10 years or more) receiv
retirement benefits no larger than if they had never worked for pay. .
widow who has continuous labor force experience must be entitled to
retirement benefit larger than her deceased husband's full benefit i
order to collect on account of her own earnings record rather than as
surviving dependent.

The midlife woman employed intermittently throughout adulthoc
and who is no longer a wife or mother fares worst under the current s
of public programs. Time out of the labor force reduces the number
years used to compute retirement benefits, resulting in lower benefi
for women who have spent some portion of their adult years in chi
care and homemaking. A previously married midlife woman usually ha
lifetime earnings far below those of her former spouse. Her retiremer
benefit, if she was married for at least 10 years, reflects her forme
dependency status as a wife. She is not entitled to an additional bene
because of her tax contributions to the system for however many yea
she was employed. The same applies to a married woman. These d
chotomous classifications mask the realities of women's multiple rol
and, indeed, penalize them.

Midlife women who have not followed a traditional male occup
tional earnings career (a majority) and who are no longer wives and/
mothers of dependent children (an increasing percentage) fall throug
the holes in the "social safety net." There are no programs available
supply financial aid to the midlife career homemaker should she becon
disabled or unable to perform her domestic occupation. The survivors
a deceased career homemaker are not entitled to benefits, either. Shou
a midlife woman find herself widowed, divorced, or separated prior

tirement age, the risk of poverty is high, while the chance for em-
loyment is low if she is not already employed.

What, then, are the forms of assistance and support for midlife
omen in need of income? There exist no federal cash transfer entitle-
ent programs that provide for women before retirement age unless
ley have dependent children, with the exception of disability insur-
nce. However, disability insurance is not paid to career homemakers
ho become disabled or chronically ill. Even if needy midlife women
ceive cash transfers from disability insurance, the benefits are usually
sufficient to boost the women out of poverty. Women with paid em-
oyment experience who become disabled and can prove recency of
nployment are entitled to benefits, but their dependents collect bene-
s only if the disabled woman can prove she is the primary wage-earner
the household. The Old Age, Survivor's, Disability, and Health Insur-
nce program seems blind to the realities of women's employment
ythms. There is a considerable need for new programs as well as
odifications to the current Social Security system.

Interest in the way women are treated under the Social Security
stem has grown in recent years. Task forces, national commissions,
nd congressional committees have been formed to examine the issues
nd offer proposals or recommendations for change (U.S. Dept. of
.E.W., 1979; National Commission on Social Security, 1981; Cahn,
78). Three variations on the Social Security tax and benefit structure
ve received considerable attention. These three proposals offer the
ost practical solutions for revising the unwieldy Social Security
stem.

The first variation proposes an individually based benefit structure.
lis structure would resemble the current one, with the exception that
rvivors' and dependents' benefits would eventually be phased out.
omen and men would be encouraged to enter paid employment as
ell as to share homemaking responsibilities. Without time spent in
id employment, a person would not be eligible for the forms of Social
curity assistance available today.

The second variation proposes changes to accommodate home-
akers who are, under the current system, not entitled to any benefits
account of their status as workers. Rather than deriving benefits from
ouses, full-time homemakers would be credited for their years of ser-
ce in the home. The credits would apply toward future retirement
nefits, which the homemaker could collect at retirement age regard-
ss of marital status. These credits would be financed through taxes on
e homemaker or on the total household income.

The third variation proposes that the total income of a couple, regardless of the actual proportion contributed by each spouse, be shared equally in calculating credits toward benefits. Under this plan, full-time homemakers would receive the same benefits as their husbands while married, accumulating these credits throughout their marital career, and keeping them if the marriage should end.

These proposals are a first step in remedying the unfair treatment of women under Social Security. But while these plans recognize that women, regardless of the type and amount of work they have performed, need basic protection like men, they do not realize that women lack the opportunities to achieve economic security through their own efforts. Innovative and diverse support systems are required to address the needs of women at midlife and after. Programs must be established to accommodate successive groups of midlife women with varied educational, marital, and employment histories—women who desire to learn new skills to enter or reenter the job market, to engage in volunteer activities as leaders, teachers, and counselors, to complete high school or college degrees, and to enhance and transform multiple role experiences into socially valued, marketable credentials.

REFERENCES

Albrecht, A. Informal interaction patterns of professional women. In B. A. Stead (Ed.). *Women in management*. Englewood Cliffs, N.J.: Prentice-Hall, 1976.

Angrist, S., and Almquist, E. M. *Careers and contingencies: How college women juggle with gender*. Port Washington, N.Y.: Kennikat Press, 1975.

Baird, L. L. Role stress in graduate students. *Dissertation Abstracts*, 1967, *11-A*, 3929.

Barnett, R. C., and Baruch, G. K. Women in the middle years: A critique of research and theory. *Psychology of Women Quarterly*, 1978, *3*, 187–197.

Barnett, R. C., and Baruch, G. K. *Role strain, number of roles and psychological well-being*. Working Paper, Wellesley College Center for Research on Women, 1981.

Bart, P. Depression in middle aged women. In V. Gornick and B. K. Moran (Eds.), *Women in sexist society: Studies in power and powerlessness*. New York: Basic Books, 1971.

Bartol, K. M., and Butterfield, D. A. Sex effects in evaluating leaders. *Journal of Applied Psychology*, 1976, *61*, 446–454.

Baruch, R., Segal, S., and Hendrick, F. A. Constructs of career and family: A statistical analysis of thematic material. *Journal of Counseling Psychology*, 1968, *5*, 308–316.

Bass, B. M., Krusell, J., and Alexander, R. A. Male managers' attitudes toward working women. *American Behavioral Scientist*, 1971, *15*, 221–236.

Bayes, M., and Newton, P. M. Women in authority: A sociopsychological analysis. *Journal of Applied Behavioral Science*, 1978, *14*, 7–20.

Bernard, J. *Academic women*. University Park: Pennsylvania State University Press, 1964.

Bernard, J. *The future of marriage*. New York: World, 1972. (a)

Bernard, J. Changing family lifestyles: One role, two roles, shared roles. In L. K. Howe (Ed.), *The future of the family*. New York: Simon & Schuster, 1972. (b)

Bernard, J. Models for the relationship between the world of women and the world of men. In L. Kriesberg (Ed.), *Research in social movements, conflicts, and change* (Vol. 3). Greenwich, Conn.: JAI Press, 1978.

irnbaum, J. A. *Life patterns, personality style, and self-esteem in gifted family oriented and career committed women.* Doctoral dissertation, State University of Michigan, Ann Arbor, 1971.

orker, S. R., Loughlin, J., and Rudolph, C. S. The long-term effects of adolescent child-rearing: A retrospective analysis. *Journal of Social Service Research,* 1979, 2, 341–355.

rim, O. G., Jr. Theories of the male mid-life crisis. *Counseling Psychologist,* 1975, 6, 2–9.

rim, O. G., Jr. *Socialization in an unpredictable society.* Paper presented to the plenary session on family and socialization, American Sociological Association annual meeting, 1980.

rim, O. G., Jr., and Ryff, C. D. On the properties of life events. In P. B. Baltes and O. G. Brim, Jr. (Eds.), *Life-span development and behavior* (Vol. 3). New York: Academic Press, 1980.

rown, C. A., Feldberg, R., Fox, E. M., and Kohen, J. Divorce: Chance of a new lifetime. *Journal of Social Issues,* 1976, 32, 119–133.

ahn, A. F. Highlights of eighteen papers on problems of midlife women. In U.S. Congress Select Committee on Aging, *Women in midlife—Security and fulfillment* (Part I). Washington, D.C.: U.S. Government Printing Office, 1978.

ohen, J. F. Male roles in mid-life. *Family Coordinator,* 1979, 28, 465–471.

oser, L. *Greedy institutions.* New York: Free Press, 1974.

oser, R. L. Role distance, sociological ambivalence, and transitional status systems. *American Journal of Sociology,* 1966, 72, 173–187.

oser, R. L., and Rokoff, G. Women in the occupational world: Social disruption and conflict. *Social Problems,* 1971, 18, 535–552.

avis, E. Careers as concerns of blue-collar girls. In A. Shostak and W. Gomberg (Eds.), *Blue collar world: Studies of the American worker.* Englewood Cliffs, N.J.: Prentice-Hall, 1964.

ay, D. R., and Stogdill, R. M. Leader behavior of male and female supervisors: A comparative study. *Personnel Psychology,* 1972, 26, 353–360.

e Beauvoir, S. *The second sex.* New York: Vintage Books, 1974.

err, C. B. (Ed.). *Work, family and the career: New frontiers in theory and research.* New York: Praeger, 1980.

uvall, E. M. *Family development.* New York: Lippincott, 1957.

lder, G. H., Jr. Family history and the life course. *Journal of Family History,* 1977, 2, 279–304.

lder, G. H., Jr. *History and the family: The discovery of complexity.* Ernest Burgess Award Lecture, Portland, Oregon, October 25, 1980. (Revised, March 1, 1981.)

pstein, C. F. Encountering the male establishment: Sex status limits on women's careers in the professions. *American Journal of Sociology,* 1970, 75, 965–982.

van, W. M., and Levin, E. G. Status-set and role-set conflicts of the stockbroker: A problem in sociology. *Social Forces,* 1966, 45, 73–83.

eatherman, D. L. The life-span perspective in social science research. Social Science Research Council, January 15, 1981.

eldman, S. D. Impediment or stimulant: Marital status and graduate education. *American Journal of Sociology,* 1973, 78, 982–994.

annon, M. J., and Hendrickson, D. H. Career orientation and job satisfaction among working wives. *Journal of Applied Psychology,* 1973, 57, 339–340.

lick, P. *American families.* New York: Wiley, 1957.

offman, E. Role distance. In E. Goffman, *Encounters.* Indianapolis: Bobbs-Merrill, 1961.

oode, W. J. A theory of role strain. *American Sociological Review,* 1960, 25, 483–496.

ordon, F. E., and Hall, D. T. Self-image and stereotypes of femininity: Their relationship to women's role conflicts and coping. *Journal of Applied Psychology,* 1974, 59, 241–243.

Gordon, N. M. Institutional responses: The social security system. In R. E. Smith (Ed.), *The subtle revolution*. Washington, D.C.: Urban Institute, 1979.

Griffiths, M. W. How much is a woman worth? The American public policy. In J. R. Chapman (Ed.), *Economic independence for women* (Sage Yearbooks in Women's Policy Studies, Vol. 1). Beverly Hills: Sage, 1976.

Grimm, J. W., and Stern, R. N. Sex roles and internal labor market structures: The "female" semi-professions. *Social Problems*, 1974, *21*, 690–705.

Gross, N., McEachern, A., and Mason, W. Role conflict and its resolution. In B. Biddle and E. J. Thomas (Eds.), *Role theory: Concepts and research*. New York: Wiley, 1966.

Hall, D. T. A model of coping with role conflict: The role behavior of college women. *Administrative Science Quarterly*, 1972, *17*, 471–486.

Hall, D. T., and Gordon, F. E. Career choices of married women: Effects on conflict, role behavior, and satisfaction. *Journal of Applied Psychology*, 1973, *58*, 42–48.

Harmon, L. W. Predictive power over ten years of measured social service and scientific interests among college women. *Journal of Applied Psychology*, 1969, *53*, 193–198.

Harragan, B. L. *Games mother never taught you*. New York: Warner Books, 1977.

Haynes, S. G., and Feinleib, M. Women, work and coronary heart disease—Prospective findings from the Framingham Heart Study. *American Journal of Public Health*, 1980, *70*, 133–141.

Haynes, S. G., Levine, S., and Scotch, N. The relationship of psychosocial factors to coronary heart disease in the Framingham Heart Study I. Methods and risk factors. *American Journal of Epidemiology*, 1978, *107*, 362–383.

Hill, R., and Hansen, D. A. The identification of conceptual frameworks utilized in family study. *Marriage and Family Living*, 1960, *22*, 299–311.

Hill, R., and Mattessich, P. Family development theory and life-span development. In P. B. Baltes and O. G. Brim, Jr. (Eds.), *Life-span development and behavior* (Vol. 2). New York: Academic Press, 1979.

Hoferek, M., and Sarnowski, A. Feelings of loneliness of women medical students. *Journal of Medical Education*, 1981, *56*, 397–403.

Holahan, C. K., and Gilbert, L. A. Interrole conflict for working women: Careers versus jobs. *Journal of Applied Psychology*, 1979, *64*, 86–90.

Howe, L. K. The world of women's work. In J. P. Rosenfeld (Ed.), *Relationships: The marriage and family reader*. Glenview, Ill.: Scott, Foresman, 1982.

Kahn, R. L., Wolfe, D. M., Quinn, R. D., and Snoek, J. D. *Organizational stress: Studies in role conflict and ambiguity*. New York: Wiley, 1964.

Kanter, R. M. *Men and women of the corporation*. New York: Basic Books, 1977. (a)

Kanter, R. M. Some effects of proportions on group life: Skewed sex ratios and responses to token women. *American Journal of Sociology*, 1977, *82*, 965–900. (b)

Karp, D. A., and Yoels, W. C. Work, careers, and aging. *Qualitative Sociology*, 1981, *4*, 145–166.

Kinsley, S. Women's dependency and federal programs. In J. R. Chapman and M. Gates (Eds.), *Women into wives: The legal and economic impact of marriage* (Sage Yearbooks in Women's Policy Studies, Vol. 2). Beverly Hills: Sage, 1977.

Komarovsky, M. Cultural contradictions and sex roles. *American Journal of Sociology*, 1946, *52*, 184–189.

Komarovsky, M. Cultural contradictions and sex roles: The masculine case. *American Journal of Sociology*, 1973, *78*, 873–884.

Kotlar, S. Intrumental and expressive marital roles. *Sociology and Social Research*, 1962, *46*, 186–194.

Kreps, J., and Clark, R. *Sex, age and work: The changing composition of the labor force*. Baltimore: Johns Hopkins Press, 1975.

Lamb, M. E. *The role of the father in child development.* New York: Wiley, 1976.

Lashuk, M. W., and Kurian, G. Employment status, feminism, and symptoms of stress: The case of a Canadian prairie city. *Canadian Journal of Sociology,* 1977, 2, 195–204.

Laws, J. L. The psychology of tokenism: An analysis. *Sex Roles,* 1975, 1, 151–174.

Laws, J. L. Work aspirations of women: False leads and new starts. *Signs,* 1976, 1, 33–49.

Laws, J. L. Work motivation and work behavior of women: New perspectives. In J. A. Sherman and F. L. Denmark (Eds.), *The psychology of women: Future directions in research.* New York: Psychological Dimensions, 1978.

Laws, J. L. *The second x: Sex role and social role.* New York: Elsevier/North Holland, 1979.

Laws, J. L. *Problems of access and problems of success in women's career advancement.* Paper presented at the NIE Conference on Attitudinal and Behavioral Measurement in Social Processes/Women's Research, Washington, D.C., 1980.

Laws, J. L., and Tangri, S. S. *Institutional sexism: Or, why there is no conspiracy.* Paper presented at the American Psychological Association annual meeting, 1979.

Levitt, E. S. Vocational development of professional women: A review. *Journal of Vocational Behavior,* 1971, 1, 375–385.

Looft, W. R. Sex differences in the expression of vocational aspirations by elementary school children. *Developmental Psychology,* 1971, 5, 366.

Lorber, J. *Trust, loyalty and the place of women in the informal organization of work.* Paper presented at the American Sociological Association annual meeting, 1975.

Mahajah, A. Women's two roles: A study of role conflict. *Indian Journal of Social Work,* 1966, 26, 377–380.

Mayer, T. F. Middle age and occupational processes: An empirical essay. *Sociological Symposium,* 1969, 3, 89–106.

Mayes, S. S. *Women in positions of authority: An analysis of changing sex roles.* Paper presented at the American Sociological Association annual meeting, 1976.

Merton, R. K. *Social theory and social structure.* New York: Free Press, 1968.

Miller, D. C. *Social security and women's lives.* Paper presented at the National Conference on Social Welfare, Boston, Mass., 1982.

Modell, J., Furstenberg, F. F., Jr., and Herschberg, T. Social change and transitions to adulthood in historical perspective. *Journal of Family History,* 1976, 1, 7–32.

Monahan, L., Kuhn, D., and Shaver, P. Intrapsychic vs. cultural explanations of the fear of success motive. *Journal of Personality and Social Psychology,* 1974, 29, 60–64.

Moore, K. A., Hofferth, S., Caldwell, S. B., and Waite, L. J. *Teenage motherhood: Social and economic consequences.* Washington, D.C.: Urban Institute, 1979.

Mudrick, N. R. Disabled women. *Society,* 1983, 20: 51–55.

Mulvey, M. C. Psychological and sociological factors in prediction of career patterns of women. *Genetic Psychology Monographs,* 1963, 68, 309–386.

National Commission on Social Security. National commission on social security: Recommendations. *Social Security Bulletin,* 1981, 44, 3–13.

Nelson, H. Y., and Goldman, P. R. Attitudes of high school students toward the gainful employment of married women. *Family Coordinator,* 1969, 18, 251–255.

Neugarten, B. The awareness of middle age. In B. L. Neugarten (Ed.), *Middle age and aging.* Chicago: University of Chicago Press, 1968.

Neugarten, B. L., and Brown-Rezanka, L. Midlife women in the 1980's. In U.S. Congress Select Committee on Aging, *Women in midlife—Security and fulfillment* (Part I). Comm. Pub. No. 95–170. Washington, D.C.: U.S. Government Printing Office, 1978.

Nevill, D., and Damico, S. Role conflict in women as a function of marital status. *Human Relations,* 1972, 28, 487–498.

Nieva, V., and Gutek, B. Sex effects on evaluation. *Academy of Management Review,* 1980, 5, 267–276.

Norton, A. The influence of divorce on traditional life cycle measures. *Journal of Marriage and the Family*, 1980, *42*, 63–69.

Oakley, A. *The sociology of housework*. New York: Pantheon, 1974.

Oppenheimer, V. K. *The female labor force in the United States: Demographic and economic factors governing its growth and changing composition*. University of California at Berkeley: Population Monograph, Series No. 5, 1970.

Parnes, H. S., Jusenius, C. L., Blau, F., Nestel, G., Shortlidge, R., Jr., and Sandell, S. *Dual careers: A longitudinal analysis of the labor market experience of women* (Vol. 4). Columbus: Ohio State University, Center for Human Resource Research, 1975.

Pearce, D. The feminization of poverty: Women, work, and welfare. In K. W. Feinstein (Ed.), *Working women and families* (Sage Yearbooks in Women's Policy Studies, Vol. 4). Beverly Hills: Sage, 1979.

Pleck, J. H. The work-family role system. *Social Problems*, 1977, *24*, 417–427.

Powell, B., and Reznikoff, M. Role conflict and symptoms of psychological distress in college-educated women. *Journal of Consulting and Clinical Psychology*, 1976, *44*, 473–479.

Pugh, D. Role activation conflict: A study of industrial inspection. *American Sociological Review*, 1966, *31*, 835–842.

Rapoport, R., and Rapoport, R. N. The dual-career family: A variant pattern and social change. *Human Relations*, 1969, *22*, 3–30.

Rapoport, and Rapoport, R. N. Early and later experiences as determinants of adult behavior: Married women's family and career patterns. *British Journal of Sociology*, 1971, *22*, 16–30.

Riley, M. W. Social gerontology and the age stratification of society. *Gerontologist*, 1971, *11*, 79–87.

Riley, M. W. Introduction: Life-course perspectives. In M. W. Riley (Ed.), *Aging from birth to death: Interdisciplinary perspectives*. Boulder, Colo.: Westview Press for the American Association for the Advancement of Science, 1979.

Ritt, L. G. The relationships between role conflict, satisfaction, and the dropout potential of college students. *Dissertation Abstracts International*, 1971, *31*(11-B), 6910–6911.

Ritzer, G. Commitment, professionalism and role conflict resolution: The personnel manager. *Dissertation Abstracts*, 1969, *29*, 4567A.

Rizzo, J. R., House, R. J., and Lirtzman, S. I. Role conflict and ambiguity in complex organizations. *Administrative Science Quarterly*, 1970, *15*, 150–163.

Robinson, J. R., and Converse, P. *Basic tables of time budget data for the United States*. Ann Arbor: Survey Research Center, 1966.

Rodgers, R. H. *Family interaction and transaction: The developmental approach*. Englewood, N.J.: Prentice-Hall, 1973.

Rosen, B., and Jerdee, T. H. Influence of sex role stereotypes on personnel decisions. *Journal of Applied Psychology*, 1974, *59*, 9–14. (a)

Rosen, B., and Jerdee, T. H. Sex stereotyping in the executive suite. *Harvard Business Review*, 1974, *52*, 45–58. (b)

Rossi, A. S. Aging and parenthood in the middle years. In P. B. Baltes and O. G. Brim, Jr. (Eds.), *Life-span development and behavior* (Vol. 3). New York: Academic Press, 1980.

Rubin, L. B. *Women of a certain age: The midlife search for self*. New York: Harper & Row, 1979.

Sarason, S. B. *Work, aging, and social change: Professionals and the one life-one career imperative*. New York: Free Press, 1977.

Sawhill, I. The economics of discrimination against women: Some new findings. *Journal of Human Resources*, 1973, *8*, 383–396.

Sieber, S. D. Toward a theory of role accumulation. *American Sociological Review*, 1974, *39*, 567–578.

Siegel, A. E., and Haas, M. B. The working mother: A review of research. *Child Development*, 1963, *34*, 513–542.

Snoek, J. Role strain in diversified role sets. *American Journal of Sociology*, 1966, *71*, 363–372.

Spreitzer, E., Snyder, E. E., and Larson, D. L. Multiple roles and psychological well-being. *Sociological Focus*, 1979, *12*, 141–148.

Stebbins, R. A. A note on the concept of role distance. *American Journal of Sociology*, 1967, *73*, 247–250.

Stebbins, R. A. Role distance, role distance behaviour, and jazz musicians. *British Journal of Sociology*, 1969, *20*, 406–415.

Sterling, B. S., and Owen, J. W. Perceptions of demanding vs. reasoning male and female police officers. *Personality and Social Psychology Bulletin*, 1982, *8*, 336–340.

Tangri, S. Determinants of occupational role innovation among college women. *Journal of Social Issues*, 1972, *28*, 177–201.

Taylor, S., and Fiske, S. T. The token in a small group: Research findings and theoretical implications. In J. Sweeney (Ed.), *Psychology and politics: Collected papers*. New Haven: Yale University Press, 1976.

Terborg, J. R. Women in management: A research review. *Journal of Applied Psychology*, 1977, *62*(6), 647–664.

Troll, L. E., and Turner, J. Overcoming age-sex discrimination. In U.S. Congress Select Committee on Aging, *Women in midlife—Security and fulfillment* (Part I). Comm. Pub. No. 95–170. Washington, D.C.: U.S. Government Printing Office, 1978.

Uhlenberg, P. Cohort variations in family life cycle experiences of U.S. females. *Journal of Marriage and the Family*, 1974, *36*, 284–292.

U.S. Bureau of the Census. A statistical portrait of women in the U.S. *Current Population Reports*, Special Studies, Series P-23, No. 58, 1976.

U.S. Bureau of the Census. A statistical portrait of women in the U.S.: 1978. *Current Population Reports*, Special Studies, Series P-23, No. 100, 1978.

U.S. Bureau of the Census. *Statistical abstract of the U.S.: 1981* (102nd ed.) Washington, D.C., 1981.

U.S. Bureau of the Census. Characteristics of the population below the poverty level: 1980. *Current Population Reports*, Special Studies, Series P-60, No. 133, 1982.

U.S. Department of Health, Education, and Welfare. Social security and the changing roles of men and women. Washington: U.S. Government Printing Office, February 1969.

Walberg, H. J. Personality-role conflict and self-conceptions in urban practice teachers. *School Review*, 1968, *76*, 41–49.

Walker, K. *Time-use patterns for household work related to homemakers' employment*. Washington, D.C.: U.S. Department of Agricultural Research Service, 1970.

Watley, D. J., and Kaplan, R. Career or marriage? Aspirations and achievements of able young women. *Journal of Vocational Behavior*, 1971, *1*, 29–43.

Weick, K. E. Careers as eccentric predicates. *Executive*, 1976, Winter, 6–10.

Weil, M. W. An analysis of the factors influencing married women's actual or planned work participation. *American Sociological Review*, 1961, *26*, 91–96.

Wolman, C., and Frank, H. *The solo woman in a professional peer group*. Working paper 133. Philadelphia: Wharton School, University of Pennsylvania, 1972.

Woods, M. B. The unsupervised child of the working mother. *Developmental Psychology*, 1972, *6*, 14–25.

Wiebarth, C. A. Feminine role conflict: The influence of models and expectations of others. *Dissertation Abstracts International*, 1972, *33*(6-B), 2828.

Chapter 6

The Psychological Well-Being of Women in the Middle Years

GRACE K. BARUCH

This chapter addresses three questions with respect to the psychological well-being of women in the middle years. What is psychological well-being? How do midlife women vary in level of well-being? What are women's sources of psychological well-being? In other words, what is it, who has it, and how did they get it? Because answers to the last two questions depend upon how well-being is defined, the conceptualization and measurement of well-being are discussed first; findings are then presented that bear on variations and sources.

WHAT IS PSYCHOLOGICAL WELL-BEING?

The American College Dictionary defines well-being as "a *good or satisfactory* condition of existence" (italics added). This definition reflects an important point about well-being—that it may be assessed by objective or by subjective indices. To know whether a person's condition of existence is *good*, a researcher could objectively measure income, housing, and so on. One might argue, for example, that Caucasian women are higher in well-being than Hispanic women because they have larger income and larger homes and are hospitalized less often. Clearly, judgments and relative standards enter into this approach, but the judgments and standards are the researcher's.

To know whether a person's condition of existence is *satisfactory*, in contrast, you must ask the person; satisfaction is in the eye of the sub-

GRACE K. BARUCH • Wellesley College Center for Research on Women, Wellesley, Massachusetts 02181.

ject. A woman's degree of satisfaction with her home, for example, may be very different from what the researcher expects on the basis of an objective index of number of rooms. studies of psychological well-being, then, rely primarily on self-reports, on people's evaluations of their lives.

Satisfaction is by no means the only dimension of their lives that people are asked about. Until the late 1950s, most studies of psychological well-being focused on symptoms of mental illness; epidemiological studies reported the incidence in communities of psychiatric symptomatology, such as anxiety and depression (e.g., Srole, Langner, Michael, Opler, and Rennie 1962). In 1957, however a "quality of life" survey carried out by the Institute of Social Research at the University of Michigan went beyond this approach to investigate, in addition to symptomatology, aspects of "positive mental health," such as happiness, satisfaction, and coping styles (Gurin, Veroff, and Feld, 1960). This chapter draws heavily on this study, and on two other national surveys also done at the University of Michigan: a replication of the 1957 study carried out in 1976 and reported in *The Inner American* (Veroff, Douvan, and Kulka, 1981) and *The Quality of American Life* (Campbell, Converse, and Rodgers, 1976). Each study was based on a national probability sample of over 2000 subjects. (As is often the case, the numbers of minority women included in these and in other studies cited were usually not sufficient to permit fine-grained analyses.)

Despite a lack of agreement about what constitutes psychological well-being—about the specific components—researchers have consistently acknowledged that well-being is not "one thing" but rather is multidimensional and requires multiple measures (Andrews and Withey, 1974; Bryant and Veroff, 1982). There is consistent evidence, for example, that one's level of negative feelings and of positive feelings are relatively independent (Bradburn and Caplowitz, 1965). One may, for example, have high self-esteem but feel anxious and unhappy, as might be true of the mother of an acutely ill child, or the wife of a coronary patient.

In *The Quality of American Life*, Campbell *et al.* focused on two major components of well-being: happiness, defined as an affective, somewhat labile state, and satisfaction, a more stable, cognitively based appraisal of how one's life is turning out relative to one's expectations and aspirations. Happiness and satisfaction were treated as separate aspects of well-being, although they are correlated with each other at about the .50 level. The 1957 Gurin *et al.* study (1960) included, in addition to happiness and satisfaction, several measures of the self-concept, as did Veroff *et al.* (1981) in their 1976 replication. The latter study had an extremely broad array of 18 well-being indices, including happiness and satisfaction, current worries, "morale" about the future, and past feel-ings of an impending nervous breakdown.[1] The authors argue that the 18 indices measure distinct components of well-being and that analyzing the patterns and correlates of each index separately therefore stays closer to psychological reality than does combining indices. Neverthe-less, it is extremely difficult to deal with so many different measures in conceptualizing the nature, patterns, and sources of well-being. For example, the answers to such questions as "How is a woman's age related to her well-being? or "How do women and men compare in level of well-being?" will differ depending upon the specific component se-lected for analysis. Moreover, many components, such as happiness and satisfaction, are typically measured by single-item scales, which are less reliable than composite measures. As Campbell stated in 1976, "We must begin to work seriously on problems of identifying the major di-mensions of the experience of well-being."

Drawing on data from the 1957 and 1976 Michigan studies, Bryant and Veroff (1982) examined the underlying dimensions of well-being—seeking a structural model to reduce "conceptual chaos."

The authors examined separately data for men and for women col-lected in 1957 and in 1976. Using sophisticated factor-analytic tech-niques, they found empirical support for a proposed three-dimensional conceptual model of well-being (Their labels refer to the negative pole): 1) *unhappiness* (negative affect), (2) *strain* (symptomatology and wor-ies), and (3) *personal inadequacy* (Poor self-concept). Women and men resembled each other in how their well-being was structured with re-spect to these three dimensions—that is, in how the components were clustered. Sex differences in structure were smaller than differences *within* each sex between the two time periods of 1957 and 1976. The unhappiness and personal inadequacy factors were independent of each other, while strain was moderately related to each. In other words, the level of a woman's self-esteem and her degree of happiness may be quite different; however, the extent of symptomatology she reports is related to each.

In a study of psychological well-being in women 35 to 55, carried out in 1979–1980, the author and Rosalind Barnett also examined the dimensions of well-being, using exploratory factor analysis (Baruch, Barnett, and Rivers, 1983).[2] The 238 subjects, all Caucasian, were ran-

[1] For a detailed description of the measures used in the three Michigan studies, the reader is referred to the three books cited.
[2] Exploratory factor analysis is distinguished from confirmatory factor analysis, which is used to test whether the data fit a proposed theoretical model. Exploratory factor analysis is a tool for investigating the dimensions underlying an array of indices: Results need to be replicated to determine whether they are generalizable or are the product of chance.

domly selected from a community in the Greater Boston metropolitan area. Four family-status groups were included: never-married, married without children, married with children, and divorced with children. All never-married and divorced women were employed; each of the two groups of married women was divided equally between employed and not employed. Six role-pattern groups of 45 each were thus formed.[3] Employed women were selected equally among those in high-, medium-, and low-prestige occupations (Siegel, 1971); nonemployed women were selected similarly according to the prestige of their husbands' occupations. Thus, certain groups were oversampled in relation to their presence in the general population. The study was designed to include women whose role patterns are of conceptual interest and of increasing social importance; results cannot be generalized to American women as a whole.

Eight measures of well-being were included: standard single-item scales measuring happiness, satisfaction, and optimism; the anxiety and depression subscales of the Hopkins Symptom Checklist (Derogatis, Lipman, Rickels, Uhlenhuth, and Covi, 1974); the Pearlin Mastery Scale (Pearlin and Schooler, 1978), measuring locus of control; the Rosenberg (1965) self-esteem scale; and a measure of self-concept developed for this study that assessed the balance of rewards and concerns (rewards minus concerns) women reported about themselves. The analysis yielded two major underlying dimensions or factors. The first factor was labeled *mastery;* scores contributing strongly to this factor were the two self-concept scales, locus of control, and the anxiety and depression sub scales. Thus, a woman with a high sense of mastery evaluates herself positively, feels in control of her life, and has low levels of depression and anxiety. The second factor that emerged was labeled *pleasure;* scores contributing strongly to this factor were happiness, satisfaction, and optimism. Comparing these dimensions to Bryant and Veroff's, sense of mastery can be seen as combining personal inadequacy and strain; pleasure is analogous to their unhappiness factor.

This two-dimensional model, mastery and pleasure, is useful in thinking about certain puzzles and dilemmas with respect to the well being of women. For example, the women Betty Friedan described in *The Feminine Mystique* (1963) reported deriving satisfaction from their attachment to husband and children, but they also reported feeling purposeless and worthless. They can be seen as doing well with respect to the pleasure dimension of well-being but not so well with respect to

---

[3]Despite screening over 6000 women, it was not possible to locate sufficient numbers of married, childless, nonemployed women. This role pattern is apparently becoming less viable, given current economic and social conditions.

heir sense of mastery. In contrast, some career women who have struggled successfully to attain prestigious positions are portrayed by the
media as asking resentfully: Where is the joy? Is this all there is to life?
These women can be seen as having a strong sense of mastery but
is feeling deficient in pleasure. As Freud's famous dictum on love
nd work suggests, different dimensions of well-being may have differ-
nt sources. For mature women in our society today, it may often prove
difficult to maintain a highly positive self-concept in the absence of
ocially valued work, and it can also be difficult to derive an adequate
ense of enjoyment from a life in which intimate relationships are
nissing.

WHO HAS WELL-BEING?

Comparing Women and Men

A question repeatedly asked about the psychological well-being of
women is: How do they compare with men? The answer, as has been
noted, depends on how one defines well-being—on which component
ne examines. Studies consistently report that women have higher rates
f psychiatric symptomatology, and especially of depression, than do
men, although they are not less happy or satisfied; there is agreement
that this difference in symptomatology is not primarily due to women's
greater willingness to report symptoms (Radloff, 1975; Rosenfield,
980). For example, Veroff et al. found that women report more difficul-
es in their lives, and more worries, than do men. Gurin et al. found that
women had less positive self-concepts, as well as higher levels of symp-
omatology. In both studies, however, levels of happiness and satisfaction
were similar; Campbell et al. also found no significant sex difference in
overall life satisfaction.

The authors of The Inner American, speculating about the reasons for
the sex differences in symptomatology, argue that women's role as nur-
turers responsible for the well-being of others—especially as primary
caretakers of children—means living with uncertainty, lack of control,
and other stressful conditions conducive to the development of symptomatology. The fate of others is uncontrollable and unpredictable; to
feel responsible for it is risky. Rosenfield (1980) argues that power relations between women and men may be key variable in explaining wom-
en's higher roles of depression.

Other researchers point to the difference in women's and men's
patterns of involvement in paid employment as critical to their relative
psychological well-being. Gove and Tudor (1973) argue that men's participation in two domains of life—paid work and the family—provide a

kind of buffer and well-being "insurance." According to their two-role theory, when life is going badly in one domain, a second valued role may provide compensatory satisfaction. This view is consistent with much recent theory and research on multiple roles (Marks, 1977; Sieber 1974; Thoits, 1983), as is discussed below.

In a review of data from six large national surveys spanning 2 years, Kessler and McCrae (1981) report a decreasing gender gap between the sexes with respect to psychiatric symptomatology and find that women's increasing labor force participation appears to account for about 20% of the variance.[4] Why and how employment may function to increase women's well-being is discussed in the section on employment below.

CHRONOLOGICAL AGE

How one expects a woman's chronological age to influence her psychological well-being depends upon how one views the feminine role. Freud's well-known comparison of women and men illustrates the traditional view of age differences perhaps even more than of sex differences: "A man of about thirty strikes us as a youthful, somewhat unformed individual, whom we expect to make powerful use of the possibilities for development opened up to him by analysis. A woman of the same age, however, often frightens us by her psychical rigidity and unchangeability. . . . There are no paths open to further development. . . . [It is] as though, indeed, the difficult development to femininity had exhausted the possibilities of the person concerned."

In the traditional conception of femininity, physical attractiveness and involvement in motherhood and in heterosexual relations are central; a decline in well-being with age would seem almost inevitable. In this view, physiological changes in reproductive functioning, in appearance, and in a woman's role as mother should threaten a woman core identity; women will differ mainly in their capacity to cope with the decline in their sources of well-being.

A contrasting view is that women's well-being, like that of men, is tied to their social identity and thus to how society views them; these in turn shape their self-concepts and their opportunities to obtain satisfaction in a variety of roles throughout their life-span. This view permits the prediction of positive as well as negative changes with age. If women

---

[4]A decreasing gender gap in symptomatology was also reported by Srole & Fischer (1980) in their 1978 replication of the Manhattan Mental Health (1957) survey. This study has been severely criticized for methodological problems, such as sample attrition (Dohrenwend, personal communication, 1982).

n's status rises within a society during the second half of a woman's fe, for example, then her later years can bring greater well-being.

Findings of relevant studies seem to depend upon when the data vere collected. Several studies carried out in the 1950s and 1960s howed women in the middle and later years to be particularly dis-ressed. In 1958 Weiss and Samuelson reported that when asked, "What re the things you do that make you feel useful or important?" a rather ubstantial proportion of women in the older age groups said that 'nothing made them feel useful and important." Lowenthal, Thurnher, nd Chiriboga (1975), in their study of four age groups of men and vomen, described "post-parental" women as strikingly low in well-eing—as wanting to grow but seeing no way to do so.

In contrast, when the 1957 Gurin et al. study (1960) was replicated in ne 1970s, Veroff et al. (1981) reported that a decline in women's self-steem with age found in 1950 was no longer evident. Overall, the uthors of The Inner American conclude that older women were better off n 1976 than in 1957. Women in the Berkeley Growth Study who were ated as relatively autonomous seemed to experience a decline in well-eing in their 40s, but when seen again while in their 50s, they were articularly high in well-being. Whether the difference in the social cli-nate of the two time periods, rather than chronological age, explains the nprovement is unclear (Livson, 1975).

With respect to satisfaction and happiness, women, like men, typ-ally show increased levels of satisfaction, but a decline in happiness, rith age. Campbell et al. (1976) suggests that one's life is an increasingly ood "fit" as one grows older, resulting in greater satisfaction, but the tense emotions associated with feelings of happiness may become rer.

MENOPAUSE AND THE EMPTY NEST

During their middle years, most women experience menopause, nd mothers experience the empty nest. Earlier theory and research on enopause and the empty nest have been criticized for focusing on omen primarily in their reproductive role, and for failing to consider at these events not only might be neutral but even might be experi-ced as positive (Barnett and Baruch, 1978; Long and Porter, Chapter 4, is volume). For example, Lowenthal et al. (1975), failing to find evi-nce of dread of the empty nest among the women in their sample who ere facing that transition, concluded that the women's anxiety must be oo deep to be tapped." Yet reinterviews 5 years later confirmed the sence of traumatic effects.

The more women as individuals and as groups are confined to their maternal role, of course, the greater the negative impact such events as menopause and the empty nest are likely to have (Bart, 1971).

Opportunities to participate in other social roles and domains of life can give the cessation of the menses and the independence of one's children a positive meaning, facilitating involvement in paid work, enhancing sexuality (Luria and Meade, Chapter 17; this volume), permitting attention to other needs. As will be discussed in the section on motherhood, being at home with small children can be much more threatening to well-being than the empty nest, which, as Campbell points out (1976), "has a reputation that is not deserved."

THE MIDLIFE CRISIS AND OTHER AGE-LINKED CONCEPTUALIZATIONS OF THE MIDDLE YEARS

The concept of the midlife crisis has recently received wide attention. While many theorists hold the generally optimistic view that growth and change continue throughout life, theories of the middle years nevertheless typically exude a certain aura of gloom. They focus on the juxtaposition in the midlife individual of a growing sense of mortality and an awareness of limited possibilities for achieving one's goals; there is an emotional, as opposed to intellectual, recognition of the biological reality that one in fact does not live forever.

The concept of the midlife crisis is typically part of a theory of adult development in which an invariant sequence of stages linked to chronological age is postulated; the "crisis" then occurs at a predictable time. For example, Daniel Levinson's (Levinson, 1978) mapping of adult development, based on the study of 44 males age 35 to 45, gives special attention to the anxiety and depression that may accompany the tendency around age 40 to reevaluate one's achievements in the light of time left to live. Successful completion of the task of resolving this crisis is thought to lead to further personal growth, new directions, and other positive outcomes. If the crisis is not resolved, discontent and depression are likely to persist into old age.

The age-linked basis of Levinson's theory has been widely criticized, perhaps most effectively by Leonard Pearlin (1975). Pearlin points out that evidence for the existence of a midlife crisis cannot rest solely on studies of middle-aged subjects, for it is possible that the experiences they report may be equally common among 25-year-olds, or among 65-year-olds. In a large national survey of adults over 21, Pearlin and his colleagues found no evidence of a "piling up" in the middle years of anxiety, depression, or indeed of unique transitions and crises. The study of midlife women by the author and Rosalind Barnett found no difference in well-being associated with age among women 35 to 55. When w pecifically asked the women about crises and turning points—their resence, their nature—no age-related patterns emerged. To the extent that an "age and stage" view of adult development is awed, so too is the concept of the midlife crisis. Another weakness in iis concept is that the theoretical, clinical, and empirical bases for it were eveloped in studies of males, who were the patients, the subjects—and ie researchers. Very little theory-based or theory-generating work has ocused on women's middle years. Perhaps for this reason one biological ex difference is typically *ignored*—the differential life expectancy of men nd women. A man of 45 who is concerned about the implications of aving only 20 or so years to live is being realistic about his life expectan-y. A woman of 45, who can expect to live perhaps 35 more years, is more kely to be concerned about living too long, with the specter of depen-ency and loneliness (Baruch, 1980). Most women now in their middle ears, moreover, did not have expectations of astounding achievement in ie adult world of work; therefore, few find their accomplishments falling iort of expectations. Rather, many midlife women in occupations simi-r to those of Levinson's male subjects are amazed and delighted at :hieving more than they imagined to be possible. In the absence of •latively imminent mortality and a sense of accomplishing less than ie's dream, the midlife crisis loses its substance.

It may be that such crises are "age-coincidental." That is, certain ihorts have experienced, and will experience, particular influential /ents at similar ages, as Glenn points out in his work on the impact of ie Great Depression (Glenn, 1975). Men born in the 1920s and 1930s, as ere Levinson's subjects, were socialized to be achievers and breadwin-ers, and they may wonder as they turn 40 about the costs of their rogress. Women of that era typically married and had children early, id thus found themselves increasingly free of child-rearing respon-bilities as they neared 40. It may have seemed, therefore, that women id their own inevitable midlife crisis, characterized by concern about ternatives to their investment in child-rearing, followed by a burst of •hievement-related fantasies and activities. But today's young women ho remain active in careers throughout their lives are unlikely to expe-ence the same issues at midlife. (Young men who were influenced by e 1960s to be less driven in their work roles are also likely to experience idlife differently from earlier cohorts.)

The likelihood that each cohort will have different normative pat-rns over the life-course gives rise to another perspective on chronolog-il age and well-being—the on-time/off-time concept. As depicted by eugarten (1970), Rossi (1980), and others (see Long and Porter, Chap-r 5, this volume), it is not so much what happens to a woman at what .e but whether it happens at the predicted or expected time that shapes its impact on her well-being. Unanticipated events are more likely to be stressful, and those occurring off time are more likely to be unanticipated. Thus, the latter should have a more negative effect on well-being. The classic example is widowhood, which should be more devastating at age 35 than at 60.

Many other factors, of course, influence a woman's ability to cope with negative events. The important point is that we learn much less about a woman's level of well-being from knowing her chronological age than from knowing how her life pattern fits that which is normative for her cohort (see Brooks-Gunn and Kirsh, Chapter 1, this volume).

SOURCES OF WELL-BEING

For both women and men, income and education are consistently found to be positively associated with most measures of well-being. Beyond these, how do particular roles that women occupy affect their well-being? Why do these roles function as they do—what specific aspects are important? These questions address variations in women's well-being and the sources of these variations.

Employment

How a woman's employment status—the simple fact of being employed or not—affects her well-being depends upon which aspect of well-being is being examined. Symptomatology scores typically do not differ significantly between homemakers and employed women (Pearlin, 1975; Radloff, 1975). As for happiness, Veroff et al. found that housewives were slightly happier; however, among women 40 to 59 in intact first marriages, there were no differences (Serlin, 1980). Campbell et al. reported no differences in happiness or satisfaction associated with employment status, with one exception: Among college-educated housewives, employed women were higher. The authors suggest that when "able" women are confined to the homemaker role, they may be more distressed than women in general. For midlife women, self-esteem may be the aspect of well-being most enhanced by paid employment. Coleman and Antonucci (1983) reported that for midlife women included in the 1976 Michigan study, employment was the only significant predictor of self-esteem.

In our study of women 35 to 55, employed and nonemployed women did not differ in pleasure—the components of which are happiness, satisfaction, and optimism; marital status, rather than employment status, was associated with higher pleasure scores. Employed women were

gnificantly higher in sense of mastery, however, indicating a more
ositive self-concept and lower levels of symptomatology. All four
oups of employed women—never-married, married with children,
arried without children, and divorced—were higher in mastery than
ere the two groups of nonemployed women—married with children
d married without children. Regardless of marital status, then, paid
mployment seems to have positive consequences for women's self-
ncept and possibly for the tendency to report psychiatric symptoms,
t employment *per se* does not contribute significantly to happiness
d satisfaction in the middle years.

In interpreting these patterns, several considerations are important.
rst, employed and nonemployed women tend to differ in marital sta-
s—non-employed women are most likely to be married. A confound-
g of effects of employment and marriage is thus inevitable unless
arital status is controlled. Second, the effects of employment are likely
vary among cohorts, and also within the midlife range. How a woman
periences being a paid worker is influenced, for example, by her so-
lization and her values, such as whether she was brought up to be-
ve that good wives and mothers stay home. Another reason that age
oups may vary in how employment affects well-being is that for wom-
 with young children, combining roles may be more stressful than for
men whose children are older and more independent.

A third consideration is that, compared with men, women are more
nstricted in the range of occupations they occupy and are less likely to
 in high-prestige occupations. Any interpretation of the effects of
ployment on women's well-being should take this difference into
ount. The prestige of an occupation affects job conditions, which in
n affect well-being (Kessler, 1982). Among the employed women in
r study, for example, occupational prestige was strongly related to
se of mastery. Since the nature of women's occupational status is
anging, patterns now found are likely to differ when more women are
ployed in prestigious occupations.

As the data on occupational prestige suggest, it is important to
nsider the quality of a woman's experience within a role, and her
itude toward that role. When a woman's preference for being a home-
ker versus being employed is taken into account, for example, home-
kers who would prefer to be employed are consistently found to be
ver in well-being than homemakers who prefer the role they occupy
arlin, 1975). (For employed women, role preference typically does
t have a significant effect on well-being. Those who prefer not to be
ployed are not significantly lower in well-being than those who pre-
 their actual pattern of paid employment.)

The Psychological Benefits of Employment

There is increasing empirical evidence to support recent theoretica arguments that employment can function to enrich a woman's sense o identity and to provide other psychological rewards, even for womer who must juggle many roles (Marks, 1977; Sieber, 1974; Thoits, 1983) For example, a study of English women showed that for those in stress ful life circumstances who did not have confidantes, being employee seemed to protect against the occurrence of psychiatric symptoms symptoms developed in 79% of such nonemployed women but in onl 14% of the employed (Brown, Bhrolchain, and Harris, 1975). Campbe (1976) found that employed women reported more pleasures in thei lives than did nonemployed women, and since the two groups did nc differ in reports of negative aspects, employment was associated with greater net balance of good over bad.

What particular components of employment may account for th positive effects that have been found? In the first stage of our study, 7 women were interviewed intensively about the rewarding and distress ing aspects of the different roles they occupied. On the basis of thes interviews, scales with equal numbers of "reward" and "concern" item were developed to assess women's experiences in employment, mai riage, and similar factors. The 238 women in the survey stage the indicated to what extent each item was either rewarding or distressing For example, in employment, rewards included a variety of tasks, good income, and liking the boss. Concerns included having too muc to do, job insecurity, and lack of opportunity for career growth. For eac role, the balance between rewarding and distressing aspects could t assessed; this "balance score" constituted an index of the quality of woman's experience in that role. The balance between rewards an concerns in employment was significantly and positively related to bot sense of mastery and pleasure.

With the use of factor-analytic techniques, the underlying dime sions of the rewarding and distressing aspects of each role were al explored. For employment, the major reward factors were *challenge* ar *social relationships;* the major concern factors were whether the job w. *dull* and whether it was a *dead end.* Scores on these reward and conce factors were significantly related to both sense of mastery and pleasur with the exception of social relationships, which did not affect master In other words, the components of employment most likely to affec woman's well-being are how challenging her job is and whether it is d and dead-ended. Gratifying social relationships at work increase h happiness and satisfaction but not her self-esteem and sense of contr What is it about the role of homemaker that affects well-bein

holars studying homemaking point to negative aspects such as the
ck of standards for performance, the lack of objective feedback, the
pendence for approval on husbands and children; there are no "entry
quirements" (Gove and Tudor, 1973; Lopata, 1971; Oakley, 1974).
udies also show, however, that the freedom to plan one's own sched-
e—being able to structure and order one's tasks, or not do any at all—
very important to homemakers, especially if the jobs they have pre-
ously held, or the jobs they feel qualified to do, lack autonomy.

In our study, the relationship between well-being and the home-
aker role was examined; the balance between the rewards and the
ncerns in the homemaker role was strongly related to a woman's
nse of mastery and to her pleasure scores. Factor analyses indicated
at the two major sources of distress for the homemakers in our sample
ere *boredom and isolation* and *not earning money*. The major rewards were
e satisfaction of *"being there"* for one's family, the *freedom from supervision*,
d the *opportunity to do tasks that fitted one's skills*. Interestingly, only the
st factor was related to a woman's well-being; the more a woman felt
warded by this, the greater her sense of mastery. Homemaking tasks
at are a good "fit" may function like paid work as a source of self-
teem.

ARITAL STATUS

One of the most consistent findings in the literature on psychologi-
l well-being is that married women are happier and more satisfied
an are those who are not married, whether the latter are never-mar-
d, divorced, or widowed (Baruch *et al.*, 1983; Depner, 1979; Campbell
al., 1976; Glenn, 1975; Veroff *et al.*, 1981; Ward, 1979). In contrast,
arriage is not associated with components of well-being other than
ppiness and satisfaction. For example, comparing never-married
men over 30 with a matched sample of married women, Gigy (1980)
und that never-married women were less happy, but their self-esteem
s no lower, nor did they report more psychiatric symptomatology. In
r study, married women were higher in pleasure, of which happiness
d satisfaction are major components, but they were not higher in
nse of mastery; that is, they did not have more positive self-concepts
lower levels of anxiety and depression.

In interpreting these patterns, several considerations are critical.
st, married women are a different group now than earlier in our
story. As is often pointed out, divorce is more accessible now, and
men who are unhappily married are more likely to remove them-
lves from the ranks of the married. Moreover, marital status is less

confounded with employment status than it once was; today's marrie
women are more likely than formerly to be employed, and as we hav
seen, employment has a positive effect on several components of wel
being. Thus, married women are now more self-selected with respect t
both marital status and employment status.

A second point is that marriage is confounded with income—ma
ried women tend to have higher family incomes than do nonmarrie
women—and income is associated with well-being. Thus, one reason f
the greater happiness and satisfaction of married women may be the
access to money.

Third, marriage also provides access to a sexual partner. Whatev
difficulties married women may experience in their sexual relationship
the availability of a sexual partner means a greater likelihood of sexu
satisfaction, and sexual satisfaction is highly correlated with overall li
satisfaction (see Luria and Meade, Chapter 17, this volume). While bot
money and sexual satisfaction can certainly be found outside marriag
they are usually more difficult to obtain, especially as women get olde

Beyond these considerations, what is it about being married, ar
about not being married, that may account for the patterns describec

In our study, factor analyses of the rewarding and distressing a
pects of marriage indicated that the major reward was *feeling emotional*
supported and appreciated, and the major concern was *marital conflict*. Th
more a woman rated emotional support and appreciation as a rewardir
part of her marriage, the higher her pleasure score and, to a less
extent, her sense of mastery. Similarly, the greater her concern abo
marital conflict, the lower her pleasure and, to a lesser extent, her sen
of mastery. The pattern of a greater effect of marital quality on pleasu
is consistent with findings already presented. Moreover, the balan
score of rewards and concerns in marriage was very strongly related
pleasure but was only weakly related to sense of mastery.

A second approach to understanding how marriage affects we
being is to ask what qualities of the *nonmarried* state are experienced
particularly difficult. Being nonmarried today may be less distressir
than it once was: There is less stigma and thus less threat to a womar
self-concept (Veroff *et al.*, 1981). Nevertheless, for many midlife wome
it is a struggle to derive sufficient enjoyment from a life pattern that do
not provide a stable, "built-in" intimate relationship with another adu
Both for never-married women and for divorced women in our stud
the central concern was *lack of an intimate relationship*. To the extent tha
woman reported distress about this, her pleasure scores were lowe
Her sense of mastery was not affected, however, consistent with tl
finding that among *married* women, rewards and concerns, and ma
riage "balance," affected pleasure more than sense of mastery.

A reasonable conclusion about marriage and well-being is that hen a married woman is free to choose her employment status and to d an unhappy marriage, being married is likely to enhance her hap-ness and satisfaction. As a source of self-esteem and protection against xiety and depression, marriage is of little help; here, a good job is the ·y.

ARENTAL STATUS

In sharp contrast to the patterns that emerged with respect to mar-age and employment, studies consistently find no evidence that being mother—parental status—enhances a woman's well-being (Barnett d Baruch, 1981; Campbell et al., 1976; Depner, 1979; Sears and Barbee, 177; Veroff et al., 1981). As Depner states, "There is little evidence that e childless are yearning for a role which they do not have."

Reasoning that the benefits of having children might show up later life, Glen and McLanahan (1981) studied women over 50, using na-nal survey data. Finding no differences in happiness or satisfaction tween mothers and childless women (with income and employment tus controlled), the authors conclude: "The best evidence now avail-le indicates that the present young adult should not choose to have ildren on the basis of expectations that parenthood will lead to psy-ological rewards in the later stages of life. The prospects for such wards seem rather dim at best."

Childless women who fear—or are warned—that they'll be sorry ater" should also be aware that a study of widows aged 60–75 shows at even for these women, who would seem to be most in need of em, children had only very slight effects on life satisfaction and other dices of "morale" (Beckman and Houser, 1982). The authors state: ven among widows over 60, the difference [having children] made to ell-being was minute compared to the quality of overall social ties."

That such a seemingly profound difference in women's lives—that tween having children and being childless—should be undetectable in effects on well-being is counterintuitive and somewhat startling. Yet ere is at least one obvious reason all too familiar to parents: Children n make one's life miserable as well as wonderful. If one groups to-ther all women who happen to be mothers, those for whom it has rked out well may be balanced by those who have had more suffering an pleasure from their role. In *Occupation Housewife*, Helena Lopata 171) argues that being a mother is made especially difficult in our lture by the lack of agreement on standards for the role, combined th the unrealistic expectation that one can mold a child to be whatever e wants. The authors of *The Inner American*, as was noted, attributed e lesser well-being of women compared to men to the difficulties and

uncertainties of having primary responsibility for child-rearing, and t
feeling responsible for how children turn out. Data reported by Lon
and Porter in this volume (Chapter 5) are relevant here: The hypothesi
that a good experience in one role compensates for problems in othe
roles is generally supported, with one exception—for women, problem
in the parent role are not compensated for by satisfaction at work.

What influences the quality of a woman's experience in her role as
mother? In a study of 68 women in western Massachusetts, aged 33–5(
Rossi (1980) found that the combination of having a large family an
being older—that is, having had children later in life—was likely t
impair a woman's sense of well-being. This combination suggests
condition of too much work and too little energy. In our study of wome
35 to 55, the balance between rewards and concerns of motherhood wa
significantly related to both mastery and pleasure. The major concer
factor was *conflict with children;* the more a woman reported distress ov·
conflict with children, the lower her pleasure score. For employed wom
en only, mastery was also significantly lower. Perhaps employed wom
en are more likely to blame themselves for problems with their childre
than are women at home, and thus to react with anxiety and loss of sel
esteem.

OTHER SOCIAL ROLES

The set of roles most often studied for both women and men is th
"traditional triad"—spouse, parent, worker. Yet these three do not e1
compass all the roles women occupy, nor are they always the mo·
important. The role of sibling has the longest time-span, for exampl·
and both sibling relationships and relationships with same-age pee·
who are not kin seem to enhance well-being in later years more than c
relationships with children (Beckman and House, 1982; Glenn, 1975
The importance of such roles as friend, neighbor, and colleague to we·
being is increasingly being documented, especially in the literature c
stress, coping, and social ties (Pearlin, 1982). All these roles have bo·
rewarding and distressing aspects that require further study.

An important role spanning many years is that of daughter, di·
cussed in detail elsewhere in this volume (see Wood, Traupmann, a1
Hay, Chapter 8; Stueve and O'Donnell, Chapter 9). Despite Nancy F·
day's grim portrait of conflict and anger between mother and adu
daughter in *My Mother/Myself* (1977), recent research shows that f
women in the middle years, the role is typically a source of intimacy a1
gratification, not primarily of obligations and difficulties (Baruch a1
Barnett, 1983; Fischer, 1981). During the intensive interview stage of o
study, women often mentioned relationships with mothers as partic

rly rewarding parts of their lives. Based on these interviews, a scale
easuring "maternal rapport" was developed for the survey stage. The
gher women's maternal rapport scores, the higher both mastery and
easure—with one exception: For divorced women, there was a nega-
/e relationship between maternal rapport and sense of mastery. Per-
aps divorced women who are particularly close to their mothers feel
mewhat more dependent than is comfortable and thus do not feel in
ntrol of their lives. Mothers of divorced women, as Barnett points out
hapter 15, this volume), too often communicate disappointment and
sapproval along with their support, and thus may undermine daugh-
rs' feelings of adequacy.

MBINING ROLES

Long and Porter (Chapter 5, this volume) point to a sex segregation
the literature on combining roles. The study of multiple roles is based
the lives of men and the multiplicity is viewed as beneficial, while
lual roles" is a woman's topic, implying a condition in which the role
paid worker is added to the normative condition of being a wife,
other, and homemaker. Ensuing conflict and guilt are assumed, re-
lting in impaired well-being.

A new version of the negative view of women's involvement in
ultiple roles is the concept of "the woman in the middle" (Brody,
81)—the middle-aged woman who must cope simultaneously with the
eds of elderly parents and of teenage children. If she is employed, her
is assumed to make her life even more difficult. As Stueve and
Donnell (Chapter 8) indicate, however, periods of simultaneous
avy demands from both children and parents are in fact relatively
re, although when they do occur, life can indeed be difficult. Even
en, however, a woman's job may be experienced more as a life-saver
an as a last straw. In our study, a major concern women had in their
le as daughter was the care of elderly parents. But only for non-
ployed women was this concern significantly related to a measure of
le strain, and only for nonemployed women did level of role strain
ve a negative impact on mastery and pleasure (Baruch and Barnett,
81). That is, employed women could be very concerned about the care
elderly parents without experiencing severe role overload and con-
ct. If they did experience role strain, it did not necessarily impair their
ll-being. But as data from our intensive interviews suggested, non-
ployed women often feel they must be endlessly available to others,
d when they do feel resentful or overwhelmed about obligations such
those to parents, they feel they have failed.

It makes a great deal of difference in our concepts of women's lives

whether involvement in a variety of roles is shown to bring mainl
overload and conflict, or to yield more benefits than costs. The wome
lowest in mastery in our study were married, nonemployed, and child
less, a finding consistent with the Long and Porter argument that if
woman's sole role is that of housewife, this represents a condition c
underload that can impair well-being. Those lowest in pleasure were th
never-married women, who also occupied only one of the major roles—
paid worker. A reanalysis of community survey data by Thoits (198:
gives a support to the view that multiple roles can provide multipl
sources of well-being; the number of roles respondents occupied, up t
seven, increased well-being, assessed by a measure of symptomatology
Like placing one's eggs in many baskets, investing in several roles
likely to mean having several sources of stimulation, gratification, an
social validation.

In our study, employed married women who had children were th
highest in well-being, taking into account both mastery and pleasur
scores, despite their busy lives. But like most women who are currentl
middle-aged, few had very young children. Mothers of young childre
who are building careers often find their multiple roles difficult to mar
age, although the strain lessens as children get older. If the age at whic
women bear children continues to rise, more midlife women will hav
young children, and this may affect the patterns of well-being of futu
cohorts. The consequences will depend in part upon social condition
such as the availability of child care. For this reason, and for man
others explored elsewhere in this volume, women in their middle yea
have an important stake in monitoring the social and economic climat
of their society.

References

Andrews, F. M., and Withey, S. B. Developing measures of perceived life quality: Resul
    from several national surveys. *Social Indicators Research*, 1974, 1, 1–26.
Barnett, R. C., and Baruch, G. K. Women in the middle years: A critique of research a
    theory. *Psychology of Women Quarterly*, 1978, 3, 187–197.
Bart, P. Depression in middle-aged women. In J. M. Bardwick (Ed.), *Psychology of women:
    study of bio-cultural conflicts*. New York: Harper & Row, 1971.
Baruch, G. *Health-related concerns and psychological well-being of middle-aged women*. Pap
    presented at the meeting of the American Psychological Association, Montreal, 198
Baruch, G. K. and Barnett, R. C. *Who has multiple role strain: The woman in the mid
    revisited*. Paper presented at the meeting of the Gerontological Society, Toronto, 198
Baruch, G. K., and Barnett, R. C. Adult daughters' relationships with their mothe
    Journal of Marriage and the Family, 1983, 45, 601–606.
Baruch, G., Barnett, R., and Rivers, C. *Life prints: New patterns of love and work for toda
    women*. New York: McGraw-Hill, 1983.

kman, L. J., and Houser, B. B. The consequences of childlessness for the social-psychological well-being of older women. *Journal of Gerontology*, 1982, *37*, 243–250.

dburn, N. M., and Caplowitz, D. *Reports on happiness*. Chicago: Aldine, 1965.

dy, E. "Women in the middle" and family help to older people. *Gerontologist*, 1981, *21*, 471–485.

wn, G. W., Bhrolchain, M. N., and Harris, T. Social class and psychiatric disturbance among women in an urban population. *Sociology*, 1975, *9*, 225–253.

ant, F. B., and Veroff, J. The structure of psychological well-being: A sociohistorical analysis. *Journal of Personality and Social Psychology*, 1982, *43*, 653–673.

npbell, A. Subjective measures of well-being. *American Psychologist*, 1976, *31*, 117–124.

npbell, A., Converse, P. E., and Rodgers, W. L., *The quality of American life*. New York: Russell Sage, 1976.

eman, L. M., and Antonucci, T. C. Women's well-being at midlife. ISR Newsletter, Institute for Social Research, University of Michigan, Winter, 1982.

ner, C. *The parental role and psychological well-being*. Paper presented at the meeting of the American Psychological Association, New York, 1979.

ogatis, L. R., Lipman, R. S., Rickels, K., Uhlenhuth, E. H., and Covi, L. The Hopkins symptom checklist. In P. Pichot (Ed.), *Psychological measurements in psychopharmacology*. Paris: Karger, Basel, 1974.

her, L. R. Transitions in the mother–daughter relationship. *Journal of Marriage and the Family*, 1981, *43*, 613–622.

dan, B. *The feminine mystique*. New York: Norton, 1963.

d, S. *New introductory lectures on psychoanalysis*. New York: Norton, 1965.

ay, N. *My mother/myself*. New York: Delacorte Press, 1977.

y, L. L. Self concept of single women. *Psychology of Women Quarterly*, 1980, *5*, 321–340.

nn, N. D. The contribution of marriage to the psychological well-being of males and females. *Journal of Marriage and the Family*, 1975, *37*, 544–600.

nn, N. D., and McLanahan, S. The effects of offspring on the psychological well-being of older adults. *Journal of Marriage and the Family*, 1981, *43*, 409–421.

e, W. R., and Tudor, J. Adult sex roles and mental illness. *American Journal of Sociology*, 1973, *78*, 812–835.

in, G., Veroff, J., and Feld, S. *Americans view their mental health*. New York: Basic Books, 1960.

sler, R. C. The disaggregation of the relationship between socioeconomic status and psychological distress. *American Sociological Review*, 1982, *47*, 752–764.

sler, R. C., and McRae, J. A. Trends in the relationship between sex and psychological distress, 1957–1976. *American Sociological Review*, 1981, *46*, 443–452.

inson, D., Darrow, C. N., Klein, E. B., Levinson, M. H., and McKee, B. *The seasons of a man's life*. New York: Ballantine, 1978.

on, F. *Sex differences in personality in the middle adult years: A longitudinal study*. Paper presented at the meeting of the Gerontological Society, Louisville, 1975.

ata, H. *Occupation housewife*. New York: Oxford, 1971.

enthal, M. F. Psychosocial variations across the adult life course: Frontiers for research and policy. *Gerontologist*, 1975, *15*, 6–12.

enthal, M. F., Thurnher, M., and Chiriboga, D. *Four stages of life*. San Francisco: Jossey-Bass, 1975.

ks, S. Multiple roles and role strain: Some notes on human energy, time and commitment. *American Sociological Review*, 1977, *41*, 921–936.

garten, B. L. Dynamics of transition of middle age to old age. *Journal of Geriatric Psychiatry*, 1970, *4*, 71–87.

Oakley, A. *The sociology of housework.* New York: Pantheon, 1974.

Pearlin, L. Sex roles and depression. In N. Datan and L. H. Ginsberg (Eds.), *Life-sp* *developmental psychology: Normative life crises.* New York: Academic Press, 1975.

Pearlin, L. *Social roles and personal stress.* Paper presented at the National Conference (Social Stress Research, Durham, N.H., October 1982.

Pearlin, L. I., and Schooler, C. The structure of coping. *Journal of Health and Social Behavic* 1978, *19,* 2–21.

Radloff, L. Sex differences in depression. *Sex Roles,* 1975, *1,* 249–265.

Rosenberg, M. *Society and the adolescent self-image.* New Jersey: Princeton University Pres 1965.

Rosenfield, S. Sex differences in depression: Do women always have higher rates? *Jourr* *of Health and Social Behavior,* 1980, *21,* 33–42.

Rossi, A. S. Life span theories in women's lives. *Signs,* 1980, *6,* 4–32.

Sears, P. S., and Barbee, A. H. Career and life satisfaction among Terman's gifted wome In J. Stanley, W. George, & C. Solano (Eds.), *The gifted and the creative: Fifty-ye perspective.* Baltimore: Johns Hopkins University Press, 1977.

Serlin, E. Emptying the nest: Women in the launching stage. *In* D. McGuigan (Ed *Women's lives: New theory, research, and policy.* Ann Arbor: University of Michig Press, 1980.

Sieber, S. Toward a theory of role accumulation. *American Sociological Review,* 1974, *39,* 56 578.

Siegel, P. M. *Prestige in the American occupational structure.* Unpublished doctoral disser tion, University of Chicago, 1971.

Srole, L., and Fischer, A. K. The midtown Manhattan longitudinal study vs. the men paradise lost doctrine. *Archives of General Psychiatry,* 1980, *37,* 209–221.

Srole, L., Langner, T. S., Michael, S. T., Opler, M. K., and Rennie, T. *Mental health in metropolis: The midtown study.* New York: McGraw-Hill, 1962.

Thoits, P. Multiple identities and psychological well-being: A reformation and test of (social isolation hypothesis. *American Sociological Review,* 1983, *48,* 174–187.

Veroff, J., Douvan, E., and Kulka, R. A. *The inner American: A self portrait from 1957–19* New York: Basic Books, 1981.

Ward, R. A. The never-married in later life. *Journal of Gerontology,* 1979, *34,* 861–869.

Weiss, R. S., and Samuelson, N. M. Social roles of American women: Their contributior a sense of usefulness, and importance. *Journal of Marriage and the Family,* 1958, *20,* 3! 366.

ocial Change and Equality
he Roles of Women and Economics

IANE E. ALINGTON AND LILLIAN E. TROLL

ODERN MYTHOLOGY

 our hunger for progress, we tend to encourage media-propagated yths that shroud the reality of women's lives and discourage efforts to iprove that reality. One of the most fundamental—and misleading—of ie current myths is that the seeds of equality sown over many genera-ons have at last flowered in response to the collective efforts of 20th-:ntury women. We argue that the facts do not provide support for the :lief that women have played a causal role as agents of change, and iat it is important to correctly identify the antecedents of social change. ur thesis is that the recent changes are rooted in the economic needs of ie nation, not in the sociopolitical needs of its women. Because of the <ternal genesis of this change, its consequences are less permanent, ss significant, and less beneficial than commonly claimed.

We propose that lasting change may occur when its source is the ellspring of human need, when it is inspired by human deprivation, 1d when its goal is the improvement of the human condition. A jour-:y through the pages of women's history shows us how temporary ıange can be when its source is external, when it is inspired by institu-onal necessity and based on economic exigencies.

The winds of change have swept through women's worlds before,)ening the doors of opportunity in response to economic conditions, 1ly to close them again when conditions change. Historically, women's

IANE E. ALINGTON • Centenary College, Hackettstown, New Jersey 07840. LILLIAN E. ROLL • Department of Psychology, Rutgers University, 39 Easton Avenue, New runswick, New Jersey 08903.

entries into and exits from the "outer world" are encouraged by appropriate mythology, propaganda, and legislation. Some doors have opened recently, but the status of women and of their achievements remains low relative to those of men. For this reason, the promise of equal opportunity is an empty one, for many women lack both the self-confidence and the social support required to open the most challenging doors. Arbitrary change has arbitrary consequences, which are beneficial in some instances, negative in others, illusory in some, and nonexistent in the remainder. As a result of this capriciousness, the world of women is often filled with conflict, inconsistency, and ambiguity, all of which can affect motivations and emotion, determining which doors women will open and how they will feel about their choices.

THE WINDS OF CHANGE

Over the centuries, courageous feminists have articulated the long ings of women with seemingly little success. The current movement has survived so far because it has provided a convenient rationale for the cultural change that whirled women out of their kitchens into newly created "pink-collar" jobs—and into newly empty classrooms.[1] Now the winds are beginning to change again: A lengthy recession and rising unemployment are taking their toll, and the antifeminist rhetoric of the New Right is thriving in an increasingly fertile social climate.

Dollars and Sense

The history of women's education is rife with unmet needs, broken promises, and reluctant compromises. To the degree that economic and social pressures have fluctuated over time, so have the quality and quantity of education available to women. Feminist movements have had seemingly little influence on the actual course of events, although feminist principles have frequently been utilized by institutions in *post hoc* "explanations" whenever they have opened their doors to women.

A ROOM OF ONE'S OWN. Many examples of scholarly excellence were found in the medieval convent, where a number of women achieved international renown. In addition to providing a physical haven, a "room of one's own," the convent served two other important functions: It provided women with independence and with authority

---

[1] After all, feminism is hardly a new concept. Christine de Pisan argued for sexual equality 500 years ago. Her opinions in regard to military tactics were more esteemed by Henry VIII than were her opinions in regard to the status of women, for he had her military treatise translated into English in her own lifetime. Interestingly, *La Cité des Dames* was translated into English last year, after being out of print for several centuries.

imone de Beauvoir (1953) tells us: "Living in a convent made women idependent of man: certain abbesses wielded great power. . . . From ie mystical relation that bound them to God [they] acquired the author-y necessary for successes which women usually lack . . . Queens by ivine right and saints by their dazzling virtue were assured a social ipport that enabled them to act on an equality with men. For other omen, in contrast, only a modest silence was called for" (p. 96).

According to Mozans (1913), women of that era were accorded this ixury because learning was, in general, held in disrepute: "the knights id barons of France and Germany were inclined to look upon reading id writing as unmanly and almost degrading accomplishments . . . nd some] regarded learning as having an effeminating effect on ien. . ." (p. 277). We can hypothesize that the low status of learning as a function of the economic structure of that period; a man did not ave to be able to read in order to wield either a plowshare or a sword.

A CHANGE OF HEART: THE NEXT 400 YEARS. With the advent of the enaissance, learning became more valued by men, and women were cluded once again (Mozans, 1913). We can assume that the fledgling chnology sired by the Renaissance was responsible for the increase in ie status of learning; now reading and writing were becoming essential the economic survival of Everyman. As a consequence of the revolu-)nary zeal of the Reformation, the convents of Europe were destroyed, sulting in "the absolute extinction of any systematic education of omen for a long period" (Mozans, 1913, p. 41). In a cruelly ironic twist fate, the convents that Henry VIII appropriated became the men's)lleges of Oxford and Cambridge. It was to be nearly four centuries :fore a systematic education would be available to Western women— id five centuries before an egalitarian educational system would exist last.

BACK TO THE DRAWING BOARD. Women's colleges appeared on the merican scene toward the end of the 19th century, created in response the universally exclusionary practices of the burgeoning colleges and ofessional schools of that era. The women's college was modeled on e only existing prototype, the medieval convent (Baker, 1976). Unlike e medieval convent, however, its clientele was limited to young wom-1, and its curriculum was far from scholarly. Even so, its goals were)ble, and its creation a monumental achievement, given the attitudes the day. Small wonder that it failed to live up to the dreams of its unders. For despite its blueprint of planned obsolescence, when sexu-equality would pronounce it unnecessary, the women's colleges did ave "promises to keep" to at least a few generations of women. And e college broke its most important promise when it failed to prepare e students for successful careers. As Baker (1976) says:

> It was a triumph of consumerism . . . it was almost as if there existed a nonaggression pact: the women's colleges would provide educated wives but not professional competition for the men of Amherst, Yale . . . and the rest; in return, the men's institutions assumed a real but paternal interest in the Sisters, serving as sources for administrators, trustees, faculty and, not least, financial support as alumnae husbands (p. 11).

The last bastions of male educational privilege continued to resis coeducation until the 1970s, when the doors of the Ivy League wer finally pushed ajar by the pressure of economic exigency. Partially re sponsible for the opening of the doors were the federal government' executive orders requiring affirmative action programs and supporte by the threat of loss of billions of dollars of federal contracts. Howeve the primary economic pressure was internal, and its source was th admissions office. Both the quality and the quantity of the Ivy Leagu applicant pool was decreasing, as many of the most able students chos coeducational public institutions (e.g., Baker, 1976). All the more rea son, then, to move boldly ahead with coeducation, borrowing feminis rhetoric to justify their revolutionary about-face!

POMP AND CIRCUMSTANCES. The other interesting educational phe nomenon of the 1970s was the sudden emergence of the "reentry" stu dent (see Schossberg, Chapter 14, this volume). The fact is that by th mid-1970s, all educational institutions were looking toward matur women to solve the increasingly serious enrollment problems caused b the changing demography of the country. According to Niebuhr (1980 the crisis higher education has been facing is of a magnitude not see since the Civil War. Apps (1980) predicted that 200–300 more college would close during this decade if current trends continued. His solu tion? "[It is time to eliminate] the longstanding, condescending 'tolera tion' [of adult students which comprise] a possible new clientele." Sinc that time, the adult student (usually female) has been recruited "agres sively" (Bowen, 1980). The part-time reentry student is, in fact, savin the day; because of her presence, college enrollment is not suffering th dreaded decline.

The adult student is a familiar, if lonely, figure trudging across th landscape of women's history; she is not a creation of this women movement. Traditional educations being unavailable to the historic counterparts of today's students, some women were self-taught whi others were trained as assistants in adulthood by male relatives. Amon the latter category are two astronomers, Caroline Herschel and Mar Kirch. The 27-year-old Herschel first began to assist her brother in h studies in 1777; her late start notwithstanding, her contributions we substantial. She discovered a number of nebulae (including Androm eda), and at 39 she became the first woman to detect a comet (Mozan

)13 pp. 182–190; Osen, 1980, pp. 71–81). Kirch, whose discovery of a
)met was never formally recognized, was also tutored in adulthood;
1e and her three sisters-in-law were trained as assistants by her astron-
mer husband (Mozans, 1913 p. 173).

The journey of other women was lonelier yet. Completely self-
1ught, Mary Sommerville discovered algebra in the pages of a fashion
1agazine at the age of 15 and was simply unable to acquire any mathe-
1atical books until she was in her 30s. As a consequence of her late
:art, academic recognition was not forthcoming until she reached her
1rly 50s (Osen, 1980, p. 110). Sophie Germain, a self-taught founder of
1athematical physics, learned differential calculus from the books in her
1ther's library and began her serious work in her late 20s, ultimately
ttracting the notice of the great mathematicians of her era, including
10isson, Fourier, and Gauss (Osen, p. 90).

Today's adult student differs from her predecessors in two impor-
1nt ways. She is highly visible today, in part because she is the subject
f a great deal of (self-serving) institutional publicity, claiming humanis-
:c concern for the welfare of the midlife woman, and in part because she
 no longer lonely; even Jihan Sadat and Joan Kennedy have joined the
:ampede for a midlife degree.

In addition, midlife students are no longer subjected to the overt
)ndescension and second-class status from which her predecessors suf-
:red as recently as a decade ago (see Schlossberg, Chapter 14, this
olume). On the contrary, now that her presence has become an eco-
omic necessity, she is the new campus sweetheart, and admissions
ffices vie for her business with two seductive promises. They have kept
1eir promise to provide her with necessary financial aid and auxiliary
ervices, such as daycare; they have failed to keep their promise, howev-
c, for long-term career development. According to H.E.W. (1980), "ed-
cational institutions, anxious to have students, allow women to follow
aditional career paths (leading to employment) at the low end of the
ay scale . . . rather then design new models that will open real career
pportunities for women."

Iow Equal is Equal?

Women have been whirled in and out of the paid work force as the
2volving doors of opportunity have turned in response to the economic
xigencies of war and peace. Their entries and their exits have been
encouraged" by means of the two-edged swords of legislation and
ropaganda—even feminist propaganda has been utilized when
ecessary.

ROSIE THE RIVETER IN WAR AND PEACE. The notable achievements of

women during World War I proved to be short-lived, for women werforced out of their jobs by the Armistice in 1918. Berkin (1979) points ou
that this ousting was egalitarian: "Women streetcar conductors anwomen judges were removed with the same dispatch." It is probably ncoincidence that the disintegration of the women's movement of that er
occurred simultaneously with the return of the newly unemployed vet
erans from the battlefields of Europe.

The effects of World War II on the employment of women wersimilar to those of the earlier global conflict. During this period of man
power shortage, a new generation of women was lured into the work
place for the first time, and Rosie the Riveter became the symbol of
million women, many of them wives and mothers. Both Germany anthe United States used propaganda extensively in their efforts to reac
this untapped labor force. Despite government-sponsored polls indicat
ing that women respond primarily to economic motivations, recruitmen
campaigns were based largely on patriotism and emotion, because th
government feared that a stress on wages would produce inflatio
(Rupp, 1979). As a consequence, slogans stressed the protection of loveones, the revenge of lost lives—and the ease of the work: "Millions o
women find war work pleasant and as easy as running a sewing ma
chine or using a vacuum cleaner." This statement proved to be true, a
least as far as a top official at the Aberdeen Proving Grounds was con
cerned; the performance of his workers "justified his hunch that a deter
mined gal can be just as handy on a firing range as over the kitchen
stove" (Rupp, 1979).

A few years later, the wind changed direction once again. Postwar
appeals to married women stressed patriotic duty and were reinforceby the "mythic imperative" (Janeway, 1971) that a woman's "place" wa
in the home. The widespread internalization of this propaganda ulti
mately culminated in the Feminine Mystique described by Friedan
(1963).

On the chance that this propaganda proved ineffective, the govern
ment further "encouraged" early retirement through its overnight elim
ination of the support services it had provided for women when thei
cooperation was required for the war effort: Child-care centers, flexibl
shift jobs, and job sharing all disappeared from the scene in 1945 (Stell
man, 1977, p. 20).

Still, nearly one-third of all women remained in the paid work force
even at the height of the Feminine Mystique, and their recalcitrance onl
reinforced earlier fears voiced by the Office of War information tha
women might not want to "go back where they belong" after the wa
(Rupp, 1979). This figure should not be surprising, for nearly 20% of a
women were in the paid work force as long ago as 1890—and this figur

is probably a gross underestimate, since farm wives were not counted (Stellman, 1977).

The fact is that the majority of women have always worked alongside men (Fisher, 1979). Even though many women were isolated from the mainstream of the marketplace when the middle-class home was "invented" some 300 years ago (Janeway, 1971), many others continued to engage in paid employment outside the home as a matter of necessity.

The persistence with which one-third or more of American women claim a niche in the paid work force, regardless of propaganda efforts and inadequate support systems, has led to the institution of "protective" legislation, which is demonstrably effective in protecting men's jobs, if not women's health. Stellman (1977, pp. 179–80) details some of the "perils of protection". Lawmakers "protect" women from holding high-paying industrial jobs—where they would have to carry heavy weights—but remain strangely silent about heavy lifting when it comes to hospital and restaurant workers, whose presence is essential and whose jobs are less remunerative. Similarly, women are barred from lead exposure—only in industrial jobs, not in the (lower-paying) pottery industry. Further, exposure to X rays is "optional" for pregnant workers in health care facilities (where women are essential), despite the fact that legislative concern generally focuses on the female reproductive system. In reference to this "fetus fetish," Stellman says there is "an aura of sanctity about the fertilized egg that apparently disappears when a child is born or matures into a working person" (pp. 179–80).

Legislation in this area is hypocritical at best, absurd at worst. Laws in regard to lead exposure are based on a 1902 study that found a sex difference in normal hemoglobin levels, leading the authors to the peculiar conclusion that women suffer from an insufficiency of iron, which makes them more susceptible to the toxic effects of lead (Stellman, 1977). This unjustified use of male norms in determining the standards for women's health is not unique; the sole American study of the effects of maternal employment during pregnancy documented the fathers' occupations—but not the mothers' (Stellman, 1977)!

Undeterred by myths, propaganda, and legislation, more and more women entered the work force, until by 1960 their numbers equaled those of the war years. Their ranks were increased largely by the many middle-class wives and mothers who were forsaking full-time homemaking for the office. What happened between 1945 and 1960? Current mythology would have us believe that the influx of married women into the marketplace was a consequence of the altered consciousness of the American homemaker (and her somewhat recalcitrant husband). It is widely believed that women simply rejected the "procreative imperative" (Harris, 1980). Inspired by the Civil Rights movement, the sexual revolution, and Betty Friedan's book (not necessarily in that order), they founded a Woman's Movement. Not only that, they made a collective decision to develop a self-actualizing life-style that was to include a meaningful career, a sensitive husband, and few (if any) children. In fact, some authors cite a deliberate increase in childlessness as a factor in the alteration of female employment patterns (Stellman, 1977),[2] even though increases in childlessness have not been found over the 20th century. Recent historical scholarship suggests that this scenario is almost entirely mythical, and that the factors that lured women away from home and hearth were economic in nature.

SLEEPING BEAUTY TO THE RESCUE. Harris (1980) cites the demand of the fledgling service-economy for "pink-collar" workers as a determining factor in the migration of married women into the corporation: "the white housewife was the service employers' Sleeping Beauty. Her qualifications were superb . . . she had been trained to take orders from men . . . she would accept temporary jobs, part-time jobs, jobs that would let her go home to cook or take care of the children . . . at the end of the 1960's [women were in] a niche specifically designed for the literate but inexpensive and docile workers who would accept 60% or less of what a man would want for the same job. . . . It is a great deception to believe that women went out and found jobs . . . these jobs found the women as often as women found the jobs."

The doors to the typing pool were flung open with enthusiasm. Doors to move lucrative enterprises remained firmly closed, however, until the might of the federal government succeeded in wedging them open far enough for a few hardy women to squeeze through. Title VII of the 1964 Civil Rights Act, incorrectly considered a triumph of feminist activism, forcibly opened the way for many women. People take Title VII for granted now, but perhaps they would be less complacent if they knew that sex was only added to this crucial piece of legislation in a bizarre attempt to block the passage of a bill that many legislators found abhorrent (Kanowitz, 1971).

Why did women migrate into the corporation just when they were needed most? Did the siren song of the women's movement lure them into seeking "liberation"? On the contrary, researchers attribute the phenomenon to the "life-cycle squeeze" experienced by many women of that generation. The children of suburbia's "pioneering" families were off to college—and a single paycheck could not be stretched far

---

[2]According to Stellman, "Birthrate data show that from at least 1910–1960, the majority of women gave birth to only one or two live-born children during their life-time . . . since 1960 . . . the vast majority of women are now mothers of at least two children and childlessness is rapidly disappearing" (1977, pp. 4–5).

nough to cover tuition (Harris, 1980; Rossi, 1980a). Inflation was rag-
ng, and women were helping to fan the fires themselves, as they fell
rey to Madison Avenue pressures to buy new furniture and better
ppliances (Friedan, 1963).

We can find little evidence that changes in women's employment
atterns circa 1960 reflected a fundamental revolution in the conscious-
ess of the American woman. Rather, we suggest, the "Movement" was
consequence of the changing work patterns of women, not an anteced-
nt; it provided women with a rationale for their changing behavior, and
t provided the corporation with a rationale for its (somewhat limited)
hange of tune.

Clearly, the climate was such that a new woman's movement was
ound to flourish. The benefits derived from women's working were
uch that their "liberation" received amused (but tolerant) support
vhere it counted. As Harris (1980) states:

> Neither the interests of big business nor of the government lay as they once
> had in a united defense of the marital and procreative imperative. . . . In an
> age of nuclear arms, high birth-rates were no longer a military priority, while
> for government and business, the immediate assured benefits of employing
> women overshadowed the long-run penalties of a falling birth-rate.

The long-term risks of a little "consciousness raising" were per-
eived as minor, probably because the state of a woman's consciousness
eems irrelevant in most important respects. Even today, N.O.W. sup-
orters find it necessary to sport "59 cent" buttons in order to advance
he cause of salary equality.[3] Even today, women have not yet suc-
eeded in their efforts to break into the executive suite—or the union
hop.

In fact, current recessionary times are not good for women or for
heir cause; pending congressional legislation that would limit their re-
roductive freedom is but the tip of the growing antifeminist iceberg.
listorically, women's rights generally suffer as a consequence of eco-
omic recession, and we are seeing many inroads into recent gains.
Academe (Gray, Nichols, and Schafer, 1981) documents the disparate
ffects of proposed cutbacks on women. Numerous programs that are
acing budgetary cutbacks or elimination are those upon which wom-
n—especially midlife women—are disproportionately dependent (see

---

It is almost laughable: The women of ancient Rome and 14th-century Toulouse were
limited by law to earning 60% of a man's salary (Stellman, 1977; Shayner, personal
communication, 1982). Modern women are now earning 60% of a man's salary and are
doing it voluntarily. A little-known but interesting fact is that women with degrees from
prestigious Ivy League institutions also earn about two-thirds the salary of their male
classmates, despite the lack of a discernible difference in occupational choice (e.g.,
Harlan, 1976).

Long and Porter, Chapter 5, this volume). Not surprisingly, the cuts that are affecting women are being made willy-nilly, without regard to cost-effectiveness. A supported-work project for long-term AFDC recipients has been abruptly eliminated, even though the program was successful—and paid for itself (Masters and Maynard, 1981).

THE EMPRESS'S NEW CLOTHES

Having looked at the transient nature of externally imposed change, we turn now to look at its superficiality. The unique constellation of events of the 1960s and the 1970s was such that the appearance of change surrounds us. The economic needs of the middle-class woman, the corporate demand for service workers, and the (accidental) passage of Title VII all played a role in the degree to which new doors were opened to women—at least in theory.

In fact, many of the most interesting doors are quite safe from assault by the fair sex; on or off a pedestal, women simply have a lower status than men, and the changes we have seen in this century have done almost nothing to alter this fact. The battle against overt discrimination is progressing well, but the war against negative stereotypes is not faring so well, and there is no indication that the future looks any brighter (Steinberg and Shapiro, 1982).

Here we have a classic example of a self-fulfilling prophecy. Because women are undervalued by others, they lack the necessary self-confidence to open the most challenging doors. And because women's work is undervalued by others, their efforts to achieve are often frustrated by the lack of necessary social support; only a woman of the most uncommon promise is likely to find support in her home, school, and community.

The Nimble Fingers Syndrome

Although some researchers report progress in the status of women, others fail to find any difference in the degree to which people judge women as less competent than men (Etaugh and Kasley, 1981). Women are still considered unsuitable for responsible management positions (e.g., Steinberg and Shapiro, 1982) and have not, in fact, made much progress in achieving such positions. Women are still employed in an "occupational ghetto" (Diamond, 1981), holding 80% of the clerical jobs, 70% of retail sales clerk jobs, and 98% of the domestic service jobs (Rones and Leon, 1979); college graduates continue to restrict their career choices to teaching and nursing (Harmon, 1981).

Women are not perceived as leaders, and their leadership behavior ꜱ not perceived as such (Denmark, 1980); further, they are perceived as ᴇss influential and less powerful than males (Wiley and Eskilson, 1982). ᵀypically, a woman's success is attributed to effort, while a man's sucᴄess is attributed to ability (Riger and Galligan, 1980). Since pay raises ꜱre based on effort, and promotions on ability (Heilman and Guzzo, ᴵ978), the negative consequences for women wishing to climb the corpoꜱate ladder are obvious.

Whatever the reasons, women and their work are universally unᴵervalued in a most mysterious manner. According to American myᴛhology, women make good typists because they have nimble fingers; ᴵnglishwomen, on the other hand, are not judged capable of tackling ᴛhe typewriters at that august establishment, Lloyd's of London. Unlike ᴛheir American counterparts, Soviet women are considered competent ᴇnough to handle a scalpel, for medicine is a relatively low-status ocᴄupation in the USSR. Soviet mythology also supports the employment ᴏf women as typists, as the second author discovered to her amuseᴍent—and chagrin. In Moscow for a conference, L.E.T. found it necesꜱary to type a few extra notes for her scheduled address; she found it all ᴏut impossible to maintain her concentration in the face of repeated ᴵnterruptions, as one person after another requested her secretarial ꜱervices.

It is reasonable to assume that these negative perceptions of women ᴍust have an influence on their own feelings of competence and value ꜱelative to men, and the data we have support the notion that women ᴵnternalize these negative biases in predictable ways. Females typically ᴵack confidence in their ability to succeed (Crandall, 1969; Stake, 1979) ꜱnd suffer undue anxiety in the face of competition (Sassen, 1980), esᴘecially when they are required to compete against males (Ingram, ᴵ980). The 'Catch-22' in this instance is obvious when we observe the ᴵact that many women fear the negative social consequences of success ᴵn male-dominated occupational fields (Vaughn and Wittig, 1979). Conꜱidering the situational and institutional barriers that feed the female ꜱense of inadequacy whenever they are required to function in a "man's ᴠorld," the wonder is that any women ever open the most challenging ᴅoors.

ᵀhe 40-Hour Day

The superficiality of recent change is clear when we examine the ᴵcts surrounding women's efforts to combine family and career responꜱibilities. There is no indication that any change has occurred at all in the degree to which women carry the heavier burden in the home, whether or not they are also in the paid work force.[4] Women's work, in or out of the home, is simply accorded less status than men's. Perhaps because it is inherently less valuable, it is supposed to be less taxing. Whatever the reason, many researchers report that a wife's employment status has little or no effect on role sharing within a marriage. Despite the luxurious appearance of the modern kitchen, today's homemakers spend more time engaged in housework than did their grandmothers (Oakley, 1974). When a wife works, she must, of necessity, reduce the number of hours she devotes to housework (Beckman and Houser, 1979). Even so she needs a 40-hour day and a 300-hour week (Troll, 1982), for her employment does not affect the percentage of household chores for which she is responsible (McCullough, 1980; Nelson, 1977). Haas (1982) even had trouble finding any subjects for her study on egalitarian marriage. The nonegalitarian marriage is the norm, even when both members of the couple are physicians (Hendricks, 1980), and labor in the home remains divided in a traditional sex-role fashion among the marriages of full-time professionals (Beckman and Houser, 1979). British (female) psychiatrists interviewed by Brook (1981) chose their profession in large part because it was one that would permit them to work part time, enabling them to carry out their family responsibilities.

Cultural attitudes in regard to the status of women are extremely resistant to change (Steinberg and Shapiro, 1982). But until they are modified, the opening of doors to women remains largely an empty gesture; most women will have neither the interest in nor the energy for fighting a long, hard battle to achieve success in rewarding, male-dominated occupations.

The Bride Wore Black

Externally imposed change tends not only to be transient and superficial but also to be capricious. Doors have been flung open, but the barricades of prejudice remain to block women's entry; women recognize the difficulties of tackling new and challenging fields when their status is such that they really do have to be "more equal than equal" in order to succeed. And they recognize the difficulties in achieving suc

---

[4]Fisher (1979) compares the work load of the modern American woman (45–70 hours per week) with that of "the Australian Aborigine women of the Pitjandjara described in 193 (as having a life of arduous drudgery, sometimes consisting of as much as four to si hours a day—a work week of twenty-eight to forty-two hours). Which, if either, is the liberated woman, I leave to the reader to decide."

ess when the status of their work is such that their support system is
arely adequate to support an effort that is merely "equal."

et Them Eat Cake

Most women know that it is difficult for anyone but Wonder
Woman[5] to "have her cake and eat it too." Most women still feel the
necessity to set priorities and make choices. As recently as 1981, the *New
York Times* described the tearful words of a young bridesmaid who could
not escape the bouquet that had been hurled in her direction by the
happy (and insistent) bride. The bridesmaid's words were illuminating
in the degree to which they show the lack of progress women have
made. "But I don't want to get married. . . . I want to go to law school!"
(Gilinsky, 1981). If men felt the necessity to make such a choice, how
many of them would have the courage and the willingness to choose law
chool?

Marriage and parenthood have negative effects on the professional
tatus (Broschart, 1978) and salary (Birnbaum, 1979) of women because
of their impact on labor-force participation. Hence, the "59-cent prob-
em" is largely explained, for fewer years of participation mean less
eniority and fewer promotions.

Tending the hearth in addition to minding the store has negative
onsequences for women—and for men, as well. Ferber and Huber
(1979) report that a husband's tendency to hold office and to publish is
decreased when his wife is also an academician. Clearly, it is not easy to
manage a home without a full-time wife; adjustments are difficult and
ostly (Burke and Weir, 1976). Somebody is going to have to pay the
piper; unfortunately it is usually the wife.

Mothers and Mentors

Successful men tend to have parents—and wives and mentors—
who encourage them and support their efforts (e.g., Levinson, Darrow,
Klein, Levinson, and McKee, 1978). We have no reason to believe that

---

Today's would-be supermoms have some awesome predecessors whom they may be
trying to emulate. According to Mozans (1913). Laura Bassi, who was a famous Italian
physicist, was the "mother of twelve children [and] she never permitted her scientific and
literary work to conflict with her domestic duties or to detract in the least from the
singular affection which so closely united her to her husband and children. She was as
much at home with the needle and the spindle as she was with her books and the
apparatus in her laboratory. . . . She was living proof that cerebral development [of
women] does not lead to race suicide. . . ."

men and women differ in the degree to which such encouragement and support is necessary, although there are clear differences in the degree to which they are available.

The experience of having a mother who works enhances a daughter's interest in—and commitment to—a career (e.g., Altman and Grossman, 1977), especially if the mother is fortunate enough to hold a relatively high-status position (Haber, 1980). Other researchers have found that a mother's attitudes toward work are important antecedents of achievement motivation, even if she is not in the work force herself. "Successful" students (in graduate and professional schools) often attribute their motivation to their mothers' attitudes; this attribution was made significantly more often by females than by males (Poumadere, 1978). "Successful" women (i.e., professionals) who organize their lifecourse (including time of marriage) around their career goals report greater maternal encouragement than that of their colleagues who fail to establish their priorities at an early age (Allen, 1980).

If a mother's attitudes are significant in the life of a young woman, a husband's attitudes are equally critical in later life. A husband's attitude toward his wife's working affects her propensity to enter the work force[6] (Perrucci and Targ, 1978), and it also affects the degree of job satisfaction she will achieve. Among 30–40-year-old women, a negative attitude on the part of the husband may be more detrimental to her satisfaction than the underutilization of her skills and the presence of preschool children in the home (Andrisani, 1978). Andrisani reports that 55–65% of all women in the sample perceived their husbands to have a negative attitude; their disapproval may ultimately have an impact on the women's performance and commitment (Scanzoni, 1979). According to Huston-Stein and Higgins-Trenk (1978), only 4–6% of husbands surveyed want their wives to work continuously and express any desire to adjust their lives to her working needs in any way, although they do want to have an intellectual companion!

Mothers and husbands are not the only influential figures in a woman's interpersonal world; a mentor may be crucial to achieving success for women as well as men (Denmark, 1980; Hennig and Jardin, 1976; Riger and Galligan, 1980; Stake and Levitz, 1979). Some researchers report that mentors who are male are necessary for success (e.g., Hennig and Jardin, 1976), but that may be due to the historic paucity of women mentors, for Goldstein (1979) found that recent Ph.D.'s of both sexes were much more productive if they had same-sex mentors. It

[6]Unless she has worked before. Previous experience with the intrinsic and extrinsic rewards of employment will overcome the disappearing attitudes of a husband, according to Hongvivatana (1976).

appears to many (e.g., Denmark, 1980; Wittig, 1979) that the current dearth of senior female academics is at least partially responsible for the dismal statistics in doctoral programs in psychology, where only 35% of the women complete the programs, as opposed to 70% of the men (Hirschberg and Itkin, 1978).

Progress—real change—will remain an elusive goal until women are routinely provided with the same support and encouragement as men—no more and no less. Until this support is forthcoming, we have no reason to believe that women will storm the doors of the executive suite. In the meantime, we can expect that many women will meet their needs for achievement in the time-honored ways, in the home and in the community and in traditional career areas (Troll, 1982a), for these means of satisfaction result in less frustration and conflict, even if they also result in fewer extrinsic rewards.

STARTING OVER

Much recent change is illusory, transient, and far from dramatically beneficial in the short run. But the changes we see today may have positive consequences for the long run, for their impact on the experience of women may result in gradual—but profound—intergenerational and interpersonal development, development of a type that is not responsive to externally imposed ideology.

Mothers and Daughters: Intergenerational Development

Troll (1975) has pointed out the striking similarities between the attitudes of different generations within a family. In her exploration of attitudes toward careers and achievement, Troll found some generational shifts consistent with the changes in women's education and job-market participation. Each younger generation showed less conventional sex-role orientation and moralism, but greater cognitive complexity, feelings of control, and overall motivation to achieve. However, women in the same family tend to resemble each other more than they resemble other women of their own generation. A grandmother with high achievement motivation tends to have a daughter and a granddaughter who are also highly achievement-oriented. It is possible, in other words, to view high achievement motivation as a family theme (Troll, 1980).

As Troll and Bengtson (1982) have pointed out, social and historical forces serve as moderator variables in family lineage transmission. Transmission is tempered when social forces are inconsistent with family values and is enhanced when they are consistent. However, family themes tend to be rather stable; as Hill, Foote, Aldous, Carlson, and MacDonald (1970) state, "While rapid pace of social change encourages new ways of expressing old values, it is largely old values that are expressed"

It appears that changes in family themes occur as a function of the family's experience within the culture, rather than as a function of cultural values and ideology *per se*. For this reason, the fact that more and more women are working today as a consequence of personal misfortune, economic necessity, or individual preference has far-reaching consequences. Today's working women are discovering the intrinsic and extrinsic rewards of the paid work force (Hongvivatana, 1976), and they are discovering the frustrations of having skills that are undervalued, underutilized, and, all too often, underdeveloped. Their employment seems to "liberate" their attitudes (Molm, 1978; Olsen, 1980). Women report that they embraced feminist principles after going to work, not before. We can expect that the increasing dissatisfaction of today's working women (Andrisani, 1978) will begin to modify family themes such that boys and girls will grow up with the realization that things could—and should—be different. We can see signs that important changes are occurring in terms of family themes; Harmon (1981) reports that the daughters she surveyed mirrored their mother's attitudes toward work in every respect—except that 98% of them expected that they would always work, with minimal time off in order to raise their children.

Late Bloomers: Interpersonal Development

Women's history is filled with stories about women for whom life began at 40—or thereabouts (see Heilbrun, Chapter 3, this volume). "Grandma" Moses' late start was somewhat excessive—at age 78—but the fact that her serious work began late is not atypical for her sex. The "late bloomer syndrome" seems to be a consequence of several different factors. In some cases, personal misfortune serves as a catalyst to new types of achievement. Margery Hurst, one of the world's only self-made female millionaires, founded the original temporary help agency in London after being deserted by her husband. Divorced women are disproportionately represented among the ranks of adult students, and they are noticeably more committed, as students and as workers, than any other group (Huston-Stein and Higgins-Trenk, 1978; Maslin, 1978, Schlossberg, Chapter 14, this volume).

One can assume that divorced women may be more disillusioned with the Cinderalla myth than any other group. In addition, however, the fact that they are self-supporting again may have pointed them with newfound motivation. Motivation rooted in the need for survival may e the crucial factor enabling these women to overcome earlier inhibiions and hesistancy. For, as Hoffman (1978) states, the roles of wife and nother mean that "they have an alternative to professional success and an opt out when the going gets rough. A full-scale achievement effort nvolves painful periods of effort and many a man would drop out if that lternative were as readily available as it is to women."

In addition, midlife achievement in women, married or not, may be function of the fact that their family responsibilities have been reluced. The Eagleton Institute of Politics (1978) published a study on vomen in public office; almost without exception these women were lder than their male counterparts at their time of entry into politics. In lmost all cases their children were over 18—and in almost all cases they vere married to supportive husbands, whose aid they claimed was esential to their success.

An extraordinary number of women who have achieved a place in he history books have achieved their eminence late in life—often beause they did not have the opportunity to indulge their passions for ersonal achievement earlier.[7] Since the number of "world class" mathmaticians among women prior to this century is only slightly higher han the number of Supreme Court judges in our own time, it is asonishing to discover that three of them achieved their renown for work hey had done in their late 30s. As we have already noted, Mary Somerille, Caroline Herschel, and Maria Kirch all achieved recognition for vork accomplished in their 30s and long afterward, at an age when their nale counterparts were resting on the laurels of youthful creativity.

As any woman knows, midlife is not without stress. But many vomen survive the trials of the "sandwich generation" with equaimity, and many report more confidence, freedom, and autonomy in he postmenopausal years (Rossi, 1980a; Baruch, Chapter 6, this volme). Most women report relief at the "empty nest" (Artson, 1978) and re, in fact, happy to have the time to engage in their own interests.

Finally, midlife achievement in women may be, in part, a conseuence of the personality change that many researchers believe is uniersal at this time. Sex-role reversals have been found among women of

Some female achievements occur early but are recognized late; Sophie Germain died (aged 55) before the University of Gottingen could award her the honorary doctorate recommended by Gauss (Olsen, 1980; p. 91). Caroline Herschel was more fortunate, for she lived long enough to experience recognition; she was elected an honorary member of the Royal Academy Society at 85 and was awarded a gold medal by the King of Prussia when she was 96 (Olsen, 1980, p. 80). Probably more women should have followed the path taken by Miranda Stuart, a.k.a. James Barry. As "James" she/he entered medical school as "Dr. Barry" she/he ultimately became the surgeon inspector-general to the British army, her secret safe until her death (Macksey and Macksey, 1975, p. 144).

45–55 years of age in the United States (Neugarten and Gutmann, 1980 and in many other cultures (Brown, 1982). Gutmann (1975) found a shif from nurturance to dominance among women, and Lowenthal, Thurn her, and Chiriboga, (1975) found an increase in assertive independence Regardless of the source of these personality changes, they do seem t occur with remarkable consistency; undoubtedly they play a role in th achievement-oriented behavior that women display in midlife. Al though the data are cross-sectional, hence open to different interpreta tions, two studies suggest that the need for achievement in womer increases with age (Vanzant, 1980) and becomes a more useful predicto as women grow older and their familial responsibilities decrease (Faver 1982).

Brave New World

When we pause long enough to appraise our current situation real istically, we will be able to plan our future more intelligently. We mus take media claims of progress with a grain of salt; the press, after all proclaimed that equality had been achieved after the passage of the 19th Amendment, even as the Women's Movement was disintegrating be fore their eyes.

True progress may occur in the days ahead in response to the articu lated dissatisfaction of women who continue to experience frustration ir the paid work force and exhaustion in their efforts to cope with two full time careers.

The legacy that this generation of mothers leaves to their daugh ters—and sons—may mean a better life ahead for men and women of a ages. Change that is inspired by human experience and the collectiv wishes of individual people will be more meaningful and more lastin, than change that has been imposed from without. In the legacy left b this generation of mothers to their children may lie the genesis of tru progress.

REFERENCES

Allen, S. Professional women and marriage. *Dissertation Abstracts International*, 1980, 41, 4736.
Altman, S. L., and Grossman, F. K. Women's career plans and maternal employmen *Psychology of Women Quarterly*, 1977, 1, 365–376.
Andrisani, P. J. Job satisfaction among working women. *Signs: Journal of Women an Culture*, 1978; 3, 588–607.
Apps, J. W. Six influences in adult education in the 1980's. *Lifelong Learning: The Adult Yea 3(10) 4–7, 30 June, 1980.
Artson, B. Mid-life women: Homemakers, volunteers, professionals. *Dissertation Abstrac International*, 1978, 39B, 3481.

aker, L. *I'm Radcliffe, fly me! The seven sisters and the failure of women's education*. New York: MacMillan, 1976.

eckman, L. J., and Houser, B. B. The more you have, the more you do: The relationship between wife's employment, sex-role attitudes, and household behavior. *Psychology of Women Quarterly*, 1979, *4*, 160–174.

erkin, C. R. Not separate, not equal. In C. R. Berkin and M. B. Norton (Eds.), *Women of America: A history*. Boston: Houghton Mifflin, 1979.

etz, N., and Hackett, G. The relationship of career-related self-efficacy expectations to perceived career options in college men and women. *Journal of Counseling Psychology*, 1981, *28*, 399–410.

irnbaum, M. H. Is there sex bias in salaries of psychologists? *American Psychologist* 1979, *34*, 719–720.

owen, H. R. Adult learning, higher education, and the economics of unused capacity. *In* Chandler, B. J. (Ed.). *Standard Education Almanac*. Chicago: Marquis Academic Media, 1980.

rook, P. The choice of career or consultant psychiatrists. *British Journal of Psychiatry*, 1981, *138*, 326–328.

roschart, K. R. Family status and professional achievement: A study of women doctorates. *Journal of Marriage and the Family*, 1978, *40*, 71–77.

rown, J. K. Cross-cultural perspectives on middle-aged women. *Current Anthropology*, 1982, *23*, 143–156.

runs-Hillman, M. Traditional and nontraditional female achievers: Factors which may account for divergent modes of expression of achievement motivation. *Dissertation Abstracts International*, 1980, *40B*, 5460.

urke, R. J., and Weir, T. Relationship of wives' employment status to husband, wife, and pair satisfaction and performance. *Journal of Marriage and the Family*, 1976, *38*, 279–287.

randall, V. C. Sex differences in expectancy of intellectual and academic reinforcement. In C. Smith (Ed.), *Achievement-related motives in children*. New York: Russell Sage, 1969.

e Beauvoir, S. *The second sex*. New York: Knopf, 1953.

enmark, F. L. Psyche: From rocking the cradle to rocking the boat. *American Psychologist*, 1980, *35*, 1057–1065.

iamond, E. E. Sex-typical and sex-atypical interests of Kuder Occupational Interest Survey criterion groups: Implications for counseling. *Journal Counseling Psychology*, 1981, *28*, 229–242.

agleton Institute of Politics: The Center for the American Woman and Politics. *Women in public office: A biographical directory and statistical analysis*. Metuchen, N.J.: Scarecrow Press, 1978.

taugh, C., and Kasley, H. C. Evaluating competence: Effects of sex, marital status, and parental status. *Psychology of Women Quarterly*. 1981, *6*, 196–203.

aver, C. A. Achievement orientation, attainment values, and women's employment. *Journal of Vocational Behavior*, 1982, *20*, 67–80.

erber, M., and Huber, J. Husbands, wives, and careers. *Journal of Marriage and the Family*, 1979, *41*, 315–325.

isher, E. *Women's creation: Sexual evolution and the shaping of society*. New York: McGraw-Hill, 1979.

riedan, B. *The feminine mystique*. New York: Dell, 1963.

ilinsky, R. M. A cloudless June day . . . *New York Times*, June 6, 1981.

oldstein, E. Effect of same-sex and cross-sex role models on the subsequent academic productivity of scholars. *American Psychologist*, 1979, *34*, 407–410.

ray, M. W., Nichols, I. A., and Schafer, A. T. The impact of the 1982 federal budget on women in higher education. *Academe*, 1981, *67*(4), 202–204.

Gutmann, D. Parenthood: Key to the comparative psychology of the life cycle? In N. Datan and L. Ginsberg (Eds.), *Life-span developmental psychology*. New York: Academic Press, 1975. Pp. 167–184.

Haas, L. Determinants of role-sharing behavior: A study of egalitarian couples. *Sex Roles*, 1982, *8*, 747–760.

Haber, S. Cognitive support for the career choices of college women. *Sex Roles*, 1980, *6*, 129–138.

Hare-Mustin, R. T., and Broderick, P. C. The myth of motherhood: A study of attitudes toward motherhood. *Psychology of Women Quarterly*, 1979, *4*, 114–128.

Harlan, A. *Career differences among male and female managers*. Paper presented at the National Academy of Management, Kansas City, Mo., 1976.

Harmon, L. W. The life and career plans of young adult college women: A follow-up study. *Journal of Counseling Psychology*, 1981, *28*, 416–427.

Harris, M. Why it's not the same old America. *Psychology Today*, August 1980, pp. 23–51.

Hendricks, J. G. Career-family management of women and men physicians. *Dissertation Abstracts International*, 1980, *41A*, 1792.

Heilman, M. E. and Guzzo, R. A. Perceived cause of work success as a mediator of sex discrimination in organizations. *Organizational Behavior and Human Performance*. 21(3) 346–357, 1978.

Hennig, M., and Jardin, A. *The managerial woman*. New York: Doubleday, 1976.

Hill, R. N., Foote, J., Aldous, R., Carlson, R., and MacDonald, R. *Family development in three generations*. Cambridge, Mass.: Schenkman, 1970.

Hirschberg, N., and Itkin, S. Graduate student success in psychology. *American Psychologist*, 1978, *33*, 1083–1093.

Hongvivatana, T. Employment decisions of married women. *Dissertation Abstracts International*, 1976, *38A*, 2923.

Huston-Stein, A., and Higgins-Trenk, A. Development of females from childhood through adulthood: Career and feminine role orientations. In P. E. Baltes (Ed.), *Life span development and behavior* (Vol. 1). New York: Academic Press, 1978. Pp. 258–298.

Ingram, R. P. The effects of locus of control and sex-role preferences on the achievement orientation of females. *Dissertation Abstracts International*, 1980, *41A*, 4337.

Janeway, E. *Man's world, woman's place: A study in social mythology*. New York: Dell, 1971.

Kanowitz, L. Title VII of the 1964 Civil Rights Act. In N. Reeves (Ed.), *Womankind: Beyond the stereotypes*. New York: Aldine/Atherton, 1971.

Levinson, D. J., Darrow, C. N. Klein, E. B., Levinson, M. H., and McKee, B. *The seasons of a man's life*. New York: Knopf, 1978.

Lowenthal, M. F., Thurnher, M., and Chiriboga, D. *Four stages of life: A comparative study of women and men facing transitions*. San Francisco: Jossey-Bass, 1975.

Macksey, J., and Macksey, K. *Book of women's achievements*. New York: Stein & Day, 1975.

Maslin, A. Older undergraduate women at an urban university: A typology of motives ego development, sextypedness, and attitudes toward women's role. *Dissertation Abstracts International*, 1978, *39A*, 2067.

Masters, S. H., and Maynard, R. *The impact of supported work on long-term recipients of AFDC benefits: Vol. 3 of the final report on the supported work evaluation*. New York: Manpower Demonstration Research Corporation, 1981.

McClelland, D. C. *The achieving society*. New York: Free Press, 1961.

McCullough, J. L. Contribution to household tasks by Utah husbands and wives. *Dissertation Abstracts International*, 1980, *41A*, 4313.

Miller, D. V., and Philliber, W. M. The derivation of status benefits from occupational attainments of working wives. *Journal of Marriage and the Family*, 1978, *40*, 63–69.

Molm, L. D. Sex role attitudes and the employment of married women: The direction of causality. *Sociology Quarterly*, 1978, *19*, 522–533.

Mozans, H. J. *Woman in science*. Cambridge, Mass.: M.I.T. Press, 1913.

Nelson, E. N. Women's work—Household alienation. *Humboldt Journal of Social Relations*, 1977, *5*, 90–117.

Neugarten, B. L., and Gutmann, D. L. Age-sex roles and personality in middle age: A thematic apperception study. In B. L. Neugarten and Associates, *Personality in middle and late life*. New York: Arno Press, 1980.

Niebuhr, H., Jr. A renewal strategy for higher education. *Continuing Higher Education*, 1980, *28*(2): 2–9.

Oakley, A. *Woman's work: The housewife past and present*. New York: Pantheon, 1974.

Olsen, S. M. Sixteen middle-class mothers view the women's movement: Its ideological relevance and psychological effects. *Dissertation Abstracts International*, 1980, *41B*,

Osen, L. M. (1974) *Women in mathematics*. Cambridge: MIT Press.

Perrucci, C. C., and Targ, D. B. Early work orientation and later situational factors as elements of work commitment among worried women college graduates. *Sociology Quarterly*, 1978, *19*, 266–280.

Poumadere, J. I. Combining family and professional responsibilities: A study of graduate and professional students' plans. *Dissertation Abstracts International*, 1978, *39B*, 6203.

Riger, S., and Galligan, P. Women in management: An exploration of competing paradigms. *American Psychologist*, 1980, *35*, 902–910.

Rones, P. L., and Leon, C. Employment and unemployment during 1978: An analysis (Special Labor Force Report, No. 218). Washington, D.C.: Bureau of Labor Statistics, 1979.

Rossi, A. Life-span theories and women's lives. *Signs: Journal of Women in Culture and Society*, 1980, *6*(1), 4–32. (a)

Rossi, A. S. Aging and parenthood in the middle years. In P. B. Baltes and O. G. Brim, Jr. (Eds.), *Life-span development and behavior*. New York: Academic Press, 1980. (b)

Rupp, L. J. Woman's place is in the war: Propaganda and public opinion in the United States and Germany, 1939–1945. In C. R. Berkin and M. B. Norton (Eds.), *Women of America: A history*. Boston: Houghton Mifflin, 1979.

Sassen, G. Success anxiety in women: A constructivist interpretation of its social significance. *Harvard Education Review*, 1980, *50*, 13–24.

Scanzoni, J. Sex-role influences on married women's status attainments. *Journal of Marriage and the Family*, 1979, *41*, 793–800.

Stake, J. E. The ability/performance dimension of self-esteem: Implications for women's achievement behavior. *Psychology of Women Quarterly*, 1979, *3*, 365–377.

Stake, J. E., and Levitz, E. Career goals of college women and men and perceived achievement-related encouragement. *Psychology of Women Quarterly*, 1979, *4*, 151–159.

Steinberg, R., and Shapiro, S. Sex differences in personality traits of female and male Master of Business Administration students. *Journal of Applied Psychology*, 1982, *67*, 306–310.

Stellman, J. M. *Women's work, women's health: Myths and realities*. New York: Pantheon, 1977.

Troll, L. E. *Development in early and middle adulthood*. Monterey, Calif.: Brooks/Cole, 1975.

Troll, L. E. Intergenerational relations in later life. In N. Datan and N. Lohman (Eds.), *Transitions of aging*. New York: Academic Press, 1980.

Troll, L. E. *Continuations: Development after 20*. Monterey, Calif: Brooks/Cole, 1982. (a)

Troll, L. E. *Being called an eminent woman psychologist*. A.P.A. address, Washington, D.C., 1982. (b)

Troll, L., and Bengtson, V. Generations in the family. In W. Burr, R. Hill, F. Nye, and I. Reiss (Eds.), *Contemporary theories about the family* (Vol. 1). New York: Free Press, 1979.

Troll, L. E., and Bengtson, V. L. Intergenerational relations throughout the life span. In B. B. Wolman, G. Sticker, S. J. Ellman, P. Keith-Spiegel, and D. S. Palermo (Eds.), *Handbook of developmental psychology*. Englewood Cliffs, N.J. Prentice-Hall, 1982.

Troll, L. E., Neugarten, B. L., and Kraines, R. J. Similarities in values and other personality characteristics in college students and their parents. *Merrill-Palmer Quarterly*, 1969, 15 323–336.

U.S. Department of Health, Education, and Welfare, Education Division. *Lifelong Learning and Public Policy*. A report prepared by the Lifelong Learning Project. Washington, D.C. *In* Chandler, B. J. (Ed.). *Standard Education Almanac*. Chicago: Marquis Academic Media, 1980.

Vanzant, L. R. Achievement motivation, sex-role, self-acceptance, and mentor relationship of professional females. *Dissertation Abstracts International*, 1980, *41A*, 4248.

Vaughn, L. S., and Wittig, M. A. Occupational competence, and role overload as evaluation determinants of successful women. *Journal of Applied Social Psychology*, 1979, *10*, 398–415.

Wiley, M. G., and Eskilson, A. Coping in the corporation. *Journal of Applied Social Psychology*, 1982, *12*, 1–11.

Wittig, M. A. Graduate student success: Sex or situation? *American Psychologist*, 1979, *34*, 798.

Yorkis, K. L. Marital status, parenting, and pursuit of graduate degrees: Their relationship to and effect on the careers of women administrators in institutions of higher education. *Dissertation Abstracts International*, 1981, *41A*, 4932.

he Daughter of Aging Parents

NN STUEVE AND LYDIA O'DONNELL

TRODUCTION

emographic changes since the turn of the century have reshaped the ntours of the parent–child relationship, considerably increasing the an of years in which children and their parents meet and interact as lults. Sixty-five-year-old mothers and fathers typically look back not ly on long and shared relationships with their sons and daughters but so look forward to shared futures lasting, on the average, 15 years or ore. In contrast to previous generations, when children often experi- ced the death of a parent during their formative or young adult years, ntemporary men and women in midlife and beyond are having to fine and negotiate what it means to be a son or daughter when one s children, or even grandchildren, of one's own.

Over the past several decades, researchers, service providers, and e public have become increasingly interested in how adult children gotiate this relationship and how they respond when parents need lp. In large part their interest reflects the dramatic and well-docu- ented increase in the number of elderly parents and a growing recog- tion of the important role children, and daughters in particular, con- ue to play in the lives of the old. There is considerable research, for ample, on the kinds and levels of support needy parents receive from spring (e.g., Cantor, 1979; Shanas, 1979a, 1979b, 1980) and on the ids of problems children encounter when they attempt to care for iously ill or disoriented parents at home (e.g., Archbold, 1978; Isaacs, vingstone, and Neville, 1972; Lowenthal, 1964). While such pressing

N STUEVE • 23 Hamilton Avenue, Ossining, New York.   LYDIA O'DONNELL • Welles- College Center for Research on Women, Wellesley, Massachusetts 02181.

and practical issues clearly merit attention, what has been overlooked i how children experience the long period of years during which parent are old but often healthy, and how they differ in the ways they fram their commitments to elderly kin. In this chapter, we examine the adul child–elderly parent relationship from the vantage point of daughter and look at how women in different social and life-cycle positions var in the ways they respond to the adult–daughter role. To do so, we drav from our own research, which entailed interviews with 81 daughters o elderly parents, as well as from relevant literature on the parent–chil tie.

Focusing on the Mother–Daughter Relationship

While sons, of course, also have elderly parents, the parent–chil relationship in later life is of particular concern to women. Wherea demographic trends call attention to the elderly parent–adult chil bond, sex-specific social changes focus our attention on the moth er–daughter tie. First, women tend to outlive men; as a result, there ar more elderly mothers than elderly fathers. As Treas (1977) documents this situation is relatively recent. At the turn of the century, there wer approximately 102 men 65 years and older for every 100 women. Thirt years later, the numbers of older men and older women were roughl equal. By 1960, however, a gap had emerged, and there were only 8 older men for every 100 women. By 1975 the gap had widened sti further: For every 100 elderly women there were only 69 elderly mer These statistics mean not only that there are more elderly mothers tha elderly fathers alive today but also that older women are more likely t be widowed and living alone. Whereas most elderly fathers can expe to live out their lives in the company of a spouse and to draw on th support and help that spouses routinely provide, elderly women are n so fortunate. In 1978 three-fourths of all men between 65 and 74 years age were married and living with their spouses, compared to less tha one-half of all similarly aged women; the disparity was even more pr nounced among those 75 years and older, with 68% of all men marrie compared to only 22% percent of all women (Soldo, 1980). Not surpri ingly, when women—and men for that matter—lose a spouse, the typically turn to their children, especially their daughters, to provide wide range of material, social, and emotional supports (Lopata, 197 Shanas, 1979a, 1979b, 1980). Indeed, many daughters pinpoint th death of a mother or father as the time when their relationship with th surviving parent changed and intensified, in part because they saw the newly widowed parent as more needy but also because the death of or arent provides a jarring reminder that parent–child relationships do ot last forever.

While demographic changes draw attention to elderly mothers, ere are also reasons to focus on daughters. In our culture, it is women ho perform most of the work entailed in managing and nurturing a mily and binding members of different generations together. For ex- nple, it is women in their dual roles as mothers and grandmothers ho help out when grandchildren are born and who act as baby-sitters ring the subsequent years. Similarly, it is typically women who, as ughters, tend to elderly parents when they are sick, provide transpor- tion to and from doctors' offices, and are on call for any emergency. It also women who, as daughters, wives, mothers, and sisters, make rangements for visits, encourage phone calls, worry about whether eir parents are lonely, and generally keep tabs on whether husbands, ns, and brothers maintain appropriate contact with older generations. oreover, this kin-keeping work has recently been called into question the increasing labor force participation of midlife daughters and, ore generally, by the cross-flow of ideas and rhetoric about women's oper roles and the value of putting the needs of family members ead of one's own aspirations and goals. Finally, unless differences in e life expectancies of men and women narrow appreciably, it is daugh- rs, more than sons, who are likely to become tomorrow's elderly par- ts and, thus, to make demands on their children for help and support old age. It is for these reasons that much of the research, as well as our n, focuses on daughters' responses to aging parents.

aling with Complexity in Parent–Child Ties

A recurring theme in much of the literature on adult development nters on the complexity and diversity of life paths and careers among er adults (Hagestad, 1981). With each passing year individuals be- me increasingly different from one another in terms of the life experi- ces they have accumulated and where they stand with respect to fferent timetables and roles. A 40-year-old woman, for example, may "launching" her teenage children or embarking on first-time mother- od, "peaking" in her profession or reentering the labor force. Com- xity and diversity are even more pronounced when we turn from dividual lives to parent–child relationships. Not only do both genera- ns bring different roles and experiences to the adult child–elderly rent relation, but over the course of their lifetimes, parents and chil- en develop their own idiosyncratic strategies and understandings as ll. By the time parents are elderly and children are in their middle

years, both generations have acquired a repertoire of beliefs and pra
tices that orient their behaviors toward one another and reflect how the
lives have been organized and connected throughout the adult year
"With the passage of time," write Hess and Waring (1978), "so muc
diversity arises in family groups that possibly no two sets of parents ar
children in the society—or even in the same family—have traveled pa
allel paths" (p. 267, quoted in Hagestad, 1981, p. 21).

While complexity and diversity have been highlighted in theoretic
and discursive accounts of parent–child relationships, they have n
been emphasized in research reports on parent–child ties. To the co:
trary, researchers have tended to portray the interactions betwee
daughters and their elderly parents in one-sidedly positive or negati
terms. On the positive side, for example, survey after survey documen
the persistence of social, emotional, and material exchanges betwee
children and their elderly parents (e.g., Shanas, 1979a, 1979b, 198
see Troll, Miller, and Atchley, 1979, for a review). Gerontologists ha
also highlighted the responsiveness of daughters in attending to pa
ents' needs and serving as care-givers when necessary (Brody, 198
Hill, Foote, Aldous, Carlson, and MacDonald, 1970). Indeed, much
the research over the past 30 years has been directed toward disprovir
the notion that family ties have withered with the advent of mode
industrial society or that families—and, in particular, children—aba
don the old. While there is recognition that the flow of goods and se
vices may shift over the course of the family cycle and vary by soc
class, distance, and the like, the major thrust of this work emphasiz
the persistence and reciprocal nature of intergenerational ties. Mor
over, in drawing such a positive portrait, many researchers have d
counted as simplistic or inaccurate such concepts as "role reversal
which implies that mothers and fathers become childlike in old age a
children are pressed into assuming a parentlike stance.

In contrast to this fairly positive image of family relations, attenti
has more recently shifted to the difficulties adult children may encou
ter in maintaining good relations with their parents. In particular, soc
scientists and policy analysts have focused on issues of *parent-caring*
term that refers to the unpaid work entailed in nurturing and meeti
the needs of an elderly parent and implies some degree of dependen
of the parent on the child (e.g., Cicirelli, 1981). A small but growi
body of ethnographic, fictional, and autobiographic accounts (Archbo
1978; Gordon, 1978; Isaacs *et al.*, 1972; Murphy, 1980) describes in de
the tensions that can be introduced into family life when children a
sume responsibility for chronically ill or disoriented parents: The wc
load increases, other family relations suffer, children's social activit
are curtailed, and the relationship between offspring and their pare

:comes strained. Current assessments of the state of the modern family
so feed into this negative view of adult child–elderly parent relations
ı marked by dependency and difficulty. It has become almost com-
onplace for gerontologists to point to changes in the family that are
:ely to make it more difficult for children to act in a caring and respon-
ble manner with respect to their aging parents. It is often noted that
ng-run declines in family size mean that while there are relatively
ore elderly parents today than in the past, there are relatively fewer
ıildren to share the burden of work and responsibility (Treas, 1977).
oreover, as parents survive to increasingly advanced ages, the chil-
en of elderly parents are more often approaching old age themselves
rody, 1979). Perhaps most visible and talked about of all is the in-
eased labor force participation of women. As opportunities and pres-
ıres for female employment increase, more and more women, it is
njectured, will be caught in the bind of weighing the needs and expec-
tions of parents against employment aspirations and commitments of
eir own. While a number of studies are now under way to examine the
mifications of such changes—especially increases in women's em-
oyment (e.g., Brody, 1981)—it is too often taken for granted that such
anges are limiting the capacity and willingness of family members to
eet traditional responsibilities toward aging parents.

There are undoubtedly both positive and negative sides to the adult
ild–elderly parent relationship, yet to focus on one side to the exclu-
>n of the other yields an incomplete and overly simplistic picture; it
scures the variety and complexity of the relationship. Children differ
ıt only in the ways they experience the aging and death of a parent but
;o in how much they are called upon to help out when parents grow
l. Following a description of the Adult Daughter Study, the remainder
the chapter addresses issues and variations that must be considered
order to develop more complex frameworks and models for under-
ınding how the child–parent relationship develops in the latter half of
ɛ family cycle.

e Adult Daughter Study

The Adult Daughter Study consisted of interviews with 81 white
ımen between the ages of 30 and 60, all of whom had at least one
ing parent 70 years of age or more.[1] The women were selected at
ıdom using annual town census listings from two communities in the

ıese interviews were part of a larger study on families and care-giving strategies funded
the National Science Foundation (NSF DAR 7910358), Laura Lein, principal investi-
tor.

Boston metropolitan area. One community housed a largely working and lower-middle-class population; the second was more affluent, and its residents were more likely to be college-educated and working at professional and managerial jobs. Women were contacted during the spring and summer of 1980; among those who met the sample criteria approximately 75% agreed to participate.

The daughters who were selected by this procedure are what we generally think of as middle Americans. All but one of the women had at least a high school education: 20% were high school graduates with no further schooling, 38% had received some technical training or completed some college, while 41% had finished 4 years of college or more. In addition, most (80%) were married and most (85%) were mothers but, as reported later, they differed in where they stood in their family cycle careers. The financial positions of these women and their families ranged from moderate to affluent. Sixteen percent reported annual family incomes of less than $20,000, 14% had incomes of over $60,000, while the incomes of most respondents were somewhere in between. Participants also differed in their ethnic heritages and religious affiliations and reflect the wide range of backgrounds commonly found in the Boston area. Forty-three percent of the women described themselves as Catholics, 23% were Protestants; 11% were Jewish, and the remaining 22% did not identify with an organized religion or church.

The parents of these women also varied considerably in terms of their ages, marital status, and early life experiences. Forty percent of the women interviewed reported that their older (or only) parent was between the ages of 70 and 74, while 30% had at least one living parent who was 80 years or more. Three-fifths of the respondents were daughters of widowed parents, with widowed mothers outnumbering widowed fathers four to one. Although virtually all of the daughters were born in this country, almost half (48%) reported that at least one of the parents was foreign-born. Not surprisingly, these older parents were generally less well educated than the daughter generation. Over one third of the older mothers (35%) had completed less than 4 years of high school, and several had received little formal schooling at all; 29% of the mothers were high school graduates, 16% had received some technical training or college after high school, and 19% had completed the requirements for a B.A. degree. The financial status of parents was more difficult to assess than their other characteristics because most of the daughters reported being uninformed about this aspect of their parents' lives. Only 21% reported knowing their parents' incomes, while an additional 41% were willing to wager a guess. About half of those who knew or guessed at parents' incomes reported that mothers and fathers lived on less than $10,000 annually, but only 15% of the daughters

ported that they were helping parents out with financial contribu-
ons, and half of these reported doing so only from time to time.

It is important to note that the women who participated in this
udy were not selected because of some special relationship they
hared with their elderly parents. They were not picked because their
arents were particularly healthy or particularly needy, or because their
arents lived especially close by or far away. Nine percent of the daugh-
rs shared a home or lived in a two-family dwelling with parents, 34%
ved either in the same community as parents or in a bordering town,
ad 30% lived more than an hour's drive away. Similarly, respondents
ere not selected because they were especially concerned about the
ging of parents or because they were heavily involved in providing
arents with help. While some of the women were, or expected to
come, their parents' primary care-givers, others anticipated that a
bling would take on most of the responsibility and work. In addition,
e participants do not solely represent daughters who get along well
ith elderly parents or daughters whose relationships are marked by
mflict and strain. Rather, they are a diverse and random sample of
hite working- and middle-class daughters of elderly parents, and they
ovide a variety of situations and experiences to examine and compare.

HE INTERLOCKING OF GENERATIONS

Perhaps the most basic question to address in identifying important
riations in the adult child–elderly parent relation is: Who are the
aughters of aging parents? Most often, we think of these daughters as a
neration "caught in the middle," women in their 40s and early 50s
ho are responsible for meeting the needs of both their elderly parents
d their adolescent children while often working at a paid job as well. If
e look at this characterization more closely, however, we see that it
aderstates the many different ways in which the life cycles and life
mmitments of adult children and elderly parents interlock. First, not
daughters of elderly parents are similar in age. Although the modal
spondent in our study was in her late 40s, 25% of the women inter-
ewed were less than 40 years old while nearly 13% were approaching
, the upper age limit in this sample. Indeed, demographic trends
dicate that an increasing number of men and women who are 65 years
older themselves still have a parent or parent-in-law alive (Harris and
ssociates, 1975; Brody, 1979). Second, not all daughters of aging parts are at similar points in their own family cycles. While the modal
spondent was a mother of teenage children, 27% of our sample were
rrently raising preschool- or school-age children and a similar percent-
e had no child-care responsibilities, typically either because they had

not yet had children or because their children had grown and left home In addition, a few midlife women had decided to remain childless Third, while clearly more daughters of elderly parents hold paid job than in previous generations, there is a wide variation in the extent o their labor force involvement and in how they strike balances betwee paid work and family roles. Although nearly 70% of the daughters w interviewed were in the labor force, half of these women worked onl part-time hours. Thirty-one percent of the sample were full-time home makers.

In large part, these variations reflect the family-timing decision made sequentially by members of each of the two generations involved How old you are when your parents turn 70 is obviously a function c how old your parents were when they started their families and you own place in the sibling hierarchy. How elderly parents fit into you family cycle then depends on the timing and spacing of your own chi dren, which, in turn, affect how and when you become involved i other roles such as that of paid worker. The members of a multigener tional family are thus interlocked in ways that reflect the aggregation c family-timing patterns and decisions made by all of the nuclear familie involved. As a result, it is not surprising that there is wide variation i the ways the life cycles of daughters and elderly parents intersect sinc normal variations in the family-timing patterns within any one gener tion, here the elderly parents, are then compounded by the differer decisions made by members of the next generation, their children. T date, however, there has been little effort to examine how these diffe ent family configurations influence the relationships between childre and elderly parents. In the next section, some of the implications different timing patterns are discussed.

The Impact of Timing Patterns

Most of us carry a standard image of how the parent–child relatio ship progresses in adulthood, an image that is accurate in many case The relationship between young adults and their parents is most oft characterized by issues of separation, with children establishing sep rate identities and households at a time when their midlife parents a still vigorous and healthy. As children settle into adult roles and ha offspring of their own, a period of rapprochement and stability is like to follow, with both parents and children remaining relatively indepe dent; Baruch and Barnett (1983) describe this period as the "era of go feelings." Finally, as middle-aged children become established and p pare to launch their own offspring into the adult world, they begin deal with the aging of their parents and the inevitability of their paren death. This is an accurate description of how the life-courses of sor

ughters and their parents are interlocked, but, as the data presented
ove suggest, many daughters are off time with respect to this stan-
rd image and encounter the aging and death of parents at earlier or
er points in their lives. Neugarten (1968), among others, suggests that
ng off time may make such transitions more difficult. A thematic
ding of the interview protocols suggests that variations in family-
ting patterns play an important role in shaping how daughters deal
th some of the psychological issues and considerations that arise
en parents grow old.

Several case studies illustrates how different family-timing patterns
pe the ways daughters frame the issues of loss surrounding the
ssibility of a parent's death. Theresa Camilli, who is in her 30s, and
tel Lindstrom, who is in her 50s, are both faced with the possibility
t their parents may not have much longer to live.[2] Yet contrast the
ferent ways they deal with their impending loss: Mrs. Camilli, when
ed to describe her parents, responded in this way:

> They are very understanding. I'd be lost without them. They've helped me
> through many, many hard times. I really wouldn't know what to do [if they
> died]. I don't even want to talk about them leaving because I just want them
> around forever. I just kind of block that right out my mind. When my father
> had the heart attack, it scared me half to death. And when my mother had
> her operation, that made me very nervous. I made it on my own with my
> husband, but there's lots of times you just can't tell a friend something, and
> you need somebody. And then I go talk to my mother. I'm very close with
> my mother. . . . If I have a problem, I know that she'll give me good advice
> and so will my father. They do not beat around the bush. They just come
> straight out and tell you what they think.

er the course of her interview, Mrs. Camilli emphasized the loss she
uld feel should her parents die at this point in her life, and her words
ressed fear and apprehension about whether she could make it on
own. The older Mrs. Lindstrom described her concerns about her
ther's death in a very different way:

> Well, the thing that concerns me most is that I hope my mother will go very
> quickly. I hope she will die and not be prodded and poked and all these
> things they have to do to you. And I hope that she won't be uncomfortable
> and not tell us about it, because she's apt to do that. And I hope that she will
> just go and not be frightened at the time. . . . If they told me that she would
> die tomorrow, I think I'd be very, very happy because I'd know that she had
> a happy life to the last moment. That's the thing that concerns me the most—
> not how soon she will go, but *how* she will go.

Mrs. Camilli was barely able to consider her parents "leaving" and
rly had not accepted the possibility of their loss, whereas Mrs.

nes have been changed to assure the confidentiality of respondents.

Lindstrom appeared resolved to the inevitability of her mother's deat and more concerned about her mother's suffering than her own. Thes differences can be linked in part to the life stages of both the daughter and their parents. Mrs. Camilli is still reliant on her parents, both psy chologically and instrumentally. She counts on her mother and fathe both for advice and for practical support in raising her four young chi dren. Mrs. Lindstrom, by contrast, is happily employed full time an busy establishing a second marriage. Although she used to confide her mother at length when she was younger, she now finds that her li is fairly stable, and she has others with whom she can talk and who a often more helpful than her ailing mother. While the two women bo maintain daily contact with their parents through phone calls and visit Mrs. Camilli looks upon these encounters as at least as important f herself as for her parents, while Mrs. Lindstrom realizes how much h mother looks forward to such contacts and continues them primarily f this reason.

Mrs. Camilli and Mrs. Lindstrom illustrate how the impact of parent's aging can differ depending upon the extent of one's psych and emotional separation from parents. Psychologists point out th some women never effectively separate, particularly from their mothe since the transition from a childlike and dependent status to equal foo ing as an adult can be difficult even under the best of circumstanc (e.g., Cohler and Grunebaum, 1981). While much of the psychologi work of separation occurs in the adolescent and young adult years, t issues often extend into later years as well. Women in their 30s in o sample were more likely than older women to still be preoccupied w establishing their own identities and disengaging from their parents. the case of Mrs. Camilli suggests, when an adult child must sim taneously deal with issues of separation and with the reality of a p ent's failing health and death, resolution can become more difficult a complex. When daughters are still emotionally dependent on their p ents, they feel especially vulnerable and threatened by signs of th parents' old age. Under these circumstances separation can be diffict and perhaps even prolonged, both for daughters who are close to a still reliant on parents and for daughters who have not resolved ambivalence and conflict with parents often associated with establish an adult identity.

Lauren Jarvis, who is approaching 40, expresses how much easie is to accept parents' old age once children come to terms with their o adult identity. She recounted her experiences with her 88-year-old ther in this way:

> I feel fairly comfortable with the way things are now . . . and I certainly hope that our relationship won't dissipate before my father dies. If he dies today, I would feel very comfortable with it—beyond the missing him—but I would

have no regrets. I've said what I wanted to say. I've expressed what I've wanted to, and so has he. It's not going to get any better. I hope it doesn't get worse. It's OK. Everything is comfortable. Now had he died, say, in my late twenties, ten or eleven years ago, I couldn't have said that. There was still a lot to be resolved.

Losing a parent when both you yourself are older and your parent is der seems more a part of the natural timing of events. In addition to eir greater readiness to accept the aging and death of a parent, adult ildren in their 40s and beyond are more likely to have friends and quaintances who have also experienced some of the difficulties sur-unding a parent's aging and who can act as role models and confi-nts. As one woman explained: "I talk with my friends about my rents because so many of my friends are in the same boat. Practically of my friends who are my age or older have gone through it."

While men and women have gained increasing control over deci-ns about whether, when, and how many children to have and often igh a large number of factors in making these family-timing deci-ns, they rarely think ahead to how their decisions will shape the ture of their involvement in an adult child–elderly parent relation-ip. While many couples may look forward to the security of having a ild to fall back on in old age, few consider the ramifications of their nily-timing patterns on the availability and willingness of children to pond should the need arise. For example, how many people who rry young and have children immediately realize that the advantages being relatively young when their children are young may turn into a advantage when they are old and find that their children are old as ll? Similarly, a growing number of couples are postponing children til they are in their 30s and even early 40s so that they have time to ablish careers and solidify marriages, but they rarely take the needs d expectations of elderly parents into account. For example, how ny realize they may be trading off time for themselves at the begin-g of the adult life course against time for themselves once children ve left home and old parents are needy? As Daniels and Weingarten 82) describe, there are long-term ramifications and trade-offs with all nily-timing patterns. With issues of timing becoming more and more atter over which couples have control, it is important to bring these nifications and trade-offs to the attention of both generations.

RENTS' NEEDS AND DAUGHTERS' RESPONSES

Just as variations in family-timing patterns shape the nature of the tionship between children and parents in later life, so do the vagaries parental health and life circumstances. No one can predict when a ent's health will decline or when an elderly mother or father will be widowed. As a result, the characterization of daughters as being "caugh in the middle," responsible for meeting the needs of both growing children and ailing parents, is inaccurate not only because of variations in ages and life stages but also because it rests on the assumption that elderly parents are typically needy and dependent. When we examine statistics on the physical and mental health status of the older generation and look at the ways daughters in our sample describe their parents, we see that many parents remain quite healthy and self-sufficient through out most of the period we call old age and that patterns of interdepen dence between the generations that are evident in the latter part of the family cycle are often patterns that developed long before parents grew old.

While older people on the average certainly have more chronic dis eases and disabilities than do young people, the majority are in good health. In 1975 interviews conducted by the National Center for Health Statistics found that almost 70% of the elderly questioned rated their health as excellent or good; only 9% described their health as poor (Kovar, 1977). Recent estimates also indicate that only about 4 to 6% of the population 65 years or older suffer from organic brain syndrom (Raskind and Storric, 1980) and only 10% show any signs of senili whatsoever (Fighting off old age, 1981). Even though these percentage are higher among the very old, our fears of senility and mental impai ment are greatly exaggerated. When we turn from mental and physic health and look at the day-to-day functioning of older people—wh gerontologists call the activities of daily living—the story is much th same. One needs-assessment survey conducted in Massachusetts foun that over half of the elderly people interviewed were self-sufficie when it came to transportation, housekeeping, food shopping, and foo preparation; over 80% were self-sufficient when it came to person hygiene (Branch, 1977). Moreover, these figures are really underes mates since many of the older people who were not classified as se sufficient actually relied on their spouses for help, and clearly, turni to one's spouse is not unique to the elderly.

These positive figures on the health and independence of the c coincide with the ways daughters in our sample described the health their parents and how much support they have been called upon provide. Not only do older people describe themselves as healthy a active, but their children do so as well. When asked, "How would y describe your parents' health?" 69 of the women interviewed answer with a label resembling the categories used in survey questionnair One-third of these daughters characterized their parents' health as cellent or very good; an additional 42% characterized it as good, wh only one-quarter portrayed the health of either parent as only fair

oor. Even fewer described their parents as disoriented, confused, se-
ile, or forgetful to the point of its hampering their daily functioning.
iterestingly, although every respondent had at least one mother or
ther who was 70 years of age or older, the majority (61%) did not think
their parents as old. In response to the question "Do you think of
our parents as young, middle-aged, old, or what?" most daughters
ooke of them as "getting older," middle-aged, or in terms of some
her more youthful-sounding category. Parents did not seem to fit the
ereotypic image of befuddled and inactive old people. Even in those
ises when daughters initially responded that they thought of their
arents as old, several quickly qualified their answers, as illustrated by
ie following response:

> Well, I guess I'd have to think of her as old, but not very old. She's youthful
> for her age. I mean, she is old, she's seventy-three. But she is certainly
> younger in her appearance and her actions than some women I've seen in
> their fifties. She's very agile and gets out and does everything and doesn't
> depend on anyone for anything. [Interviewer: What makes you think of her
> as old?] Well, that's a good question. I guess the fact that I know she's old. I
> really don't think of her as old, but middle-aged seems more what I am—I'm
> fifty-three. So I really couldn't say that she was middle aged. . . . I guess I
> think of her as "getting older," perhaps that would be more correct.

is possible to interpret the unwillingness of some daughters to label
eir parents as old as a defensive response, a denial of both their own
d their parents' aging. However, given the descriptions of parental
alth and the national figures cited above, a more likely explanation is
at in many cases their parents have, in fact, remained vigorous and
tive despite their advanced chronological ages.

It is therefore not surprising that the majority of daughters were
ily minimally involved in what could be termed "parent-caring" at the
ne of the interview. On the basis of a thorough reading of the inter-
ew protocols, we scored the respondents on the extent to which they
ere involved in providing instrumental support to their parents. More
ecifically, we rated respondents on whether they provided no, some,
substantial help (score = 0, 1, or 2, respectively) with the following
ven tasks and activities: personal care and hygiene, household chores,
ands, transportation, financial management, institutional interac-
ns (e.g., dealing with Medicare forms), and actual financial contribu-
ns. Out of a possible score of 14, respondents received scores ranging
m 0 to 12. Two out of every five daughters, however, received scores
0, meaning that they provided no regular help with the activities of
ily living, and only one out of every five received a score of 5 or
her.

For the most part, these relatively low scores reflect the fact that the

parents of the women interviewed were free of major physical and men
tal impairments that would call for prolonged and intensive time invest
ments on the part of children. Good health, however, is not the whol
explanation. First, many of the illnesses associated with aging are chror
ic in nature. In living with a chronic illness such as arthritis or diabetes
older people learn to adapt and make do. Instead of major weekly shop
ping trips, parents go to the local store several times a week; instead c
cleaning the entire house at once, they clean one room at a time; instea
of mowing the law in one afternoon, they spread the chore out ove
several days. Putting a premium on their own independence, parent
learn how to live within their limitations. Second, although the elderl
are more likely than their children to have serious illnesses, more fre
quent hospitalizations and surgery, and longer recuperative period:
many do, in fact, recover. While daughters may be quite involved du
ing intensive periods of need, parents often get back on their feet agair
Paula Bird's situation is fairly typical.

> My father had pneumonia from Thanksgiving until after Christmas. He had
> it and we didn't know it. He was falling a lot. I was going over, doing his
> breakfast dishes, getting some type of lunch for him and seeing that some-
> thing was cooked for dinner, because I knew he was falling and he was
> weak. I though, Gee, what are we going to do? Finally, since my sister had
> had pneumonia the month before we said, "Dad, I think you ought to go to
> the doctor." And sure enough, he had pneumonia.
>   It was scary. It was before Christmas and we were very, very busy. I had
> to go over every day because I am the only one in my family who is "not
> working." . . . It was a drastic change, and he became very dependent on
> me. He was very weak. He was falling asleep all the time. But the pneumonia
> took care of itself, and now he's better.

While to this point we have emphasized how many parents rema
in good health throughout most of their lives, it is undeniably true th
many elderly people get seriously or terminally ill. In such circui
stances, parents typically turn first to each other and then to their ch
dren for care (Cantor, 1980; Lewis, Bienenstock, Cantor, and Schne
wind, 1980; Shanas, 1979b, 1980; see also case studies reported in se
help books, such as Silverstone and Hyman, 1976). The vast majority
children are at their parents' beck and call when catastrophic illness do
arise, whether it means traveling to be on hand for a parent's serio
operation and recuperation, being there when a parent is dying,
helping a parent make funeral arrangements and adjust to widowhoo
    There is considerable variation, however, in how much and wl
types of care children are called upon to give to parents, both in cases
dire emergency and in borderline situations where parents are becomi
more frail and needy. There is also variation in how graciously daug
ters accept the role of helping parents and adapt their lives to fit paren

ıeds. First, daughters from working-class backgrounds are more likely
▸ live with or near their parents and to have built up patterns of interde-
ındence and helping out, which more easily slide into patterns of
ırent-caring when the need arises. By contrast, middle-class daugh-
rs, particularly women who have left home to attend college, are more
ɛely to have drawn strict boundaries between their own nuclear fami-
ʲs and those of their parents and to have constructed lives that are
·parate from those of their parents and siblings. Working-class daugh-
ɩs are therefore more likely to find themselves in circumstances that
ıll them into parent-caring, circumstances (such as living in the same
ʲighborhood or town) that are in turn shaped by a value system that
ınphasizes interdependence and the responsibility of one nuclear unit
 the extended family for another. For such daughters, taking care of a
ıil or ailing parent is virtually taken for granted, as illustrated by the
llowing case study.

> Nora Dubchek lives two miles away from her widowed father. She works
> part time as a hairdresser, and her husband is a self-employed gardener.
> When she was first asked if her father had come to rely on her, she replied,
> "No. No. Only when he doesn't feel well. You know, I will sometimes take
> him to the post office, or drive him here, or go over and do a few things in the
> house." When asked how often she saw her father, however, she went on to
> say, "Oh, I see him every day. I was there this morning. This morning I did
> the dishes for him because he has a bad hand. And I just talked to him."
> Later in the conversation, it came out that Mrs. Dubchek did many other
> things for her father—she tends to home repairs, makes sure his house is
> properly cleaned, takes him places in bad weather, and nudges her brothers
> and children to make regular visits. She has thought about her father's ad-
> vancing age and the possibility that at some point he may not be able to live
> alone. She anticipates becoming more involved in his life, even to the point
> of establishing a joint residence.

 the case of Mrs. Dubchek and other working-class women like her,
ɾents are seen less as presenting problems and complicating their lives
ɑn as being a part of their immediate family; parents' needs are part of
ɛ fabric of daily life.

   Middle-class daughters, by comparison, are less likely to integrate
ɾents into their lives to this extent or to provide parents with the type
 support Mrs. Dubchek takes for granted. They typically made fewer
ʲits to parents, even when they lived in the same metropolitan area.
ɦen we compared working- and middle-class women in terms of the
ɩount of instrumental aid they reported providing to parents, we
ınd that a disproportionate number of working-class daughters were
ɩong the most heavily involved. More specifically, whereas one-fifth
 the women with only high school or vocational training received the
ʷest possible instrumental score, almost half (45%) of the women with

at least college educations did so; whereas half of the less educate
women received instrumental scores of 4 or higher, only 15% of thei
better educated counterparts were this involved.

Even among the working class, however, it is not always daughter
who are called upon for help. Just as elderly spouses turn to each othe
for assistance with routine chores, they also look to one another in time
of illness and need (Johnson, 1980; Lewis et al., 1980; Stueve, 1982). Eve
in cases where parents call on children, one child is often singled out a
primary care-giver rather than responsibility being equally share
among siblings. In our research, daughters typically reported providin
more assistance than their brothers, proximate daughters tended to pro
vide more help than respondents who lived farther away, and olde
and youngest daughters seemed to take more responsibility for elder
parents than women who held middle positions in the sibling line
Thus, while most studies (including this one) suggest that daughters ar
the major providers of instrumental support to needy parents, still man
women do not expect to be called upon for more than occasional a
sistance because they know that a sister (or, less often, a brother) wi
step in instead. As one respondent with several brothers and sisters pu
it, "It's not that my oldest sister would *feel* most responsible but that th
responsibility would fall on her because she would be the most access
ble (should my parents need help)."

In addition, it is not uncommon, particularly in middle-class fam
lies, for parents to look to friends and neighbors for help rather than t
family, especially if children live far away and a community of age-pee
is available. Some older people, particularly those who are affluer
enough to buy homes in retirement communities and who are a
customed to living apart from their children, prefer to hire service
when necessary or to engage in reciprocal exchanges with friends rath
than becoming dependent upon offspring. Carol Post, whose paren
moved to a condominium limited to people 50 years and older, de
scribed some of the advantages of this living arrangement:

> My parents have a huge network of friends and people to bring them what
> they need. I mean if one of them is in the hospital, the other one gets invited
> out for every meal or people bring in things. People are just tremendously
> supportive. They'll drive you to the hospital to visit. My parents have a
> whole network there.

What differentiates this respondent from more interdepende
working-class women is the notion that parents can be taken care of l
people other than family members. This is a notion that appears to l
shared by both daughters and parents. A middle-class daughter is mo
likely to assume that her parents would hire a housekeeper or, if nece
sary, a private-duty nurse than expect her to perform such tasks. N
only are parents seen as having the financial resources to purchase th

ervices they need, but they are also perceived as having become ac-
ustomed to making arrangements without resorting to children. If both
arents and children are used to maintaining boundaries between their
espective households and leading separate and independent lives, they
re less likely to look to one another for help if something goes wrong.
Middle-class parents may hesitate to disrupt their children's lives and at
mes may actually prefer the less emotionally charged strategy of hiring
elp or relying on their informal networks. However, middle-class par-
nts, like working-class mothers and fathers, expect their children to be
vailable in serious situations, and their children acknowledge this
aim.

One such serious situation that arises is the death of a parent,
aving a widowed mother or, less commonly, father alone. After an
nitial period of intense involvement, children may pick up some of the
sks previously performed by the deceased parent. Mothers may call
pon their sons and sons-in-law, for example, for advice on financial
atters and taxes; fathers may look to their daughters and daughters-in-
w for help with housekeeping and the like. Children report making
eater efforts to stay in touch, either by dropping in more often or by
oning, since widowed parents are often thought to be lonely. The
fferent patterns of interaction characteristic of working- and middle-
ass families, however, persist. Working-class daughters continue to
ace a greater emphasis on integrating their widowed mothers and
thers into their lives, whereas middle-class daughters tend to do what
ey feel is necessary to help a widowed parent re-establish a life of his
her own.

In discussing the health and life circumstances of parents, it is diffi-
lt to strike a proper balance, to avoid presenting a picture that is either
erly optimistic or too narrowly focused on the problems of old age.
ur point is not that elderly parents never become dependent upon
ughters. Some parents need a lot of help a lot of the time, especially
ose who are very old or who are seriously or terminally ill; some
rents need a lot of help some of the time—for example, during spells
sickness or following the death of a spouse. However, when we
nsider the number of years adult children now have to relate to parts who are elderly, it is fair to say that the adult child–elderly parent
nd is best thought of as an extension of the relationship that devel-
ed during early parts of the family cycle.

OMEN'S CHANGING ROLES

Thus far, we have argued that the image of daughters as being
aught in the middle" is inaccurate both because daughters differ in
eir own ages and family stages when they are faced with their parents'

old age and because old age is an extended period of time during which most mothers and fathers remain active and healthy. In looking forward to how the adult child–elderly parent relationship will be shaped in the future, one additional question that must be addressed is: What is the effect of women's increasing labor force participation? To date, this remains a largely unanswered question. While a substantial amount of research has focused on the implications of women's employment on family interactions during the child-rearing years, less evidence has accumulated on the relationship between women's employment and interactions with older generations. Here again, it is easy to oversimplify the issue. It is often assumed either that employed women are pressed into relinquishing responsibilities to elderly parents or that the needs of elderly parents place undue constraints upon their daughters' workplace involvements. Our interviews with midlife women suggest that the relationships are more complex and that we must look at employment in light of what we have learned about the nature of the adult child–elderly parent tie.

First, there are many circumstances and situations in which women employment is of negligible importance. Whether or not employment constrains the amount of care-giving daughters provide to parents is moot point if parents are healthy and managing on their own. Similarly employment makes little difference if daughters live several hundred miles away, since face-to-face contact is limited whether or not a woman is employed. Employment also makes little difference if parents and daughters have become accustomed to independent lives and daughters are not relied on as the first line of defense against the day-to-day problems of old age.

Second, there any many situations in which daughters have learned to maneuver around employment, especially if their schedules are flexible or they work part-time hours. Among daughters who lived within an hour's drive of parents, part-time employees actually visited parents more often than either full-time workers or full-time homemakers, and they provided more instrumental assistance when parents lived very close by. Clearly, many of the ways daughters assist parents can be accommodated into a part-time work routine. Reassuring phone calls can be made before or after work hours, errands can be run on weekends, and so on. In addition, in cases of necessity, women make effort to accommodate paid work to the needs of parents. Approximately two fifths of the employed women we interviewed had taken time off from work to aid parents, yet most often the time required was minimal—for example, an afternoon to take a mother to a doctor's appointment—and the women did not see it as interfering with their responsibilities on the job. For those women who had been employed for long periods of time atterns of mutual assistance were often developed before parents grew ld.

Third, women's decisions about whether and how much to work ypically take into account a number of factors—financial considerations, the needs of children and spouse, volunteer work and other commitments, and, in some cases, the needs of parents. About 10% of the women in our sample mentioned that their parents' failing health and reliance upon them was one factor in their decisions to postpone or terminate employment or to limit their work hours. For example, one woman quit her full-time job in part so she would be more free to visit her recently widowed father, who lives several hours away. However, there were a number of other factors involved that reinforced this decision. She was also tired of the pressures her job entailed and was looking forward to starting a family and being a full-time mother. She quit her job as much in anticipation of pregnancy as she did because of her father. Another woman postponed going back to work because she was heavily involved in helping her widowed parent with day-to-day housekeeping, doctors' visits, and the like. Additional factors entering into her decision, however, were her satisfaction with being a full-time homemaker and her ambivalence about leaving a young teenage daughter at home alone. As these examples illustrate, it was usually a composite of factors, rather than the needs of aging parents alone, that influenced daughters' employment decisions, and even the women themselves had difficulty in ranking their relative importance.

In some cases, however, it does appear that employment—especially full-time employment—makes a difference. Among daughters who lived within an hour's drive of parents, full-time employees provided less instrumental assistance and visited parents less often than other part-time workers or full-time homemakers. Not surprisingly, full-time employment placed greater constraints on those forms of parent–child interaction that require more time and energy: Visits were more affected than contacts by phone. To what extent a decline in face-to-face contact is experienced as a loss either by daughters or by parents unclear. For example, in returning to the labor force, daughters may e trading the social contact with parents for social contact with fellow workers. Parents, likewise, may offset the decline in daughters' visits by increasing contacts with neighbors and friends; alternatively, they may miss the more extensive contact with kin since they are at a time in their lives when other forms of social participation may be constrained. Among the women we interviewed, employment-related cutbacks never meant that daughters stopped seeing their parents but rather that they decreased their visits incrementally from daily to several times a week, from bimonthly to monthly, and so on. In addition, there is evidence that some employed daughters cut corners with parents in other ways as well. Special favors may be shaved; employed daughters may not be quite as available to listen to a mother's problems or talk on the phone several times a day; they may suggest taking a cab rather than offering to chauffeur; they may still be willing to run errands or take a parent to a doctor's appointment, but everyone is more constrained to a tight schedule. What difference this trimming makes in the lives of daughters and parents remains unclear and merits further investigation.

Employment can also serve as a legitimate excuse to pass on some of the work involved in keeping a parent comfortable to an unemployed sibling, although some unemployed siblings are less willing to accept this excuse than others. One woman, for example, complained that her brother and sisters expected her to fill in and be on call for her widowed mother since she was the only one "not working." As she herself was currently raising young children and involved in a number of community activities, she sometimes felt she was doing more than her share.

Finally, there is the matter of cohort differences. The present daughter generation is composed of members of several different cohorts, each of which has faced the impact of women's changing roles at a different point in the life cycle. What paid work means to a woman in her 30s today and what kind of balance she strikes between paid work and family roles may be quite different from how a woman in her 50 orders her priorities. With growing numbers of midlife women in the labor force, it will be important to pay attention to such cohort differences in our efforts to understand the ramifications of women's employment on family ties in the years to come. In light of these considerations, it becomes apparent that assessing the impact of employment on daughters' responses to aging parents is no simple matter. Just as we are beginning to develop more complex models for understanding how women strike balances between their work and family roles in the early part of the family cycle, we will need equally complex models in examining the work–family interface in the latter half of the family cycle as well.

CONCLUSION

In this chapter, we have examined the adult child–elderly parent relationship from the vantage point of daughters and discussed some of the ways daughters differ in how they respond when parents grow old. Our analysis suggests that while most women's lives are touched by the aging of parents, simplistic stereotypes, such as that of daughters being "caught in the middle," distort our understanding of parent–child relationships in later life.

In closing, there are three further considerations that warrant attention. First is the matter of women's involvements with other elderly kin

Women may be pressed into a care-giving role not only by the needs of their own mothers and fathers but also by their parents-in-law and other elderly kin. For example, at the time of the interviews, among married respondents with at least one parent-in-law still living, three-quarters reported that at least one parent-in-law was 70 years or older. The question of how and when women become involved in the care of elderly mothers- and fathers-in-law merits its own discussion and cannot be adequately treated here. Suffice it to say that while some respondents were quite involved in helping out their husbands' elderly parents, most often this responsibility was assumed by a sister-in-law.

Second, there is the question of whether women with elderly kin feel caught in the middle, whether they find that being a daughter or daughter-in-law conflicts with their roles as wives and mothers or interferes with their efforts to pursue careers. This again is a difficult and complex matter, one that can only be touched upon here. A number of the women interviewed felt pulled by the competing demands of some combination of parents, children, spouses, employment, and other activities. These pulls were experienced not only by employed women but by busy homemakers as well. When parents do need help, it can be draining and time-consuming; even in the best of circumstances, it can be emotionally difficult to watch a parent grow old. Adult children do worry about their parents, and their worries range from concern over whether parents will have an accident while they are vacationing in Florida, to whether a widowed mother will be able and willing to make it on her own, to whether an elderly relative will take a turn for the worse and have to be placed in a nursing home. Elderly kin can and do complicate the lives of daughters, but so do husbands, children, grandchildren, and younger relatives. These complications are part of family life, a part that a growing number of midlife women are now experiencing and fitting into the rest of their lives.

Finally, while the current generation of daughters is accommodating to the needs of aging parents, it is less clear what will happen when these women are elderly mothers themselves. For example, will they want the same things from their daughters as their mothers now want from them? Can they reasonably expect the same kinds of help and attention from daughters that their mothers expect and receive from them? Given the decisions of more men and women to limit the size of their families, how many elderly mothers and fathers of the future will have daughters to call on and rely upon at all?

REFERENCES

Archbold, P. G. *Impact of caring for an ill elderly parent on the middle-aged or elderly offspring caregiver.* Paper presented at the 31st Annual Scientific Meeting of the Gerontological Society, Dallas, November 1978.

Baruch, G., and Barnett, R. C. Adult daughters' relationships with their mothers: The era of good feelings. *Journal of Marriage and the Family*, 1983, 45, 601–606.

Branch, L. G. *Understanding the health and social service needs of people over age 65*. Center for Survey Research, University of Massachusetts and the Joint Center for Urban Studies of M.I.T. and Harvard University, 1977.

Brody, E. M. Aged parents and aging children. In P. K. Ragan (Ed.), *Aging parents*. Los Angeles: The Ethel Percy Andrus Gerontology Center, 1979.

Brody, E. M. "Women in the middle" and family help to old people. *Gerontologist*, 1981, 21, 471–480.

Cantor, M. H. The informal support system of New York's inner city elderly: Is ethnicity a factor? In D. E. Gelfand and A. J. Kutzik (Eds.), *Ethnicity and aging*. New York: Springer, 1979.

Cantor, M. H. *Caring for the frail elderly: Impact on family, friends, and neighbors*. Paper presented at the 33rd Annual Scientific Meeting of the Gerontological Society of America, San Diego, November 1980.

Cicirelli, V. G. *Helping elderly parents*. Boston: Auburn, 1981.

Cohler, B. J., and Grunebaum, H. U. *Mothers, grandmothers, and daughters*. New York: Wiley, 1981.

Daniels, P., and Weingarten, K. *Sooner or later: The timing of parenthood in adult lives*. New York: Norton, 1982.

Fighting off old age. *Time*, February 16, 1981, p. 54.

Gordon, M. *Final payments*. New York: Ballantine, 1978.

Hagestad, G. O. Problems and promises in the social psychology of intergenerational relations. In R. W. Fogel, E. Hatfield, S. B. Kiesler, and E. Shanas (Eds.), *Aging: Stability and change in the family*. New York: Academic Press, 1981.

Harris, L., and Associates. *The myth and reality of aging in America*. Washington, D.C.: National Council on Aging, 1975.

Hess, B. B., and Waring, J. M. Parent and child in later life: Rethinking the relationship. In R. M. Lerner and G. B. Spanier (Eds.), *Child influences on marital and family interaction*. New York: Academic Press, 1978.

Hill, R., Foote, N., Aldous, J., Carlson, R., and MacDonald, R. *Family development in three generations*. Cambridge, Mass.: Schenkman, 1970.

Isaacs, B., Livingstone, M., and Neville, Y. *Survival of the unfittest*. London: Routledge and Kegan Paul, 1972.

Johnson, C. L. *Obligation and reciprocity in caregiving during illness: A comparison of spouse and offspring as family supports*. Paper presented at the 33rd Annual Scientific Meeting of the Gerontological Society of America, San Diego, November 1980.

Kovar, M. G. Elderly people: The population 65 years and over. In National Center for Health Statistics, *Health, United States: 1976–1977*. Washington, D.C.: United States Government Printing Office, 1977.

Lewis, M. A., Bienenstock, R., Cantor, M., and Schneewind, E. *The extent to which informal and formal supports interact to maintain the older people in the community*. Paper presented at the 33rd Annual Scientific Meeting of the Gerontological Society of America, San Diego, November 1980.

Lopata, H. Z. *Women as widows: Support systems*. New York: Elsevier-North Holland, 1979.

Lowenthal, M. F. *Lives in distress: The paths of the elderly to the psychiatric ward*. New York: Basic Books, 1964.

Murphy, D. *Wheels within wheels*. New York: Ticknor and Fields, 1980.

Neugarten, B. L. The awareness of middle age. In B. L. Neugarten (Ed.), *Middle age and aging*. Chicago: University of Chicago Press, 1968.

Raskind, M. A., and Storric, M. G. The organic mental disorders. In E. W. Busse and D. G. Blazer (Eds.), *Handbook of geriatric psychiatry*. New York: Van Nostrand Reinhold, 1980.

hanas, E. Social myth as hypothesis: The case of the family relations of old people. *Gerontologist*, 1979, *19*, 3–9. (a)

hanas, E. The family as a social support system in old age. *Gerontologist*, 1979, *19*, 169–174. (b)

hanas, E. Older people and their families: The new pioneers. *Journal of Marriage and the Family*, 1980, *42*, 9–15.

ilverstone, B., and Hyman, H. K. *You and your aging parent*. New York: Pantheon, 1976.

oldo, B. J. America's elderly in the 1980s. *Population Bulletin*, 1980, *35*, whole volume.

tueve, A. The elderly as network members. *Marriage and Family Review*, 1982, *5*, 59–87.

reas, J. Family support systems for the aged: Some social and demographic considerations. *Gerontologist*, 1977, *17*, 486–491.

roll, L. E., Miller, S. J., and Atchley, R. C. *Families in later life*. Belmont, Calif.: Wadsworth, 1979.

Chapter 9

Motherhood in the Middle Years
Women and Their Adult Children

VIVIAN WOOD, JANE TRAUPMANN, AND JULIA HAY

The mother–child relationship may well be the most salient and enduring relationship in human experience, and its importance does not stop when the child reaches adulthood. When Troll (1972) asked adult women and men of a wide age range to describe a person they knew, mothers and fathers were spontaneously referred to more frequently than any other persons. Baruch and Barnett (1983) found in a recent study that midlife women generally have very positive feelings about their mothers, and indeed their sense of well-being was tied to the quality of that relationship. Further, mothers relate to their offspring as adults for a much longer period than they relate to them as children (Goldberg and Deutsch, 1977, p. 317), and the time period during which mother and child relate to each other as adults is increasing. As Hagestad (1981) has pointed out, increased life expectancy is producing longer-term intergenerational bonds and, increasingly, the possibility that parents and children will grow old together. And because women generally outlive their husbands, it is mostly mothers and daughters who grow old together, often one or both having been widowed or divorced.

In this chapter[1] the focus will be upon the relationship between

Support for the development of this chapter and for carrying out the reported research was received from several sources: Administration on Aging Grant No. 90-A-1230 to the Faye McBeath Institute on Aging, University of Wisconsin-Madison; a project assistantship funded by a Ford Foundation grant to the Women's Studies Research Center, University of Wisconsin-Madison; and funds from the The Andrew W. Mellon Foundation grant given by Radcliffe College for research by Dr. Traupmann at the Henry A. Murray Research Center of Radcliffe College.

VIVIAN WOOD • School of Social Work, University of Wisconsin, Madison, Wisconsin 53706.   JANE TRAUPMANN • Family Development Center, Cambridge, Massachusetts, and 39 Pond Street, Natick, Massachusetts 01760.   JULIA HAY • Wisconsin Family Studies Institute, 1906 Monroe Street, Madison, Wisconsin 53711.

women and their adult children from the mother's perspective. The concern is with the relationship but the emphasis is on its meaning and consequence for the mother. For professionals concerned about the well-being of older people, it is of more than academic interest to understand what leads to the maintenance of good relationships between mother and child. Women, because they usually outlive their husbands, often find themselves in need of help in the later years of their lives. Studies indicate that the most likely source of help is their children, particularly their daughters (Shanas, 1979).

Because of the salience of relationships to older parents, gerontologists have given some attention to this area in their studies of old age. Much of the existing research, however, has not been systematic or explicit with regard to many dimensions. Studies often do not differentiate between sons and daughters or between fathers and mothers, and the ages of either the parents or the children are often not given. Furthermore, gerontologists' studies have focused primarily on proximity, social support, and help patterns, rather than on the quality of the relationships between elderly parents and their adult children (Rosow, 1965; Gibson, 1972). These studies generally have emphasized the positive aspects of the relationship—namely, that one or more of the older parents' children live nearby, and that they interact regularly and help each other in times of need.

The problem aspects of the relationship at this stage of the older generation's lives have for the most part been neglected. Incidents of elderly parents abused by their adult children, which have recently appeared in the media, suggest that this relationship can be fraught with problems and can lead to tragic results. Exploratory research in this area suggests there is parent abuse, but its prevalence and severity are still unknown (U.S. House of Representatives, 1980).

Because of the scientific neglect of what McCall and Simmons (1966, p. 202) have referred to as the "career of a relationship," the existing literature provides little understanding of the factors that influence the development and maintenance of the mother–child relationship as the child moves into and through adulthood. With the focus largely on infancy and childhood, the developing relationship of the mother with the child once he or she becomes an adult is little understood. There is some research on early-middle-aged parents launching their children into young adult roles; a hiatus in the research exists, however, between this stage and the point when parents are elderly and the children are middle-aged (Troll, Miller, and Atchley, 1979). What happens in the intervening 20 or more years? It seems highly unlikely that the relationship remains static, but we have very little knowledge of how changes in the lives of the mother and of the adult child affect the relationship. The offspring's becoming a parent automatically makes the mother a grand

mother. How do the mother's and the child's new roles affect the relationship? Does the fact that both the mother and the offspring are now
parents change the relationship? Is the impact different for mother–daughter and mother–son relationships? In these days when multiple generations are alive at the same time, often the mother will also be
the daughter of elderly parents; thus, the mother and her offspring will
share the fact that each of them is fulfilling both the parent and child
roles at the same time. Does the mother's relationship with her offspring
change when her parents die, she loses her daughter role, and becomes
the oldest generation in her family?

In sum, research on the mother–child relationship, with a few
important exceptions, has focused on the early years and has neglected
critical issues concerning the relationship after the child becomes an
adult. When mothers and offspring first relate to each other as adults,
the former are usually in their early middle years. This is apt to be an
important period developmentally for the mother as well as for the
child. Not only must mothers learn to relate to offspring as adults, these
"women in the middle" (Brody, 1981) are adjusting to the empty nest
and perhaps becoming mothers-in-law and grandmothers. Moreover,
mothers of this age may be dealing with developmental changes as
profound and diverse as going back to school (Traupmann, 1981), reentering the labor force, working out different relationships with their
husbands, and helping their elderly parents deal with the problems of
old age. Finally, there is the added dimension of integrating with these
activities the new realization that their own lives are finite, that they too
may find themselves old, feeble, and in need of care one day.

FRAMEWORKS FOR STUDYING ADULT FAMILIES

Models of socialization that imply a one-way flow of influence have
not been found to be very useful as a framework for examining the
mother–adult child relationship. Early students of adult intergenerational relations were generally concerned with values and behaviors
transmitted from older to younger generations, usually from parent to
child (see Troll and Bengtson, 1979, for a discussion of transmission
research). These studies showed that there is substantial but selective
intergenerational continuity within the family. Parent–child similarity
(which is considered evidence for transmission) is most noticeable in
religious and political areas, least in sex roles and life-style characteristics. Yet, as Troll and Bengtson (1979) point out, systematic theory in
this area remains undeveloped and generalizations remain tentative.
Formulations of socialization as a process of bilateral negotiation seem to
offer a more fruitful perspective for looking at such transmission phenomena. According to this approach, "relations between generations

are seen as a continuous bilateral negotiation in which the young and the old exchange information and influence from their respective positions in developmental and historical time" (Bengtson and Black, 1973, p. 207).

Findings from Fischer's (1981) research support the notion of continuous negotiation. She found that a daughter's marriage and becoming a mother led to a reordering of the mother–daughter relationship on both symbolic and interactional dimensions: Mothers and daughters reevaluated each other at the same time that they became more involved in each other's lives. For daughters, marriage was a way of demonstrating to their mothers a new adult status; becoming mothers themselves gave the daughters a new appreciation of their mothers' parenting role. With regard to interaction, married daughters with children had significantly more frequent contact with mothers than did married daughters without children.

Hagestad (1981) expands the notion of "continuous negotiation" with her discussion of historical changes in the family cycle, which have been brought about in part by increased life expectancy. Adults in the family, she points out, "now confront each other in relationships for which there is no historical precedence and minimal cultural guidance while they individually find themselves in life stages that also have few culturally shared expectations attached to them" (p. 25). Examples of these uncharted relations are a mother and a daughter who are both old and widowed at the same time; or the woman who becomes a step-grandmother when her daughter marries a divorcee with children from an earlier marriage. Hess and Waring (1978, p. 242), in a similar discussion of intergenerational relations among adults, conclude, "Clear normative prescriptions are lacking at the same time that choices of what to do are expanding." As Hagestad (1981, p. 25) has pointed out, adults in these ambiguous new relationships to a large extent have to negotiate and "create the structure and meaning of their bonds."

While the idea of continuous negotiation as "a process through which shared expectations are created" makes good sense, research for studying ongoing relationships faces tough methodological problems. The methodological issues of studying the development of an *individual* over time have been pointed out by developmental psychologists, with partial resolution of some issues through the use of cross-sequential methods (Schaie, 1970). Studying a *relationship* over time undoubtedly introduces new complexities that are yet to be dealt with. Not only does the relationship itself change with the passage of time, but also the two parties to the relationship dyad are changing; furthermore, these changes occur within a changing social milieu. (See Troll and Bengtson, 1979, for a discussion of these issues.)

DIMENSIONS OF RELATIONSHIPS IN ADULT FAMILIES

The study of an ongoing relationship at any stage in the life cycle requires a determination of the salient issues or dimensions of the relationship. This is complicated because some issues may be relevant to only one stage while others are pertinent to all or several stages, as Neugarten (1968) has pointed out in her essay on *individual* adult development. Bengtson (1982) has outlined four problem areas that family members often mention in regard to interaction between adult generations: (1) the challenges presented by changing roles and expectations accompanying growing up and growing old; (2) issues of autonomy and dependency—issues that seem to predominate when the child is young and again when the parent is old; (3) a just balance of giving and receiving between generations or, put another way, the issue of maintaining equity; and (4) the maintenance of continuity in the family and the avoidance of, or dealing with, disruptions such as those caused by divorce or death.

There has been research about each of these problem areas but its usefulness for understanding the mother–adult child relationship is limited. For example, many studies, such as Lowenthal and Chiriboga's (1972) study of the "empty nest," focus on one or the other member of the dyad—either the mother or the child—rather than on their relationship. Research on interaction and exchange of help between generations (Hill, Foote, Adlous, Carlson, and MacDonald, 1970; Shanas, Townsend, Wedderburn, Friis, Milhoj, and Stehouver, 1968; Sussman and Burchinal, 1962) has been largely descriptive and has been only peripherally concerned with the effect of such exchanges on the relationship between parent and child. Such research indicates that most older persons have at least one adult child living nearby with whom they interact regularly and exchange help when needed (see, for example, Shanas, 1979). The parents do most of the visiting and helping when the children are young adults, but the pattern is often reversed when parents move into advanced old age, particularly if they become ill and disabled. This research has emphasized that children do keep in touch and aid their older parents if needed. But researchers generally have not asked about children who fail to keep in touch and their reasons for lack of contact, leading Hagestad (1981) to suggest that it is time for such studies.

Schorr (1960) points out a gender difference in the mother–adult child relationship. He suggests that the widowed mother–daughter relationship is smoother and closer than the mother–son relationship. Because females in families have been primarily responsible for care-giving and household tasks, mothers and daughters can reciprocate these services, but mothers and sons often cannot. Sons are more likely to provide instrumental help such as financial assistance and advice—services mothers usually cannot return. The reciprocity of the mother–daughter relationship produces a more balanced relationship, while the one-way flow of the mother–son relationship tends to cause imbalance and often dependency. Data from our own study on differentiation in the relationship of mothers to their daughters and to their sons will be presented later in this chapter.

We turn now to a closer examination of two of the issues—dependency and equity—which Bengtson (1982) has designated problem areas.

Dependency

The mother–child relationship is unique in that dependency *is* so central—dependency of the infant and young child on the mother in the early years, a renegotiation of that dependency in the child's adolescence, typically a trading back and forth of the dependent role during the mother–adult child "middle period," then the possibility of increased dependency of the mother on the adult child in her old age.

Dependency, as a dimension of the mother–adult child relationship, is undoubtedly different from dependency in the mother–young child relationship, but the distinction has not been considered in much depth in the literature. Dependency is a major issue in old age; in literature on this period, however, the concept of dependency is used in many ways. In a monograph on dependency in old age, for example, the editor (Kalish, 1969) points out that the term *dependency* is used to refer to an interpersonal relationship, a condition, a personality characteristic, and a particular example of behavior. In this chapter, of course, we are concerned with dependency in the mother–adult child relationship. If we say that the mother is dependent on her daughter, for example, we imply that the daughter gives more than she receives in the relationship. Interrelated elements such as the sense of obligation, duty, and the norm of reciprocity muddy the picture and make clear distinctions difficult. The fact that dependency in old age is a sensitive topic further complicates the tasks of examination; while the dependency of the young child on the parent is normative, there is ambiguity concerning the dependency of the parent on the adult child. In addition, there are sensitive political implications embedded in the issues of dependency for women. Power, and thus powerlessness, are always factors in relationships in which one person necessarily depends on another. Most research has ignored these touchy issues when looking at family relationships. However, as women, often both daughters and mother

themselves, strive to understand their relationships better, this area is
no longer being ignored (Dinnerstein, 1976; Matthews, 1979; Rubin,
1979).

What have life-span scholars to say about dependency in adulthood? Rosow (1965) claims that the fact that children see and help their
older parents has been seen by many researchers as evidence of good
relationships based on affection and positive sentiments. He argues that
this should not be assumed but should be a question for investigation,
pointing out that children may maintain these ties out of a sense of
obligation that may strain rather than strengthen affectional bonds.
Blenkner (1965), in contrast, claims that a sense of duty enhances relationships between adult children and older parents, and Cicirelli's (1980)
research tends to support this idea.

Another body of research suggests an intriguing picture of the effects that feelings of obligation may have on mother–adult child relationships. On the one hand, research by Adams (1968b) and Lopata
(1973) shows that widowhood, which often creates a state of increased
need for the mother with resultant feelings of obligation on the part of
her children, may strain the relationship. On the other hand, divorce of
adult children, which may involve increased dependence of the younger
member of the dyad, may actually lead to an improved relationship
between the mother and her divorced child (Hagestad, Smyer, and
Stierman, 1983). A shift or an imbalance in dependency may be detrimental to the relationship. The importance of both parent and adult
child maintaining independence has been stated by anthropologists
Clark and Anderson (1967):

> A good relationship with children in old age depends, to a large extent, on
> the graces and autonomy of the aged parent—in short, on his ability to
> manage gracefully by himself. It would appear that, in our culture, there
> simply cannot be any happy role reversals between the generations, neither
> an increasing dependency of parent upon child nor a continuing reliance of
> child upon parent. The mores do not sanction it and children and parents
> resent it. The parent must remain strong and independent. If his personal
> resources fail, the conflicts arise. The child, on the other hand, must not
> threaten the security of the parent with requests for monetary aid or other
> care when parental income has shrunk through retirement. The ideal situa-
> tion is when both parent and child are functioning well.

Bengtson (1982, p. 92) agrees, arguing that "much of the drama of
intergenerational relations concerns issues of autonomy on the one
hand and dependency on the other." Kerckoff (1966), in a study of 135
couples, found that those who had the lower levels of mutual support
activities with their children had higher morale, noting that both dependency on children for living arrangements and propinquity of offspring
appeared to contribute to unhappiness in later life. In other words, high

morale was associated with relative independence of the two genera
tions. But, as Kerckoff suggests, there is no way to identify the directior
of causality in these findings since an elderly parent's low morale may
require the offspring to provide assistance, rather than the assistanc
fostering low morale. Johnson and Bursk (1977) found that poor healtl
and poverty contribute to dependency, and the greater the dependency
the more likely parents and children are to have negative feelings to
ward themselves and toward each other. It is important to note tha
mothers much more often than fathers are at risk of being dependent or
children. While 52% of women 65 and over are widowed, only 14% o
older men are. And women are more highly represented among the
aged poor than are men.[2] Thus, men more often than women have
spouse to depend on in later life; women, on the other hand, usuall
must turn to their children for care and assistance. So it is more often
mother's dependency than a father's that strains the relationship be
tween parent and adult child.

Matthews (1979), in looking at dependency and the balance of ex
change in elderly mother–adult child relationships, focuses on the ide
of power. Matthews argues that the current structure of the "modifie
extended family" does not give the old widowed mother a viable pos
tion in this group. The old mother, she suggests, is in a subordinat
position in her family because she is very likely to have only her off
spring as a source of support and needed services, and at the same tim
may have very little to offer in return. From the exchange theory per
spective that Matthews uses, the old mother with few resources ha
little power in relation to her offspring, creating an imbalanced relatior
ship. While the likelihood is high that the old widow's offspring hav
other sources of rewards and help, she may depend only on the relatior
ship with her children for rewards, particularly if she has always bee
family-centered. The importance of maintaining good relationships wit
her children is great and explains the necessity for complying with he
offspring's definition of her position in the family. Matthews gives ex
amples of how the children's treatment of their mother—unconsciously
perhaps—emphasizes her subordinate position. They drop in to see he
at their convenience, for example, but she is never made to feel free t
visit the children unannounced. Old mothers of the future, with mor
education and more advantageous economic positions, are less likely t
be dependent on children in later life. Indeed, one can imagine childre

---

[2]In 1978 36% of nonmarried older women had incomes below the poverty level, as cor
pared with 27% of nonmarried older men; only 8% of older men and women in coupl
had incomes below the poverty level (U.S. Department of Health and Human Service
1981).

nd grandchildren vying for invitations to the elderly widow's retirement condominium complete with swimming pool and other amenities.

In summary, many investigators consider dependency a key dimen-
ion in the "career" of the mother–adult child relationship. Dependency
is particularly salient when the child is an adolescent and is striving for
autonomy, and again when the mother is old and is attempting to maintain her independence. The mother–child relationship seems to be at its
est during the mother's middle years, when both parent's and child's
autonomy is unthreatened and both are capable of reciprocating care
and assistance.

Maintenance of Equity

The second key issue to be discussed here is related to what Bengt-
on (1982) called "a just balance of giving and receiving between genera-
ons." Family theorists have suggested that the norm of reciprocity
(Gouldner, 1960) is one of the most powerful of social forces sustaining
intergenerational ties for the middle-aged and their elderly parents.
Sussman (1976) describes this as an implicit bargain struck between the
generations such that the daily maintenance, provisions for education,
and general caring during the child's infancy and early years will be
reciprocated with similar services and caring in the parents' later years.
In the words of a mother of three boys now in their 30s, "My sons are
my old-age insurance."

There is disagreement among theorists, however, as to the effectiveness of the reciprocity norm for ensuring intergenerational care for
the elderly. Clark (1969) points out that social reciprocity is temporal in
nature. Because our culture is strongly oriented to present and future,
past services rendered or aid given does not bind the recipient for very
long to a request for reciprocity. Is a sense of fairness or equity apparent
between mothers and their adult children? Or is the current generation
of older mothers feeling a distinct lack of reciprocity for their long labors
of child-rearing?

A recent study of middle-aged and older women (Wood and Traupmann, 1980) sheds some light on these questions. A total of 187 mothers
were interviewed about their feelings as mothers and as daughters. The
interview was part of a large multidisciplinary study of women aged 50
to 93 conducted by the Faye McBeath Institute on Aging of the University of Wisconsin-Madison. The sample for the larger study was composed of 240 randomly selected women living in five different areas of a
small midwestern city. The theoretical framework for this research was
equity theory (Walster, Walster, and Berscheid, 1978), a social psychological theory concerned with fairness in interpersonal relations. Equity

theory states that individuals in equitable rather than inequitable relationships are happier and less distressed and are more likely to remain
in the relationship. Inequities in either an overbenefited or an underbenefited direction can be distressing, though the degree of distress for
those feeling they are getting more than they deserve (overbenefit) is
less severe than for those who feel they are getting less than they deserve (underbenefit).

There has been criticism of equity theory when applied to intimate
relationships, largely because it offends people's ideas of what such
relationships should be like. Many people believe that in relationships
based on love and family ties, people are not aware of what they give
and get but, rather, love unconditionally (e.g., Fromm, 1956), and that
an awareness of the patterns of give and take would surely spell the
relationship's demise (e.g., Murstein, Cerreto, and MacDonald, 1977)

Other theorists take the opposite view, that it is only through a
relationship based on the equality of contributions and of rewards that
intimacy flourishes (e.g., Scanzoni, 1972; Lederer and Jackson, 1968). It
may be that an awareness of the implicit bargain surfaces *only* when an
imbalance becomes acutely apparent—as when, for example, the wife
who has put her husband through medical school later finds him unin-
terested in her, or the mother who has struggled to raise four children
finds that they all settle thousands of miles away and only send birthday
cards once a year.

Miller (1976) suggests another twist to the issue of fairness in family
relations. She hypothesizes that women are socialized to accept less
than "a fair shake" from life. These expectations lead women to feel
distinctly guilty when they are the recipients of nurturance or special
kindnesses because they feel they do not deserve such benefits. Mothers, they believe, should be givers but not receivers.

The questions investigated in the Wisconsin study were whether
women would report an awareness of the fairness of exchanges that go
on in their family relationships and, if so, whether fairness or equity in
these family relationships was important to them. If the reciprocity
norm is operating with mothers and their adult children, it was expected
that women who feel content and happy with their sons and daughters
would report a sense of fairness about the relationship overall. Those
who feel distressed—angry, resentful, or guilty about their relationship
with their adult children—would report a distinct lack of fairness.

Most crucial to a test of the reciprocity norm, however, is a comparison of the perceived fairness in the childhood *and* in the parenthood of
the same individuals. Do men and women who have been generously
overbenefited in childhood then raise their own children in a similar
manner by giving so much that they then place themselves in an underbenefited position? And conversely, do underbenefited children go on

underbenefit their own offspring 20 years hence, thus putting them-
elves in an overbenefited position when their children show kindness
nd concern? In other words, is a repetition of the equity/inequity condi-
ons across generations the pattern we would be most likely to encoun-
r in a study of today's older generation?

An equally plausible prediction, elaborated by family theorists,
ikes just the opposite position (see Boszormenyi-Nagy and Spark,
973). Men and women who were underbenefited in childhood attempt
undo the inequity by overbenefiting their own children, thereby put-
ng themselves in an underbenefited position in adulthood with respect
their children. Examples of this cross-generational undoing abound in
opular folklore—the poor uneducated cleaning woman who works at
ree jobs to put her son through college, or the immigrant father who
icrifices in order to set his son up in business.

Since most of the respondents in the Wisconsin study were both
aughters and mothers, it was possible to examine equity/inequity ef-
cts across two generations. Respondents were asked to reflect on their
lationships with their adult children and with their parents. The ques-
ons asked were modified versions of standard equity questions used in
revious equity/intimacy research. (See Traupmann, Petersen, Utne,
d Hatfield, 1981, for a description of the development of these mea-
ires.)

First, after a series of questions about children and a brief introduc-
on to conceptualizing the complexities of family life in terms of "give
d take," respondents were asked the following question:

> When you think about all you did and do for your children and the joys and
> frustrations of raising them . . . and . . . all that they did and do for you and
> their joys and frustrations from their life with you, how do things "stack
> up"?
> 1. They got a much better deal.
> 2. They got a somewhat better deal.
> 3. They got a slightly better deal.
> 4. We got an equal deal.
> 5. I got a slightly better deal.
> 6. I got a somewhat better deal.
> 7. I got a much better deal.

Much later in the interview, after a series of questions about par-
its, the following question was asked:

> When you think about what you did for your parents and what you got from
> them and . . . what they did for you and got from you, how do things "stack
> up"? [The same 7-point scale for responses was used.]

The respondents were first placed in one of three groups on the
isis of relationships with children: (1) women who felt their children
ot a better deal—or who felt *underbenefited*, (2) women who felt the deal

was *equitable,* and (3) women who felt they got a better deal than their children or who felt *overbenefited.* A similar grouping was done in regard to their relationships with their parents.

The results were as follows: Most women felt a sense of fairness in both their relations with children and their relations with parents. Over two-thirds of the women reported that the relationship with their children was equitable, and nearly two-thirds reported the same about their relationship with their parents.

Second, most of those who felt relations were inequitable, whether they reported from the perspective of daughter or from that of mother, thought children generally got the better deal in relation to their parents. Of the daughters who perceived themselves inequitably treated, almost twice as many (64% compared to 36%) felt they, not their parents, had gotten a better deal. When the respondents changed their perspective to that of mother, the pattern of inequities remained in favor of children. Over twice as many mothers (68% vs. 32%) felt their children had received a better deal in the relationship than they had.

Turning to the cross-generational question either of repetition of inequities experienced in childhood or of the undoing of childhood inequities, an interesting pattern emerges. Those overbenefited as children tend to *repeat* that pattern with their own children (62% vs. 38%). Those underbenefited as children tend to report *undoing* that pattern with their own children (73% vs. 27%).

The Consequences of Inequities with Parents

If a sense of fairness or unfairness exists between mothers and adult children, how does it affect what they are willing to do for each other? One would expect that the underbenefited would have concluded in their own adulthood that their parents deserved little if anything from them now, since the balance had been tipped in the other direction for so long. Conversely, the overbenefited might feel a strong sense of obligation to repay the generous favors they received in childhood. In order to explore the consequences of inequities, women were asked to reflect on how the responsibility for care of their aging parents had been divided between them and their siblings, using the following question:

> In some families one son or daughter is primarily "in charge" of caring for aging parents. In other families these responsibilities are shared among the sons and daughters. How was it in your family?
>
> 1. Others (brothers, sisters, etc.) were solely in charge. I gave them no help or almost no help.
> 2. Others (brothers, sisters, etc.) were primarily responsible but I helped some.
> 3. We shared the responsibilities more or less equally.

4. I was primarily responsible but got some help from others.
5. I was solely in charge, I got no help or almost no help from others.

The results were surprisingly inconsistent with expectations. Of the women who felt underbenefited with respect to their parents—those expected to take little responsibility for parents in old age—a much greater percentage (57% vs. 26%) were taking primary responsibility for them than those in the overbenefited group were doing. Those in the overbenefited group either let others take responsibility (39%) or shared the responsibility with siblings (35%).

A word of caution: The data are complicated by the fact that some women had two living parents, some had only one living parent, and for the majority both parents were dead. Thus, some respondents, in answering the questions about their parents, were talking about ongoing relationships while others were speaking retrospectively of past relationships.

Given that qualification, the inconsistency between the reported inequities in older women's relationships with their parents and the parent care-giving they are subsequently prepared to do poses further interesting questions. Are parent–child relationships different from most relationships? Are the norms of expected behavior in the parent–child relationship so strong that what one *should* do overrides what one feels like doing? Are the patterns of the relationship so set when the children are young that they are not easily changed?

The reasons our respondents gave for keeping in contact with their parents had some relevance to these questions. Using scales developed by Adams (1968a), we asked women to assess the importance for them of different reasons for keeping in close contact with aging parents. The list of reasons included "feelings of obligation," "I need their help," "they need my help," and "enjoyment." Underbenefited women, we found, were most likely to place emphasis on a sense of obligation or on the fact that their parents needed them as the reasons for keeping in touch. The overbenefited women—those who thought they'd gotten the best of the deal in the relationship with their parents—were most apt to say they kept in touch with their parents because *they* needed their parents. These results suggest that early relationship patterns tend to persist, and that in some cases the norms of expected behavior override more immediate feelings.

THE CONSEQUENCES OF INEQUITIES WITH ADULT DAUGHTERS AND SONS

We have seen that feelings of inequity with parents in adulthood may affect one's sense of responsibility for care-giving and even one's feelings about simply keeping in touch with parents. What is known

about the consequences of inequity with sons and daughters in adult
hood? First, we found evidence that contradicts Miller's (1976) predic
tion that women prefer inequitable (underbenefited) rather than equita
ble relationships with their adult offspring. The happiest and leas
distressful relationships were the equitable relationships, followed firs
by the overbenefited and then by the underbenefited relationships. Als
noteworthy is the fact that the curve for daughters diverges at the tw
inequity points from that for sons, suggesting that there may be mor
distress associated with inequities with daughters than with inequitie
with sons, though the interaction was not statistically significant. Thi
differential distress between daughters and sons emerges clearly (and i
statistically significant) in the women's pattern of resentment about in
equity. Women express virtually no resentment toward sons, regardles
of whether their sons have treated them fairly or unfairly. However
resentment is expressed toward daughters who have given their moth
ers less than the mothers feel they deserve. This supports Gunhil
Hagestad's observation (cited in Troll et al., 1979, p. 97) that middle-age
mothers expect more interaction and help from their daughters and ar
upset when they do not get them. On the other hand, they expect mucl
less from their sons and are delighted with anything they get.

In sum, there does not seem to be a simple relationship betwee
feelings of equity in cross-generational relations and the way these rela
tionships are subsequently maintained. Equitable relationships seem t
be the predominant type and can be comfortably maintained in late
adult life. However, when feelings of inequity arise early on, a mor
complicated set of consequences seems to ensue that is not so readil
predictable from a simple equity theory framework. Inequities in th
overbenefited direction are more often attributed to children and ar
more likely to be replicated in the next generation than are inequities i
the underbenefited direction. However, overbenefited feelings do nc
seem to motivate subsequent care-giving behavior. Remarkably, it wa
those who felt underbenefited who more often took responsibility fc
care of parents in old age.

OTHER ISSUES

Dependency and equity were considered as independent concep
in this discussion. It should be apparent, however, that the two con
cepts are related. Dependency refers to a situation in which one membe
of a dyad receives more from the other member than he or she gives i
return. Equity, on the other hand, refers to the reaction of either mem
ber of the dyad in terms of whether he or she thinks the particul
balance of give and take is fair. These two concepts and related on

ich as obligation, duty, and reciprocity need further conceptual clarifi-
ition and deserve further study.

An important issue with regard to the mother's old age is whether
ie offspring's dependency on the mother in childhood has allowed the
iother to build up "credit," which is repaid in old age with care from
er child when needed. Johnson (1978), in an analysis of what contrib-
tes to a good relationship between older mothers and their daughters,
iund that the relationship the pair developed over many years and
irough many crises appeared, from the perspective of both the mothers
id the daughters, to have great relevance for the current quality of that
lationship. One research question to be resolved regarding the quality
: the mother–child relationship when the mother is old is whether the
ist long-term relationship or the current situation of the older mother
is greater effect.

One might also conjecture that the *objective* balance between depen-
ince and autonomy in the relationship is often less important than the
bjective reaction—whether both the mother and the child feel there has
:en a fair and equitable give and take in the relationship. A relationship
iat seems imbalanced and unfair to an outsider may be seen as per-
ctly fair and satisfactory to the parties involved. Relationships that
ay be most problematic are those in which one member of the dyad
ews the relationship as equitable and the other does not—for example,
ie son who takes for granted the scrimping and saving of his widowed
iother to put him through medical school and who then, as a successful
iysician, is ashamed of and avoids his mother.

SUMMARY

We have pointed out the neglect by researchers of the mother–child
lationship after the child becomes an adult. We referred to the increas-
g duration of this relationship as life expectancy has increased. We
iinted to the importance of understanding the development of this
lationship over time and to the special significance of the relationship
mothers in their advanced old age. Failure to study this relationship
ims in part from the lack of adequate frameworks for doing so, a
:uation that appears to be improving as students of intergenerational
lationships turn their attention to the quality of relationships between
irents and their adult children.

We examined in detail two dimensions of the relationship that the
erature suggests are salient to our understanding of this bond: depen-
 incy and equity. Data from our own study of older women and their
lationships to their parents and to their adult children were included
order to shed light on equity in mother–adult child relationships.

Attention was directed to the relationship between dependency and equity and to the need for conceptual clarification.

References

Adams, B. N. *Kinship in an urban setting*. Chicago: Markham, 1968. (a)

Adams, B. N. The middle-class adult and his widowed or still-married mother. *Social Problems*, 1968, *16*, 51–59. (b)

Baruch, G., and Barnett, R. Adult daughters' relationships with their mothers: The era of good feelings. *Journal of Marriage and the Family*, 1983, *45*, 601–606.

Bengtson, V. L. A generation gap? Research perspective on ways that generations interac In J. P. Rosenfeld (Ed.), *Relationships: Marriage and family reader*. Chicago: Scott Fore man, 1982.

Bengtson, V. L., and Black, O. Intergenerational relations: Continuities in socialization. I P. Baltes and W. Schaie (Eds.), *Life-span developmental psychology: Personality and s cialization*. New York: Academic Press, 1973.

Blenkner, M. Social work and family relationships in later life with some thoughts on fili maturity. In E. Shanas and G. Streib (Eds.), *Social structure and the family: Generation relations*. Englewood Cliffs, N.J.: Prentice-Hall, 1965.

Boszormenyi-Nagy, I., and Spark, G. M. *Invisible loyalties*. Hagerstown, Md.: Harper Row, 1973.

Brody, E. "Women in the middle" and family help to older people. *Gerontologist*, 1981, 2 471–482.

Cicirelli, V. *Age differences in adult children's feelings of closeness toward parents: Effects of fili obligation and partial dependency*. Paper presented at the annual meeting of the Amen can Psychological Association, Montreal, 1980.

Clark, M. Cultural values and dependency in later life. In R. Kalish (Ed.), *The dependenci of old people*. Ann Arbor: University of Michigan, Institute of Gerontology, 1969.

Clark, M., and Anderson, B. *Culture and aging*. Springfield, Ill.: Charles C Thomas, 196

Dinnerstein, D. *The mermaid and the minotaur*. New York: Harper & Row, 1976.

Fischer, L. R. Transitions in the mother–daughter relationship. *Journal of Marriage and t Family*, 1981, *43*, 613–622.

Fromm, E. *The art of loving*. New York: Harper & Row, 1956.

Gibson, G. Kin family network: Overheralded structure in past conceptualizations family functioning. *Journal of Marriage and the Family*, 1972, *34*, 13–23.

Goldberg, S., and Deutsch, F. *Life-span individual and family development*. Monterey, Cali Brooks/Cole, 1977.

Gouldner, A. The norm of reciprocity: A preliminary statement. *American Sociological R view*, 1960, *25*, 161–179.

Hagestad, G. O. Problems and promises in the social psychology of intergeneration relations. In R. Fogel, E. Hatfield, S. Kiesler, and E. Shanas (Eds.), *Aging: Stability an change in the family*. New York: Academic Press, 1981.

Hagestad, G. O., Smyer, M. A., and Stierman, K. Parent–child relations in adulthood: Th impact of divorce in middle age. In R. Cohen, B. Cohler, and S. Weissman (Eds Parenthood as an adult experience. New York: Guilford Press, 1983.

Hess, B., and Waring, J. M. Parent and child in later life: Rethinking the relationship. In M. Lerner and G. B. Spanier (Eds.), *Child influences on marital and family interactior* New York: Academic Press, 1978.

Hill, R., Foote, N., Aldous, J., Carlson, R., and MacDonald, R. *Family development in thr generations*. Cambridge, Mass.: Schenkman, 1970.

nson, E. S. "Good" relationships between older mothers and their daughters: A causal model. *Gerontologist*, 1978, *18*, 301–306.

nson, E. S., and Bursk, B. Relationships between the elderly and their adult children. *Gerontologist*, 1977, *17*, 90–96.

lish, R. Introduction. In R. Kalish (Ed.), *The dependencies of old people*. Ann Arbor: University of Michigan, Institute of Gerontology, 1969.

rckoff, A. C. Family patterns and morale in retirement. In I. H. Harper and J. C. McKinney (Eds.), *Social aspects of aging*. Durham, N.C.: Duke University Press, 1966.

derer, W. J., and Jackson, D. D. *The mirages of marriage*. New York: Norton, 1968.

pata, H. Z. *Widowhood in an American city*. Cambridge, Mass.: Schenkman, 1973.

wenthal, M. F., and Chiriboga, D. Transition to the empty nest: Crisis, challenge or relief? *Archives of General Psychiatry*, 1972, *26*, 8–14.

tthews, S. H. *The social world of old women*. Beverly Hills: Sage, 1979.

Call, G., and Simmons, J. L. *Identities and interaction*. New York: Free Press, 1966.

ler, J. B. *Toward a new psychology of women*. Boston: Beacon Press, 1976.

rstein, B. L., Cerreto, M., and MacDonald, M. G. A theory and investigation of the effect of exchange orientation on marriage and friendship. *Journal of Marriage and the Family*, 1977, *39*, 543–548.

ugarten, B. Adult personality: Toward a psychology of the life cycle. In B. Neugarten (Ed.), *Middle age and aging*. Chicago: University of Chicago Press, 1968.

sow, I. Intergenerational relationships: Problems and proposals. In E. Shanas and G. Streib (Eds.), *Social structure and the family: Generational relations*. Englewood Cliffs, N.J.: Prentice-Hall, 1965.

bin, L. *Women of a certain age*. New York: Harper & Row, 1979.

nzoni, J. *Sexual bargaining: Power politics in the American marriage*. Englewood Cliffs, N.J.: Prentice-Hall, 1972.

aie, W. A reinterpretation of age-related change in cognitive structure and functioning. In L. R. Goulet and P. B. Baltes (Eds.), *Life-span developmental psychology: Research and theory*. New York: Academic Press, 1970.

orr, A. L. *Filial responsibility in the modern American family*. Washington, D.C.: Social Security Administration, 1960.

anas, E. Social myth as hypothesis: The case of the family relations of old people. *Gerontologist*, 1979, *19*, 3–9.

anas, E., Townsend, P., Wedderburn, D., Friis, H., Milhoj, P., and Stehouver, J. *Old people in three industrial societies*. New York: Atherton Press, 1968.

ssman, M. The family life of old people. In R. Binstock and E. Shanas (Eds.), *Handbook of aging and the social sciences*. New York: Van Nostrand Reinhold, 1976.

ssman, M., and Burchinal, L. Kin family network: Unheralded structure in current conceptualizations of family functioning. *Marriage and Family Living*, 1962, *24*, 231–40.

upmann, J. *Women in midlife: The choice of continuing education*. Paper presented in the symposium Middle-Aged and Older Women and Achievement: Process and Implications, at the meeting of the American Psychological Association, Los Angeles, September 1981.

upmann, J., Petersen, R., Utne, M., and Hatfield, E. Measuring equity in intimate relations. *Applied Psychological Measurement*, 1981, *5*, 467–480.

ll, L. *Salience of family members in three generations*. Paper presented at the meeting of the American Psychological Association, Honolulu, 1972.

ll, L., and Bengtson, V. L. Generations in the family. In W. Burr, R. Hill, F. Ivan Nye, and I. Reiss (Eds.), *Contemporary theories about the family* (Vol. 1): *Research-based theories*. New York: Free Press, 1979.

ll, L., Miller, S., and Atchley, R. *Families in later life*. Belmont, Calif.: Wadsworth, 1979.

U.S. Department of Health and Human Services, Social Security Administration, Office c
    Research and Statistics. *Income and resources of the aged, 1978* (SSA Publication C
    13–11727). Washington, D.C.: U.S. Government Printing Office, October 1981.

U.S. House of Representatives, Select Committee on Aging (96th Congress, First Session,
    Elder abuse: The hidden problem (Comm. Pub. No. 96–220). Washington, D.C.: U.S
    Government Printing Office, 1980.

Walster, E., Walster, G. W., and Berscheid, E. *Equity: Theory and research.* Boston: Ally
    and Bacon, 1978.

Wood, V., and Traupmann, J. *The aging women project: Final report.* Unpublished manu
    script, University of Wisconsin, 1980.

Black Women in the Middle Years

EANNE SPURLOCK

WHO ARE WE?

According to the U.S. Bureau of Census (1980), Afro-American women the 35–54 age range represented 1.23% of the total population in 1979. Black women between the ages of 55 and 60 represented less than .5% of the population.

Like all groups of people, there is diversity among us. Because a greater percentage of us are from poverty backgrounds, we are likely to age quickly and are vulnerable to disorders that are related to poverty. For example, we are likely to have had poor or limited access to adequate health care services, and to face middle age with concern about our physical health. If we have had limited formal education, we are still likely to be working at lower level, low-paying jobs, or, burdened with physical and mental health problems, we survive with welfare assistance and/or Social Security disability payments. Not all of us, though; some of us struggle out to work daily even though feeling poorly.

Those of us who were born into families that were relatively free of economic crises are more likely to have had reasonably adequate health care. Even so, we may be experiencing concern about current physical health problems. Many are likely to be taking medication for hypertension, a common disorder among the Afro-American people. We may be troubled about the flare-up of arthritis or complications of diabetes, or other chronic physical disorders. Some of us are bothered with the physical signs of menopause; others experience no untoward physical reactions and have a sense of freedom.

JEANNE SPURLOCK • American Psychiatric Association, 1700 18th Street, N. W., Washington, D.C. 20009.

Having been motivated to pursue formal education, some of us have become reasonably financially secure in our chosen careers. In some professions, we find ourselves stuck at the lower levels of pay scales even though our responsibilities have expanded during the course of employment.

We are represented in politics, in both elected and appointed positions. Some of us have become nationally known in various fields; for others, the fame of yesteryear has faded, and some are yet struggling for recognition in their middle years. So it is in academe, journalism, and any number of other professions. Perhaps a greater number of us are invisible to the broader community.

We are never-married, married, separated and/or divorced, and widowed. Our coloring is black, brown, "high yellow," and even lighter. Some of us may be more preoccupied about our weight, age spots, and dry skin than we were about color in our adolescence. At middle age, many of us are more concerned about the thinning of our hair than about its texture. Others are taking the physical signs of middle age in stride, and fret little, if any, about the natural youthfulness of some of our sisters. We are represented in the statistics of the depressed and the well-adjusted. Some of us are involved in midcareer changes; others are adjusting to early retirement. We are represented among blue- and white-collar workers, as well as among the self-employed in both stable and unstable businesses.

Our sources of entertainment are varied. For some of us weekly bowling is a must; others struggle to play a decent game of tennis. Some of us are not so physically active and seek entertainment in sedentary activities. Because of financial restrictions and/or fear of night travel, television is the primary source of entertainment for many.

As most of the foregoing examples show, we respond to middle age no differently than women of the majority group in the United States. These examples also show the need to counteract concepts stereotyping Afro-American women. However, our position of double jeopardy—our race and our gender—often accounts for differences when we are compared to white women. Some of us bring to middle age the painful memories of overt racial discrimination and continue to maintain a stance of assertiveness, if not militancy. Others of us appear to have become masters at denial.

The range of differences has been observed in both personal and professional contacts, and within the author's family structure. The differences were also reflected in the answers to a questionnaire that was circulated informally to a small sample of black women (50 in number).

The differences and similarities among us are outlined in more de-il in the sections to follow. Sketches from the professional literature nd a view from the popular press precede a series of vignettes from the ens of Afro-American women poets and writers. Descriptions of vari- us intrafamilial relationships are extracted from personal and profes- ional experiences. Subsequent sections focus on the men (or absence of nen) in our lives, the range of our economic status, our involvement (or ck of involvement) in the women's movement, and patterns of adapta- on or maladaptation.

EHAVIORAL SCIENCE AND BLACK WOMEN

The absence of specific references to black women of middle age in a umber of widely read publications of black behavioral scientists is strik- g. Aging, middle age or midlife, and menopause are topics not to be und in the index of Staples's (1973) *The Black Woman in America*. Al- ough the entries that focus on other topics such as "marriage," "ma- iarchal structure," "role, female" can relate to the period of middle ge, this particular phase of life is not specifically referred to in the text. ckson's (1973) excellent review of the role of Afro-American women es not specifically address life phase differences. However, a number class and educational differences addressed by Jackson are of signifi- nce in the middle years. She challenges the premise that black women ave had greater opportunities for varied occupations than white wom- and suggests that only two kinds have been available for the most rt—(1) the traditional female profession of teaching, and (2) domestic nployment, the latter "almost solely reserved for Black females in the uth."

Ladner (1972) discusses the black female-headed household, vis-à- s the roles necessary for the black women to play: "Today Black wom- play highly functional and sometimes autonomous roles within the mily and society because the same economic and social conditions hich allowed for the emergence of a female dominated society during avery still perpetuate this type of family structure." According to dner, black women are perceived dualistically—the pillar of strength rsus the symbol of immorality. This duality renders the black woman able to compete with white women, a condition which has until re- ntly accounted for many of the problems and conflicts of black wom- . It should be emphasized that Ladner sees this problem primarily as a ing of the past: "the new thrust toward Black consciousness and Black entity have allowed for the development of an internal set of stan- rds by which many Black women have begun to judge themselves. erefore, the conflict which was caused because of the incongruity tween white versus Black identification models has lessened, and

white conceptions of womanhood have ceased to have the same rele
vance they once had" (p. 42).

Illustrations of Ladner's premise can be found in a number o
areas—from the selection of campus queens to the latest fashions i
various fields of advertising. Those of us with broad facial features, dar
complexions, or short hair can see similar images in fashion magazines
in campus publications, and/or on the television screen. This is not t
suggest that a positive sense of self is dependent upon the externa
environment, but it serves to underscore the importance of cultura
beliefs and mores.

In their 1968 publication, *Black Rage*, Grier and Cobbs describe i
narrow, if not biased, language the black woman's effort to cope wit
her negative image, as defined by the broader society: "Letting yout
go, beauty go, and sex go, they narrowed their vision to the most esser
tial feminine function—mothering, nurturing, and protecting their chi
dren" (pp. 53–54). The Grier-Cobbs premise does not stand up if on
carefully surveys the various groupings within the black female popula
tion, or even within a single group. This author thinks it unlikely tha
"beauty products" are important only to nonblack women. The depa
ture of a woman's mate is not necessarily accompanied by her "le
ting . . . sex go" and restricting herself to the mothering role. In advan
ing their premise, Grier and Cobbs overlooked the scores of blac
middle-aged women, of matronly and striking appearance, who a
involved in an ongoing relationship with a male companion, or thos
who are actively involved in church and/or other community project
This author suggests that the narrowness of vision is more that of Gri
and Cobbs rather than that of the women they describe.

The rearing of her children's children, whether as her own or as he
grandchildren, is commonly experienced by black women. As wit
women in other groups, these experiences may or may not be studde
with conflict. Lawrence (1975) provided several vivid illustrations
generational relationships that are conflicted in her account of the nu
turing figures and noxious elements of an inner-city community. Th
child is often caught up in the mother–grandmother antagonisms.

> When separation and loss are devastating, anger is severe. The nurse has
> brought a 20 year old mother, Ms. Jones, into the well-baby station for
> consultation with the psychiatrist. The woman was accompanied by two-
> year-old twins, a boy and a girl. The twins would talk to everyone in the
> house but the mother. The mother had been accused of "battering" her
> seven-year-old daughter, Patsy, who had then been removed to a small state
> school. During the consultation, the twins rarely made physical contact with
> the mother. As the mother talked . . . the girl twin began to cry. . . . One of
> the conference participants said to the mother, impatiently, "Pick her up."
> "What do you want me to do, pet her?" retorted the mother. "That's what

ruined my Patsy. My mother pet her." "You mean that your mother petted her more than she pet you," the psychiatrist proposed. "My mother didn't raise me. She sent me to my grandmother's when I was a baby." This mother had little insight into her own feelings of abandonment at this time; nor of their significance in her relations with her children. (Lawrence, 1975, pp. 72–73)

owever, as Lawrence points out, grandmothers often comfortably ᴀare in the nurturing process and reinforce that which is provided by e parents. In their longitudinal study of the impact of family structure ᴀd functioning on the mental health of children, Kellam *et al.* (1978) so illustrate the positive role played by grandmothers in one-parent ᴍilies. In addition, Furstenberg (1976) has found that the preschool ᴛildren of black adolescent mothers whose relatives (particularly the ᴀternal grandmothers) participated in child-rearing functioned at a ore advanced level than those preschoolers who were not cared for ᴀrt-time by relatives.

That so many black female-headed households exist is related to the crease in the divorce rate in the black population and to the apparent nited opportunity that black women have for remarriage (Staples, ʹ78). Barriers to remarriage, especially the diminishing number of ᵛailable black men, are related to the existence of such households.

ᴋᴏᴍ ᴛʜᴇ Pᴇɴs ᴏꜰ Bʟᴀᴄᴋ Wʀɪᴛᴇʀs

Black women in their middle years are portrayed both ster-ᵊtypically and as diverse in contemporary writings. Guy-Sheftall (1979) ᵊtes the diversity and complexity of black women in the poetry created ᵛ Gwendolyn Brooks. Brooks's poem "Sadie and Maude" (1962) viv-ly illustrates the breadth of the diversity.

> Maude went to college.
> Sadie stayed at home.
> Sadie scraped life
> With a fine-tooth comb.
>
> She didn't leave a tangle in.
> Her comb found every strand.
> Sadie was one of the livingest chit
> In all the land.
>
> Sadie bore two babies.
> Under her maiden name.
> Maude and Ma and Papa
> Nearly died of the shame.
>
> When Sadie said her last so-long
> Her girls struck out from home.

(Sadie had left as heritage
Her fine-tooth comb.)

Maude, who went to college,
Is a thin brown mouse.
She is living all alone
In this old house.

The tone of loneliness that is experienced by Maude is again suggested
in another Brooks poem, "A Sunset in the City" (1962).

Already I am no longer looked at with lechery or love.
My daughters and sons have put me away with marbles
    and dolls,
Are gone from the house.
My husband and lovers are pleasant or somewhat polite
And night is night.
It is a real chill out,
The genuine thing.
I am not deceived, I do not think it is still summer
Because sun stays and birds continue to sing.
It is summer-gone that I see, it is summer gone
The sweet flowers in drying and dying down,
The grasses forgetting their blaze and consenting to
    brown.

A mechanism for dispelling loneliness or an expression of a driving
ambition for leadership, possibly arising from an unsatisfactory marriage—these are themes that Mary Carter Smith (1970) satirically presents in "Clubwoman."

Chairman of many committees
At club meetings she's a must—
But her spouse scrambles eggs for his supper
And her furniture's covered with dust.

For some black women, middle age, as portrayed by black writers,
reflects the psychology of oppression. The need for and the protective-
ness of silence is penned by Barbara Chase-Riboud (1979) in her novel
Sally Hemming. The author sets the stage in which Sally, at age 56, views
the census taker at a distance and reflects on the past: "Her silence was
what had kept her alive and sane in this world where everything had
been taken from her except these last two sons. And even they knew
little about her life. Slaves revealed as little as possible about their origins
and background to their children. It was an old trick. Not to speak was
not to put into words the hopelessness of having no future and no past"
(p. 14).

The continuing pattern of "holding back" is described in a lighter
vein by Mari Evans (1971) in "When in Rome." The experiences of

cribed in the poem are commonplace among the scores of domestic
orkers, who, in their middle years, continue in the only kind of work
ey know.

> Mattie dear
>> the box is full
> take
>> whatever you like
> to eat . . .
>>> (an egg
>>> or soup
>>> . . . there ain't no meat).
> there's endive there
>> and cottage cheese. . .
>> (whew if I had some
>> black-eyed peas . . .)
> there's sardines
>> on the shelves
>> and such
>> but
>> don't get my anchovies . . .
>> they cost
>> too much!
>> (me get the
>> anchovies indeed!
>> what she tink she got—
>> a bird to feed?)
> there's plenty in there
> to fill you up . . .
>>> (yes'm. just the
>>> sight's
>>> enough!)
> (. . . Hope I lives till I get home
>> I'm tired of eatin'
>> what they eats
>> in Rome . . .)

And a return to a somber tone in Gloria Gayles's (1979) "Sometimes
Women Only." In the last stanza, she writes:

> sometimes
> as women only
> do we weep
> we are taught to whisper
> when we wish to scream
> assent
> when we wish to defy
> dance pretty
>> (on tiptoe)
> when we would raise circles of dust
> before the charge

INTRAFAMILIAL RELATIONSHIPS

Information obtained from the returns of the questionnaire pre viously referred to, although only suggestive, parallels that reported by other investigators (Ladner, 1972; Staples, 1973, 1978) and observed in professional and personal life experiences of the author.

In response to a question about support networks, respondent listed family members as central figures. Significantly, this respons characterized the unmarried as well as the married women. For exam ple, a 35-year-old divorcee lives alone but is very much a part of he brother's family of five; a 50-year-old never-married educator holds similar position in her married sister's family. It has been the experienc of the author that many single adults who live alone are integral mem bers of a family system, as are single adults who share a household with a family unit. The importance of the extended family was pinpointed in the frequent identification of the grandparents as the primary care givers during the respondents' childhood years.

It is of some significance that the church was often identified as a important unit in the current support system. Fellow church member were viewed as the extended family by some. This view of the churc was held both by women who had continued an affiliation with th denomination with which they were identified as children and by th converts to another denomination.

Stack (1974) has written of the successful development and utiliza tion of kin networks among lower-class black women in urban commu nities. There is no question that such systems have reinforced strength and permitted survival for many in the networks. Indeed, in the exper ence of this author, this pattern is not confined to the working poor bu is commonly utilized throughout each socioeconomic class. The value o networking has been addressed and utilized by a number of black wom en's civic and social groups.

For most people, middle age brings about changes in intrafamili relationships. It is no different for black women. Some relationship have improved; others have been terminated. One 50-year-old moth of three daughters reported that she now has a positive mother–daugh ter/friend relationship with each of her young adult children. The earli relationships were studded with conflict, especially during the storm adolescence of the middle child. Of significance, too, was the change i the nature of her relationship with her husband. After years of episod philandering, he was now, at 58, continuously emotionally committe to his family.

For some women, middle age is equated with loss and with disrup tion of some family relationships. When marriages break up and the e

usband becomes involved with a much younger woman, middle age
in be a painful period. The pain is often compounded by financial
ifficulties, reinforced by the ex-husband's inability or unwillingness to
ssume responsibilities for child support. This kind of situation often
ys the groundwork for difficulties in the divorcee's relationship with
er children, whatever their age. On the other hand, for those women
ho feel secure about themselves as a person, the middle years are
ewed as a new beginning; the divorce is a relief and paves the way for
nprovement of some intrafamilial relations.

Middle age has been a time of remarriage for some women, and for
first marriage for a smaller number. Such marriages mean the begin-
ng of many new relationships with the spouse's family. New relation-
iips and the modification of the old also develop as children marry and
andchildren are born. A number of factors will determine the nature
' the changes. Some mothers (and fathers) like their children-in-law
id easily establish rapport. In contrast, if marriage of one's child is
ewed as a loss, the relationship is likely to be in some jeopardy.

Because of the greater vulnerability of black men to poor health, a
ack women is likely to face middle age as a widow or to face the added
sponsibilities of a chronically ill spouse. Again, the nature of the
anges, if any, in the intrafamilial relationships is dependent upon a
imber of variables. The stability/instability of the family's economic
atus is not the least important.

For many black women, middle age is another period of mother-
g—now, the mothering of her grandchildren or children of her sib-
igs or members of the extended family. Women in the lower so-
economic bracket are more likely to bear the responsibility for the care
the children of their adolescent daughters. Women at every so-
economic level are likely to assume at least partial responsibility for a
andchild as the young mother struggles alone or with her husband to
nake it." Again, the nature of the relationships varies and sometimes
rallels the character of the earlier mother–child ties.

IE ABSENCE AND PRESENCE OF THE MEN IN OUR LIVES

Staples (1978) notes that the "black underclass is prevented by in-
rnal colonialism from achieving success in marriage" (p. 82) and that
ack women have fewer opportunities than their white counterparts for
marriage. A sizable percentage of middle-aged black women, who are
so a part of the underclass, are without husbands (although there may
 men in their lives). This pattern may also be characteristic of middle-
ass women in their middle years. The diminishing number of available

black men who are viewed as potential mates by the divorced, widowed, or never-married black woman has been attributed to a number of factors. Staples (1978) writes: "With 25 percent of Black males unemployed, it is not surprising to find a disproportionate number of them in prisons and the military or narcotized by drugs. But the most significant social trend is the spiraling mortality rate of Black males" (p. 86). According to 1980 Bureau of Census data, 125,000 deaths of black men took place in 1978, as compared to 124,000 in each of the previous 3 years, and as compared to 108,000 in 1960.

For some married women in their middle years the marriage is a union in name only. Staples suggests that "high status Black males often view women as property and impose rigid rules of sexual fidelity for their wives, while participating themselves in a number of extramarital affairs" (p. 84). The middle-class woman may be more likely to tolerate this behavior and seek to maintain the marriage because a divorce might well result in the modification of her middle-class status. She might elect to become involved in an affair herself, or to be celibate.

For other married women, their middle years have brought a closer union with their husbands of some 20–30 years. Some, after years of discord, and even after periods of separation, become friends again and enjoy doing things together.

Within each socioeconomic grouping there are men who are abusive and others who are considerate and supportive. The woman in the life of the abusive man is likely to be the victim of his anger and frustration, generated by his own victimization in the broader society. Some of the men in the lives of middle-aged women are younger; some are in the same age range; others are much older. There appears to be a lessening of criticism directed toward the woman who elects to form a relationship with a younger man, and clearly this kind of relationship occurs within all socioeconomic groups. Men from other racial groups play an integral role in the lives of some black women. No longer are "acceptable" interracial unions confined to individuals in the entertainment fields (if they ever were), as illustrated by Lewis (1978).

Economic Status

In our excellent historical review of the employment of black women from 1910 to the early 1970s, Jackson (1973) points out that "Black women have traditionally occupied positions of lower status than is true of Black men, assertions to the contrary notwithstanding" (page 255). Staples (1978) cites significant statistics from the United States Women's Bureau: "1,500,000 people were employed in private household work in 1970. Almost two-thirds of them were Black. The medial income for full ime, year-round household workers was approximately $1,800 per year. . . . Two out of three are at least partly self-supporting and one out of eight is head of a family." Ladner (1975), too, provides supportive evidence for Jackson's view in her citation of 1973 data for the year-round civilian labor force. The annual income of the black female worker was at the bottom of the heap when compared to her white counterparts, and to black as well as white men.

Black women have shared the benefits of the affirmative action and equal opportunity programs with black men, white women, and members of other minorities. It is often suggested that the gains made by black women have been greater than those experienced by black men. An argument sometimes used to support this notion is that hiring agents seize the opportunity to meet two goals of affirmative action policy by hiring a black woman, who is a "double minority." However, the tenacity of discriminatory patterns has prevented such a practice in many settings. Jackson (1973) cites an example:

> I, myself, have experienced several Southern situations where my educational attainment surpassed that of White female employees. Usually the racial undertones were onerous. In one specific local community mental health center, several educated Black females were categorically rejected for positions as nurses and social workers by the director (a psychiatrist of foreign birth), despite their over-qualifications. . . . The inexperienced and racially-prejudiced director catered to [the] White female prejudices . . . [that] it was too difficult for them to view any Black female in any working relationship exclusive of domestic service. The director assumed that the Blacks ought to understand that and wait until the attitudes of the Whites had changed. (p. 234)

Even with ongoing discriminatory practices, black women have become more visible in various professions, businesses, and other male-dominated careers and vocations. Ladner (1975) cautions that this new visibility is open to misinterpretation. The small number of black women who hold positions of status, or who have made considerable advancement in the world of work, "have had little effect on the status of the average black woman" (page 76). According to a report of the U.S. Department of Commerce, Bureau of Census (*The Social and Economic Status of the Black Population in the U.S.: An Historical View, 1970–78*), "The occupational changes for Black women from 1949 to 1970 . . . were mainly in the white collar and service groups."

The overwhelming majority of black women arrive at and live through the middle years burdened by economic problems. For them, the message penned by Langston Hughes (1970) in his poem "Mother to Son" conveys their feelings. For them, life "ain't been no crystal stair," nor do they expect it to be in their middle years, but they will keep on climbin'."

THE WOMEN'S MOVEMENT: INVOLVEMENT VERSUS NONPARTICIPATION

The history of Afro-Americans is studded with references to the efforts of women in activities directed toward liberation of black people—both women and men—as well as of all women. Walker (1976) notes the activities of Sojourner Truth at women's rights meetings, and the active campaigning of others, directed toward full emancipation for black women. The encounters that black women have had with sexism have not been infrequent and are as much a part of contemporary times as they were during the height of the abolitionist movement. However, black women in general have not been active in the contemporary women's movement, nor have they shown much enthusiasm for the movement.

A question regarding support of the women's movement was included in the survey questionnaire. Responses were mixed. One respondent wrote, "The racist history of the Women's Movement and the plight of Blacks negates my being a member." Some noted only partial support; others responded affirmatively and with no words of exception. Some black women have expressed the feeling that efforts directed toward the women's movement would dilute those that are still needed in the arena of the civil rights struggle. Others, stunned at the accusations that the advancement of black women has stunted that of black men, have hotly refuted these charges, and have encouraged support of the women's movement and the ratification of the Equal Rights Amendment as furthering the liberation of men as well as women. Jackson's (1973) call has a tone of urgency:

> Black women must increase their participation in the racial and feminist liberation movements, and they can find no better role models than Sojourner Truth and March Church Terrell. Their direct participation in the women's liberation movement is very critical, so that there will be no question of Black women being left out in the kitchen or the nursery. The "heat" should be placed upon those White Women who persist in believing that Black women do not wish to be liberated! (p. 255)

The labeling of the women's movement as white, middle-class (and possibly middle-aged, in view of the limited attention given to the needs of elderly women) has limited the interest that black women have shown. Beal (1970) is as discouraging of black women's involvement as Jackson has been encouraging. It has also been suggested (Hare and Hare, 1972) that black women's inactivity in the movement is not necessarily related to lack of interest and/or objections to the stated goals, but is due to their having been denied policy-making roles—"white women always dominate in coalitions and are always in charge" (p. 180). They also note that "it appears to some that white and black women are in

ace to change places. The white woman is trying to escape the drudgery
of the home for rewarding employment outside, while the black woman
still longs to escape the labor force and to get into the home."

Walker (1976) cites words of wisdom in an address given by Fannie
Jackson Coppin, a black teacher, social worker, and lecturer. The date of
the address is significant; it was given at the Woman's Congress of 1894:

> Not till race, color, sex, and condition are seen as the accidents and not the
> substance of life; not till the universal title of humanity to life, liberty and the
> pursuit of happiness is conceded to be inalienable to all; not till then is
> woman's lesson taught and woman's cause won—not the white woman's
> nor the black woman's nor the red woman's but the cause of every man and
> every woman who has writhed silently under a mighty wrong. (p. 361)

COPING PATTERNS AND BREAKDOWNS

Not unlike women of other groups, scores of black women face and
move through middle age free of major conflicts. They just "keep on
keeping on" For some, development continues; witness the growing
number who are returning to school as reentry students, to begin or
complete college or postgraduate education. The experiences of a friend
of the author provide a vivid illustration.

> E.J., who had returned to college as a part-time student when her youngest
> was in upper elementary school, graduated at age 45. She states that reentry
> was not the easiest experience in her life. The encouragement and support
> she received from her family (husband and two children still at home) helped
> in the binding of her anxiety. She went on to graduate school and now holds
> a responsible administrative position.
>
> At first glance, one would assume that E.J. is an exceptional person. So
> she is, but she is not alone. A survey of black women students—all reentry
> students—at a state university in a midwestern city, reveals many similar
> situations. (Jones, in press)

Those of us who have experienced conflicts of significance have, in
many instances, developed successful behavioral patterns to stem the
tides of discomfort and unrest. For many (maybe more at the lower
socioeconomic levels), a flight into religion and strict morality have been
the routes taken. Novelist Toni Morrison's (1970) description of Pauline
Breedlove (in *The Bluest Eye*), a mother of two, who had been verbally
and physically abused by her husband, is a graphic example: "All the
meaningfulness of her life was in her work. For her virtues were intact.
She was an active church woman, did not drink, smoke or carouse,
defended herself mightily against Cholly (her husband) . . ." For a mul-
titude of black people, church services have been "a place to discharge
frustration and hostility so that one could face injustice and hardship the

rest of the week" (Comer, 1972, p. 16). Of equal importance is the feeling of belonging that is fostered in the black-oriented religious services.

Some of us have utilized defenses that have been maladaptive. Many of us have continued a lifelong tendency to be passive-aggressive; others have been given to hypochondriasis or somatization. A sizable number of us have continued to direct considerable energies to efforts to control others in our immediate environments. It is as if these maneuvers help to bind our anxiety generated by our powerlessness. A 53-year-old widowed mother of eight tended to accentuate her efforts to inject her comments and guidance in every contact (most of which she initiated) with her adult children. She recalled that the broadening of this pattern coincided with her perception of her entry into middle age, a period that she equated with losses.

Depression of incapacitating intensity has either become more commonplace in black women or is more frequently diagnosed. In the author's experience as a clinician, there has been more than a hint that many of these women, some of whom are driven to overeat and/or to drink too much, seek initial help from a primary care physician and are treated symptomatically. Thus, the core problem is not addressed.

It has been reported that involutional melancholia is higher in women from low-income groups and those in low-prestige occupations (Ford, 1975). Since the majority of black women are in such groupings, it might be assumed that this disorder is commonly experienced by them. However, it is also noted by Ford that "minority ethnic groups are relatively less evident in the psychiatric population during the involutional years" (p. 1027). It is possible that black women are not properly diagnosed and/or not treated, or are treated by physicians other than psychiatrists.

As previously pointed out, black women are likely to be more susceptible to specific physical disorders because of poor and limited health care services. Findings relevant to this point were described at a Mini consultation on the Mental and Physical Health Problems of Black Women (1975). For example:

> The effects of hypertension are particularly significant for Black women: while it occurs less frequently among Black women than among Black men, it attacks Black women with greater severity. Heart failure is very common. . . . Physicians' figures indicate that hypertension is probably the primary cause of death for Black women between the ages of 40 and 45. (p. 1)
>
> Invasive cancer . . . has two times greater incidence than that occurring in the white population. . . . (p. 11)
>
> Poverty works to deny adequate medical attention for the Black victim of breast cancer. (p. 11)

SUMMARY

In the preceding pages, emphasis has been placed on the diversity among us, as well as on the differences and commonalities when we are compared to white women. For the most part, what we bring to middle age depends upon how life has dealt with us before and how we have dealt with life.

Most of us are a part of a family unit, even if we live alone and the family members are our adoptive kin. Our relationships with the men in our lives are varied. We may be lonely at times, or a great deal of the time, but some of us are vibrant most of the time.

We are dirt-poor, and we are affluent. We work at blue-collar and white-collar jobs; we are represented in most of the professions. We are on welfare, and we are independently well off. We are Democrats, Independents, and Republicans (in alphabetical order); some of us have never voted. A few of us have been publicly rewarded for our achievements and our contributions to the betterment of black people and the society at large; some of us are unknown and unsung heroines. Some of us are sick, so very tired, and defeated at middle age. The more fortunate among us have successfully overcome obstacles or had few to circumvent, and are content in our middle years.

REFERENCES

Beal, F. M. Double jeopardy: To be black and female. In R. Morgan (Ed.), *Sisterhood is powerful*. New York: Random House, 1970.

Brooks, G. A sunset in the city. In *Selected poems*. New York: Harper & Row, 1963.

Cannon, M. S., and Locke, B. Z. Being black is detrimental to one's health: Myth or reality? *Phylon*, 1977, *38*(4): 408–442.

Chase-Riboud, B. *Sally Hemmings*. New York: Viking Press, 1979.

Comer, J. P. *Beyond black and white*. New York: Quadrangle Books, 1972.

Evans, M. When in Rome. In J. David and M. Watkins (Eds.), *To be a black woman: Portrait in fact and fiction*. New York: William Morrow, 1971.

Ford, H. Involutional melancholia. In A. M. Feldman, H. I. Kaplan, and B. J. Sadock (Eds.), *Comprehensive textbook of psychiatry/II*. Baltimore: Williams and Wilkins, 1975.

Furstenberg, F. F. *Unplanned parenthood: The social consequences of teenage child bearing*. New York: Free Press, 1976.

Gayles, G. Parade. In R. P. Bell, B. Guy-Sheftall, and B. J. Parker (Eds.), *Study black bridges: Visions of black women in literature*. Garden City, N.Y.: Anchor Books, 1979.

Grier, W. H., and Cobbs, P. M. *Black rage*. New York: Basic Books, 1968.

Guy-Sheftall, B. The women of Bronzeville. In R. P. Bell, B. Guy-Sheftall, and B. J. Parker (Eds.), Sturdy black bridges: Visions of black women in literature. Garden City, N.Y.: Anchor Books, 1979.

Hare, N., and Hare, J. Black women 1970. In J. M. Bardwick (Ed.), *Readings on the psychology of women*. New York: Harper & Row, 1972.

Hughes, L. Mother to son. In A. Bontemps and L. Hughes (Eds.), *The poetry of the Negro 1746–1970*. Garden City, N.Y.: Doubleday, 1970.

Jackson, J. J. Black women in a racist society. In B. S. Brown, B. M. Kramer, and C. V. Willie, *Racism and mental health*. Pittsburgh: University of Pittsburgh Press, 1973.

Jones, J. S. The mature woman's re-entry into college. In press.

Kellam, S. G., Esminger, M. E., and Turner, R. J. Family structure and the mental health of children. In S. Chess and A. Thomas (Eds.), *Annual progress in child development*. 1978

Ladner, J. A. *Tomorrow's tomorrow: The Black woman*. Garden City, N.Y.: Anchor Books, 1972.

Ladner, J. A. The women. *Ebony*, 1975, *10*, 76–81.

Lawrence, M. M. *Young inner city families: Development of ego strength under stress*. New York: Behavioral Publications, 1975.

Lewis, S. D. Black women/white men: The "other" mixed marriage. *Ebony*, 1978, *3*, 37–42

Miniconsultation on the mental and physical health problems of black women. In *Mental and physical health problems of black women*. Washington, D.C.: Black Women's Community Development Foundation, 1975.

Morrison, T. *The bluest eye*. New York: Pocket Books, 1970.

Smith, M. C. Clubwoman. In A. Bontemps and L. Hughes (Eds.), *The poetry of the Negro 1746–1970*. Garden City, N.Y.: Doubleday, 1970.

Stack, C. B. *All our kin: Strategies for survival in a black community*. New York: Harper & Row 1974.

Staples, R. E. *The Black woman in America*. Chicago: Nelson Hall, 1973.

Staples, R. E. Black family life and development. In L. E. Gary (Ed.), *Mental health: A challenge to the black community*. Philadelphia: Dorrance, 1978.

U.S. Bureau of the Census. *Statistical abstract of the U.S.: 1980*. Washington, D.C.: U.S. Government Printing Office, 1980.

Walker, E. The Black woman. In M. M. Smythe, *The Black American reference book*. Englewood Cliffs, N.J.: Prentice-Hall, 1976.

Chapter 11

Problems of American Middle-Class Women in Their Middle Years
A Comparative Approach

BEATRICE BLYTH WHITING

How shall we define the middle years cross-culturally? Halfway between birth and death? Then life expectancy becomes a key variable. In most of the world, few women live to what we consider old age—identified here as retirement age. Their stages of life are defined by women's reproductive capacities. Thus, a female is a child until puberty, seldom nubile for long as early marriage is frequent, childbearing until menopause. Women who live past menopause may enjoy a few productive years before infirmities make it impossible for them to contribute to the daily routines of living.

In most of the Third World and later-developing countries, the major stages of a woman's life are characterized as (1) prereproductive, (2) reproductive, (3) postreproductive but productive—contributing to the survival of herself and others, and (4) postproductive—no longer able to make a contribution, dependent on others for survival. In these societies, the transition between the reproductive and the postreproductive stages usually occurs at menopause. If a woman does not have the ability to control conception and birth, her reproductive years continue until she is no longer fertile. Abstinence, abortion, and infanticide are the alternatives when there is no other means of birth control. In this

BEATRICE BLYTH WHITING • Laboratory of Human Development, Harvard University, Cambridge, Massachusetts 02138. Material in this chapter was originally prepared for the seminar series "Women in Their Middle Years" funded by The Social Science Research Council, 1978–1979.

perspective, the middle years as we know them are a new phenomenon, lengthened by a woman's ability to voluntarily end her reproductive career. For most American women the reproductive years are now terminated before menopause, and consequently, our women have a longer period to be productive before the aging process leads to dependency

Since the middle years are not identical chronologically, it is difficult to compare women's lives across cultures, especially the lives of women of the Third World with those of American women, defined in this volume as "in their middle years." On an average, the latter are probably in actual physiological age at least 10 to 15 years younger. Even if it were possible, however, to identify comparable physiological stages, the comparisons would be meaningless if one did not consider this period in relation to the entire life cycle, and to preceding life experiences.

In attempting to embark on a study of women's lives across cultures, it is necessary to identify universal dimensions for comparison We need a theoretical framework that isolates universal aspects of life experience. I will present as a framework a list of the needs or wants assumed to be shared by the members of all populations across all ages Accepting the fact that these universal needs must be satisfied by every culture to ensure the mental and physical health of its members over the life-span, we can then contrast the ways in which different societies attempt to meet them. The list of needs is familiar to students of human development, but in our child-centered society we have concentrated on concern for the fate of infancy and the childhood years.

I will not consider here the physical needs and their fate. These pose problems being faced by the environmentalists and the epidemiologists studying infectious and lethal diseases (DeLorey, Chapter 12, and Parlee, Chapter 13, in this volume). The consideration here is of psychological needs necessary for mental health. The basic assumption is that men and women, all human beings, have five fundamental needs or wants that we will label psychological. Included are (1) the desire to reproduce oneself, to have offspring that carry on one's family line; (2) the need for physical contact that from infancy onward reduces anxiety and fear and provides comfort; (3) the need for social, cognitive, and with puberty, sexual stimulation; (4) the need for support from other human beings who are responsive to one's overtures; and (5) the need to predict events in the physical and social world (Whiting, 1980). These are not needs in the sense of being essential for physical existence but rather wants and desires that we assume are necessary for psychological well-being.

A brief review of the fate of these psychological needs during the reproductive and postreproductive years in some Third World societies will help to place the problems of American middle-class women in

erspective. The aim is to define the needs operationally, to assess the
uccess of American middle-class culture in meeting these needs, and to
valuate some of the attempts that are being made to revise life-styles to
ope with existing deprivations in the postreproductive years.

Sociobiologists have focused their attention on the first need; they
ave been concerned with the necessity of all species to reproduce them-
elves to ensure survival. As a proximate mechanism they assume that
ach individual member of a species wishes to have offspring, and that
e or she selects either a strategy in which each strives to optimize
productive success by having as many children as possible (r strategy)
r a strategy that calls for concentrating on ensuring the well-being of a
w children (k strategy) (Trivers, 1972). American middle-class families
ave adopted the latter strategy, some women opting out of having any
ildren and attempting to satisfy the assumed need by investing in kin,
e offspring of close relatives.

Our society has recognized the second need, the desire for physical
ntact.Research on primates, infants, and children has documented the
sychological problems that ensue when infants are deprived of this
ntact. The young of a species need a secure warm body to cling to
hen exploration of the world is too frightening. Such body contact is
mforting and quieting and often encourages needed rest. During in-
ncy and early childhood the maternal figure responds with reciprocal
elings of well-being as she holds her infant.

In general, however, the fact that the need continues throughout
e life-course is overlooked, one more indication of the child-centered-
ss of our society.

Our society is just beginning to recognize this continuing need of
ntact, as evidenced by all the new types of therapy that encourage
uching, the new cult of communal bathing and the new, more crowded
tting behavior in social gatherings, and the new types of furniture that
courage close body contact.

From a comparative point of view, our society has been on the
privation side of this need. Our babies sleep by themselves rather
an with their mothers; clothes separate them from skin contact. Our
ildren sleep alone rather than with other children or with adults. We
and apart when talking to each other (Hall, 1959). American men are
rticularly deprived in that physical contact with other men has been
nsidered taboo except in the athletic arena. We are startled when we
ter hospitals in Kenya and find old people sleeping together or babies
traction sharing a crib. We are confused when Kenyan village friends
nd someone in to sleep with a field researcher to comfort her when
e shakes with malaria-induced chills.

A cross-cultural study of sleeping arrangements suggests that in

most of the Third World countries adults do not sleep alone. As in
Tarong, Luzon, and Juxtluhuaca, Mexico (Whiting, 1963), even the elderly have sleeping companions, children sent to share the bed of their
grandparents.

Middle-class women in our culture seldom sleep together, nor do
adult men; to many, such behavior would be an indication of sexual
aberration, the individuals labeled as homosexual, indicating all too
clearly that sleeping arrangements in our middle-class society are associated primarily with sexual behavior. "Sleeping with" is a euphemism
for sexual behavior in our culture. Comparatively speaking, we are extreme in our neglect of the need for physical contact.

We are on the opposite extreme when it comes to our belief in the
need for stimulation. However, the emphasis has been on the needs of
infants and children and until recently has stressed cognitive stimulation. Child psychologists recommend all types of equipment, toys,
games, and books to aid in the intellectual development of children.
Mothers are encouraged to learn how to expand their children's concepts. At present, there is a shift to an interest in social stimulation as
well, perhaps a rationalization for the new preschools for infants and
toddlers. This type of stimulation is not recent in most of the world
where there are large, extended, or polygynous families or close-knit
communities; social stimulation is part of the life experience of young
children brought up in daily association with boys and girls of all ages
and with a variety of adults.

We cannot understand the fate of these needs in the postreproductive years without considering what has taken place during the previous
years. In our society, research has focused on the needs of the young.
How does our society meet the needs of women in the reproductive
years that precede the "middle years?" Much has been written about the
deadening quality of a housebound woman in an isolated nuclear family. Here we recognize a problem. The daily routine is remarkably simila
from day to day. There may be little novelty, little stimulation from othe
adults, male or female. The ever-repeating daily routine may lead to
physical and emotional exhaustion that cannot be overcome even in the
evening when the one adult with whom there is daily contact return
home. Here, too, the interaction may be habitual, ever the same.

How is the need met in other societies? In some cultures, such a
that of the Indian women of Khalpur described by Minturn and Hitch
cock (1966), religious rituals bring welcome variation to an otherwise
uneventful life, restricted by rules of purdah, requiring married wome
during their childbearing years to remain inside the walls of the famil
compound. Weddings, birth ceremonies, the celebration of the gods an
godlings are a source of stimulation, requiring planning and the comin

ogether of women from different courtyards. They are a source of renewal and energy. Melissa Lewellyn-Davies has described a similar
reak in the normal routine of Masai women in Kenya as they plan and
rganize the ceremonies that take place at the time of important transi-
ons in women's lives (1978). The Mixtecan women of Juxtluhuaca,
Mexico, join together to provide the food for the fiestas for their patron
saints, working hard but obviously enjoying the chance to interact with
ther women (Romney and Romney, 1966).

What is required is some sort of community or religious organiza-
on, too often lacking in modern middle-class American life. Sociability,
interacting with a variety of individuals, is a source of stimulation that is
more easily provided in extended families with three or four generations
sharing living space, or in a well-run polygynous homestead where
there is friendly interchange between co-wives, or between sisters-in-
law in patrilineal groups where brothers bring their wives to live on their
father's homestead. Face-to-face communities that share work and ritu-
ls provide a variety of social experiences for women in both the re-
roductive and postreproductive years.

Robert White (1959) has written most persuasively about the third
universal need, the need for effectance. In its most primitive form it has
been studied in the behavior of the developing infant as it explores away
om home base, manipulating the physical world, seeking responses
om other human beings. The sense that one can effectively interact
with the physical and social world leads to a feeling of competence, a
sense of personal worth.

Again, this need has been recognized in children and adolescents
ut forgotten in women. The young mother is creative in a biological
sense, but in our society her feeling of competence may be confined to
recognition of success in child-rearing. In this arena, confidence is easily
undermined by the beliefs propounded by many psychologists, social
workers, and the writers of manuals on child-rearing. They assume that
the mother is all-important to her child's development, solely responsi-
le for the molding of its development, capable of making irremediable
istakes during the first 5 years of her child's life; such a belief is an
unrealistic burden for the reproductive woman. If confidence depends
n success in such an impossible assignment, ill-conceived since there
e so many other determinants of the child's development, the moth-
's sense of competence and personal worth are in peril, built on a
vulnerable foundation.

A well-run household can give satisfaction, but the challenge is not
eat with all the modern technology and the plethora of processed and
packaged foods. Perhaps the ease with which modern households can
 run leads to a desire to complicate the routine, to include a myriad of

outside activities for all the family members. Then the complicated scheduling requires executive ability. The whole frantic plan may be invented to break out of the house and use unchallenged organizational skills.

In many societies, women have arenas outside the home in addition to child-care and maintenance activities. In agricultural societies such as those of sub-Saharan Africa, a woman may spend four or five hours working in her garden or selling produce in the market, returning to her home with a sense of having contributed productively to her family' well-being, more receptive to her children than the housebound mother (Whiting, 1980). Although the economic rewards to be gained are un doubtedly a prime motive for working mothers, the need for another sphere in which to develop a sense of competence and productivity i obviously an important incentive.

The fourth need, the need for support, has become a recognized one for adults as well as children in the last decade. The nature of support groups and social networks is a popular subject in research Social scientists are returning to interest in an old subject dressed in new labels. All humans need the support of other individuals and group but it would seem that for a period we were focusing our concern on more individualistic aspects of life.

The young middle-class mother who lives in an isolated nuclear family lacks the type of support enjoyed by a woman in a well-run extended or polygynous society or in one that has close-knit microcom munities. I do not believe in being romantic about the joys of the ex tended family; it has many drawbacks—one trades autonomy for sup port. However, our isolated nuclear family is at one end of a continuum of types of social structures furnishing support systems for childbearing women. I know of no other society where, up until very recently when infant daycare and toddler preschools have been introduced, there has been so little help for women caring for young children. The isolated middle-class woman suffers from lack of instrumental and emotional support as well as from loneliness for adult company.

Belonging to a support group, having a network of friends, requires social skills, patterns of sociability. These skills involve greeting behav ior, knowledge of how to initiate and sustain friendly interaction, how to join with others in group activities, how to share—behaviors now labeled social competence by child psychologists. To master these skills one must be attuned to the needs and reactions of others, able to predict their responses to your behavior, able to attend and respond to their communications, willing to share intimacies, hopes, fears, and disap pointments. In our culture these traits have been labeled feminine, de pendent, intuitive, sensitive, and are identified as occurring proportion tely more frequently in women than in men. The label has carried with t denigration. Why men are forbidden by our culture to have these haracteristics is a research question in itself, perhaps to be explained istorically. There are indications now that these taboos are becoming ess widespread, perhaps no longer required in the modern industrial ge.

Both historically in this country and in the Third World, there are ocial systems that allow for intimacy among both adult males and emales. The age-graded societies of sub-Saharan Africa constitute one f the best examples. Young men who have been initiated into manhood ogether maintain close friendship bonds throughout life.

That American women are more skilled than men in the ability to stablish support groups is suggested by the reported reaction of men vhose wives or friends have joined groups. They express an interest in elonging to a group but their habits of interaction are primarily instru- nental, tinged with competition and friendly aggression and joking. hey find the serious, intimate exchange of women embarassing. They o not easily adopt the habit of mutual emotional help and the exchange f confidences. Cultures certainly differ on the degree to which men orm solidarities. American Protestant middle-class men of Yankee de- cent are extreme, as their ethos proscribes seeking help or engaging in ntimate exchanges with other men (Mathai, 1979). Such behavior is onsidered dependent and feminine, suggesting the interaction of others and children.

How does one come by the skills that enable one to belong to a upport group? Research on women's networks suggests that skills are arned early, from mothers who have well-developed social interaction atterns with both same-sex and cross-sex groups. Most frequently, ese mothers have lived in the same community for many years. Aber- ethy (1973) has shown that young women coming from such homes nd transferred to new environments are better skilled than women om less stable backgrounds in setting up new networks. This research nplies that those who grow up in motile families, the experience of any of the American middle class, have less well-developed social ills. Perhaps we have taken too lightly the teaching of these skills.

The last need, the sense of being able to predict the behavior of the nysical and social world, is less clearly universal, more subject to spe- fic cultural belief systems. Societies vary in the degree to which indi- duals feel competent not only to predict but to control these worlds; ey vary in the degree to which they accept their perceived ability or ability to shape fate and the degree to which they feel the necessity for edicting and controlling. For many societies the locus of control is in e supernatural, and a human being's fate is in the lap of the gods. An acceptance of fate leads to less torment on the part of mothers, less self-blame for the undesirable behavior of children, a greater ability to accept the frustrations of life. Middle-class America has been taught to believe in personal efficacy, and, as discussed above, our women during the confining years of childbearing, blinded by this belief, blame themselves unduly for some of their failures.

Accepting, then, that these five needs are present at all stages in the life-course and observing that societies differ in the cultural forms that meet these needs during the reproductive years, we are ready to address the particular problems of American middle-class women in their middle or postreproductive years. What is the fate of these needs during this period and how are women attempting to revise the cultural forms they find unsatisfactory?

Our strategy for meeting the first need, investing in a few children, has drawbacks. The loss of one child is probably more devastating when the average number of offspring per reproductive middle-class woman is less than three. The focus of attention on one or two children may lead to an overcommitment, risky for both parents and child. The overconcerned and overprotective mother of the reproductive years finds it difficult or impossible to relinquish control of her children. Too often an ambivalent relationship develops. On the one hand, she wishes to be free of feelings of responsibility; on the other, she remains emotionally bonded. Since she has invested so much in her two or three children, her unrealistic expectations and unattainable standards for success may lead to loss of self-esteem and depression, impairing her relations both with her children and with her grandchildren.

We are only beginning to explore the consequences of choosing not to have children, although in Western societies, unlike most of the Third World, the role of maiden aunts and bachelor uncles has been accepted as within the cultural norm. Investing in adopted children is found in many parts of the world. Anthropologists have begun to explore in depth the adoption patterns in the Polynesian and Micronesian Islands and in West Africa. Social scientists are monitoring the outcome of the American middle-class women who eschew childbearing. To date there are few hard data on which to base an opinion, but there are no data suggesting that these women are as a group suffering from severe deprivation. A new strategy may be in the making, reducing the expense of parental investment by sharing the cost in time, money, and emotion among kin.

For women in our culture, the need for physical comfort, for body contact, has been satisfied in the childbearing and early marital years by contact with infants and children and, depending on life-style, by sleeping arrangements of husbands and wives. We have suggested that these

eeping arrangements are associated with sexual behavior. What hap-
ens when there are no small children left at home and the desire for
xual relations with one's spouse is less intense, less frequent? Is there
new perception of the function of sharing the same bed or is there
ithdrawal from physical contact? What of the divorced, never-married,
widowed woman? (See Luria and Meade, Chapter 17, this volume.)
ow will she satisfy her need for physical contact in a manner accept-
le to our present middle-class norms?

As we have noted, there is a growing awareness of the deprivation.
ere appears to be an increase in same-sex embracing, less anxiety
out being labeled sexually aberrant. As noted above, there are new
erapies that involve touching, new patterns of bathing, and in gener-
, a loosening of all the taboos on physical contact and awareness. The
sire for sexual stimulation that has been associated in our culture with
e desire for physical contact is also being elucidated, and is recognized
present in postreproductive and postmenopausal women. There is a
volution in progress in our sexual mores. Most controversial, perhaps,
the growing acceptance of masturbatory and homosexual forms of
tisfaction.

Most attention in the literature and research on women in their
iddle years has been focused on the need for new arenas for develop-
g a sense of competence and personal worth, a need for new activities.
ere is also concern about the need for new support networks. A new
t of questions is being addressed by women in their middle years who
ve the desire for new activities and new associates.

As we have seen, many women in the Third World have had work
tside their homes in agriculture, animal husbandry, marketing, or
me industries. Their sense of personal worth and competence has not
sted exclusively on the success of any one child. In their postreproduc-
e years these women can now spend more hours in the arenas outside
e home. They are freer to move into the community, their reproduc-
e capacities no longer threatening to those who guard the sanctity of
nily honor based on sexual fidelity.

The West African market women, especially the wholesalers who
vel distances to buy and arrange for trucking in goods from outlying
tricts to the central markets, are often cited in the literature for their
mpetence and economic success. In traditional Kikuyu cultures of East
rica, postreproductive women joined the council of senior women
d took over the supervision of ceremonies and responsibility for the
neral welfare and behavior of younger women. Older women in many
ieties gain political power, recognized for their wisdom in decision-
king. In many societies, postreproductive women have careers as
dwives, herbalists, and shamans. Some become priestesses and re-

ligious functionaries. In sum, these women pursue careers already star
ed during the childbearing years or enter into new careers open
women of their age grade.

A look at the present scene in the United States shows that the
seem to be two predominant life-styles for postreproductive wome
One life-style is followed by those who adjust to the middle years
accepting their roles as wives, mothers of teenagers and grown childre
and grandmothers of their children. They concentrate their energies
the needs of their husbands and their children, no matter what the
age, hopefully venturing forth on some new social activities, seekir
volunteer jobs that are not too demanding, and hoping to be able
enjoy the role of a benevolent grandmother. They are frequently four
among travelers and shoppers. Their feelings of competence and se
worth are dependent in large part on the careers of their husbands ar
children and the density of the support groups they have already dev
oped. If they have skills in establishing and maintaining friendship
they are better equipped to follow non-career-oriented life-styles.
though this was once the most prevalent life-style among Americ
middle-class women, census data suggest that it is becoming le
frequent.

The second life-style is that of women who have already embark
on careers, have never given them up during their child-rearing yea
or are attempting to return to former career interests or initiate ne
ones. These women are becoming more numerous. It is their needs th
will be the concern of the rest of this chapter. Of particular concern is
group of women, a cohort that may not exist in the new generatior
who have dedicated years almost exclusively to child care, and wh
when the children reach a stage in schooling that makes them less d
manding, have decided to seek employment. The psychological nee
for stimulation, and for a sense of competence and personal wor
combine with economic motives to influence this decision. In their hu
ger they often overcommit themselves. Inexperienced in predicting t
demands of a job and the length of time projects take, wanting to pro
their competence, they tend to demand too much of themselves,
promise more than they can deliver. Their lives become frenetic. Th
suffer from too much rather than too little stimulation.

Prior to these new commitments, they have attended, often in co
pulsive detail, to the needs of their husbands and children. Now th
energies are redirected, and if they have undertaken full-time e
ployment or study, they return to the home tired and unable to contir
the type of nurturance that has nourished and reinforced their h
band's needs for food, comfort, and intimacy. As they increase conta
with the outside world, they set up new social networks and trans
their nurturance to colleagues, fellow students, and workers. Left

nd are the husbands, who are less able to branch out and form new
tworks.

There is evidence that the men whose wives seek new careers and
t up new networks feel deserted. Frequently they turn to other,
unger women for the intimacy and support that they are only able to
tablish with a sexual partner. It is the hypothesis here that the turning
another woman is more an attempt to satisfy these needs, frequently
eled dependent, than a desire for sexual novelty and pleasure. This
ed of men for dependence is also suggested by the frequency of di-
rce following the birth of the second child (Hetherington, Cox, and
x, 1975), behavior that can be interpreted as the husband's response
feelings of having been displaced in his wife's nurturant sphere by
o babies, a feeling of deprivation and loss.

A woman in her middle years, faced with divorce, is often devas-
ed, not understanding what has happened. Research is needed to
rify the components of the situation that has led to separation. It is
rticularly important to contrast the women with part-time and full-
ie commitments outside the home, to contrast women whose hus-
nds receive emotional support from other individuals as well as from
:ir wives, to contrast men with varying degrees of dependency needs
d women with various degrees of ambition and habits of nurturance.
: need to explore the decision-making process of women when they
cide on the type of commitment to make outside the home.

Of the women who choose to stay home, their satisfaction with life
uld be explored, and their embeddedness in social networks in rela-
n to their talents for sociability. We need to discover which women
ve the ability and opportunity to play the role of a grandmother, and
must identify the behavior that brings with it a new sense of compe-
ice.

Are these problems of the middle-aged woman universal, and if so,
w have other cultures met men's and women's changing needs? The
nsition in women's lives in the postreproductive years appears to be
iversal, but some societies have cultural forms that ease the transi-
n. Polygynous societies have an advantage. The middle-aged wife is
led by a younger co-wife who takes over part of the household re-
nsibilities, the nurturant care, and the satisfaction of the sexual de-
s of the husband, releasing the senior wife to pursue a career as a
leswoman or a more productive farmer. She is not divorced for her
v interests but remains the executive woman in the homestead, shar-
her husband with his junior wives. The senior wife often has a
cial relationship with her husband that develops in her postchild-
ring years. Large extended households also offer possibilities for a
ldle-aged woman to start on a new career. We are all familiar with the

Indian women who come to the United States in their middle years study, leaving behind husband and children, knowing that they will cared for by relatives in the large family compounds.

Several possible solutions to our problems suggest themselve Would it not be possible for women desiring new areas of competence both work and continue in a more nurturant role if there were more ha time employment opportunities? Could not men be reeducated to me some of their needs for dependency outside their sexual partners? Cou not some of the taboos on bodily contact and intimacy that have r stricted men's lives be aired and through scrutiny dispelled? Could n women be encouraged to examine their ambitions, to analyze their ove commitments, and to monitor the degree to which they are deserting t men who have learned to depend upon their nurturant initiations? implement such changes in life-styles, it is necessary to convince bo men and women that there are benefits to be gained. By contrasting t lives of men and women from different subcultures in our own societ investigating the satisfaction of their needs during the various stages the life-course, we may be able to identify those patterns that seem offer the best insurance against feelings of loneliness, abandonmer and exhaustion, and to encourage feelings of personal worth, comfoi and support.

Already it is coming to be recognized that women who choose have few children must have arenas for developing a sense of comp tence beyond the confines of child care and household maintenanc There is growing recognition that men and women need to share in macies with individuals besides their marital partners, that they ne support networks beyond the family. There is growing recognition the need to reestablish microcommunities that share activities. Less tention has been given to how one reaches these goals. We have n given enough thought to the management of the pace of life. If v develop cognitive skills to the exclusion of social skills, if we do not lea concern for others beyond ourselves and our children, we will be equipped to be members of such a community. (Whiting, 1978). We m also realize that career lines for men and women who choose to invest children and in community living may require a shorter work day, lea ing time and energy for nurturance and sociability. For many societies the Third World this combination of work and community living wa way of life, too often terminated when entrance into the industr world, with its compulsion for the 8-hour day, put an end to the hot needed for nonwork activities. We need time and energy to ensure t we can satisfy all our psychological needs.

Our focus is on the problems of women in their middle years, their choice of life-style must be synchronized with that of men. O ust be wary of the backlash against the women's movement that ems, in part at least, to be the reaction of men who fear desertion. Our search should monitor the success of the various life-styles of sub-oups in our culture in meeting the universal psychological needs of th men and women.

:FERENCES

ernethy, V. D. Social network and response to the maternal role. *International Journal of Sociology of the Family*, 1973, *3*: 386–392.

ll, E. T. *The silent language*. New York: Doubleday/Anchor, 1959.

therington, E. M., Cox, M., and Cox, R. *Beyond father absence: Conceptualization of effects of divorce*. Paper presented at the meeting of the Society for Research in Child Develop-ment, Denver, 1975.

welyn-Davies, M. Two contexts of solidarity. In P. Caplan and J. M. Bujra (Eds.), *Women united, women divided*. London. Tavistock, 1978.

thai, P. A. *The myth of the self-sufficient Yankee. Support systems of white Angle-Saxon Protestants in New England*. Thesis presented to the Faculty of the Graduate School of Education of Harvard, 1979.

nturn, L. and Hitchcock, J. *The Rajputs of Khalapur, India* (Six-Culture Series, Vol. 3). New York: Wiley, 1966.

mney, A. K., and Romney, R. *The Mixtecans of Juxtluhuaca, Mexico* (Six-Culture Series, Vol. 4). New York: Wiley, 1966.

vers, R. L. Parental investment and sexual selection. In B. Campbell (Ed.), *Sexual selection and the descent of man 1871–1971*. Chicago: Aldine, 1972.

ite, R. W. Motivation reconsidered: The concept of competence. *Psychological Review*. 1959, *66*, 297–333.

iting, B. The dependency hang-up and experiments in alternative life styles. In J. M. Yinger and S. J. Cutler (Eds.), *Major social issues: A multidisciplinary view*. 1978.

iting, B. Culture and social behavior: A model for the development of social behavior. *Ethos*, 1980, *8*(2).

PART III

Enhancing Well-Being

Iealth Care and Midlife Women

ATHERINE DeLorey

TRODUCTION

:alth care for midlife women in the United States of the 20th century is omplex blend of myth and reality viewed against a backdrop of rapid :ial change. The myths that have evolved concern women's roles, ecifically older women's roles, and also include menopause, an event it occurs most often at midlife. Until recently, little information has en available concerning the health or health care of midlife women.)st research on women's health at midlife is clinically oriented and umes that menopause is the most important aspect of women's lives l health. Although this has changed somewhat in recent years, in 't due to the impetus of women's groups such as the Menopause llective in Cambridge, Massachusetts, and the National Women's alth Network, much needs to be changed before we have research t validates women's experiences as well as providing them with the irmation that they can use to make appropriate decisions for their n health.

Any discussion of health care for midlife women needs to take 'ount of the structure and beliefs underlying the way this health care irovided—that is, how the health care system functions. Health pro-ers as well as health planners, for the most part, are outsiders observ-an alien culture, the culture of midlife women. As they attempt to derstand and interpret women's health needs, these observations are ored by the biases and preconceptions of a biomedical model perspec-:. The biomedical model of health care, based on the biosciences, sees

HERINE DeLorey • Women's Health Research Institute, Boston, Massachusetts 02113.

most health problems as exemplifying a direct cause–effect relationship
Health issues are then diagnosed and treated as scientific abstraction
although, because they involve social beings, they occur in a sociocu
tural context. The biomedical model tends to use restricted definitions (
health status without regard for social definitions; it assumes that phys
cians, who are the primary purveyors of health, are experts who a.
neutral providers, dispensing their product unaffected by social, cultu
al, or political forces (Mishler, Amarasingham, Hauser, Liem, Osherso:
and Waxler, 1981).

Because the existing system of care is based on this biomedic
model, there is in reality no "health care system," but rather a "medic
care system," which by definition perceives life in medical terms. Th
system, bounded by societally and culturally imposed ideas of womer
roles, relies on myths and stereotypes to govern the way health care
provided for women.

These myths and stereotypes impose restricted roles on women
all points throughout the life-span; women are classified as products
their reproductive system and its hormones, and normal life develo
mental stages or transitions are defined as medical issues. Therefor
women must then enter the medical care system for essentially norm
health events such as contraception, care during pregnancy and birt
ing, or information about midlife transitions.

As women age, medicine continues to view them as controlled
the endocrine system, and consequently, medical care for midlife wo
en continues to be dominated by attention to hormonal factors. Ma
events that occur at the same time in life as hormonal changes are r
caused by hormonal changes. Association is not causation. Howev
many health aspects of midlife are seen as resulting from the cycli
hormonal transitions of menopause. Thus, we have midlife wom
being given estrogen to control hot flashes or to prevent and/or amel
rate thinning of the bones (osteoporosis) when life-style changes such
improved nutrition or more exercise may be as effective. This is parti
larly relevant for the cohort of women who are 40 to 60 years old tod
the older women of tomorrow. These midlife women of today are
women who were given diethylstilbestrol to maintain pregnancy,
high doses of estrogen in the first contraceptive pills, and high dose:
estrogen at menopause, so they could be, as one physician promis
"feminine forever" (Wilson, 1961).

Within recent years there has been an increased interest in
status and health of midlife women. What has been the impetus for t
interest? During the latter part of the 20th century, midlife women h
become increasingly visible partly because of their greater numbers
well as their changing social roles. When any subgroup within the po

ion becomes more visible or noticed, for whatever reasons, the health
tus of that group takes on added interest to the larger population.

Some of the demographic and social shifts that have altered the
sibility of midlife women include a decreased birth rate coupled with
overall decreased maternal mortality rate, an increased expected life-
an at all age levels, and changes in the structure of the work force.
om 1900 to 1975 the birth rate dropped from 32.2 live births (per
ousand population) to 18.4 (Department of Commerce, 1975), while at
e same time the maternal mortality rate decreased from 69.5 (per
0,000 live births) in 1920 to 15.2, a decrease of 98% (Bureau of the
nsus, 1975). The life-span for women has increased at all ages, a result
changes in maternal mortality, medical response to infectious disease,
d early detection of noninfectious diseases. Because the maternal
ortality rate for women over 40 has consistently been nine times great-
than for women under 30 (Bureau of the Census, 1975), the decrease
maternal mortality has had a great impact on life-expectancy statistics
women 40 and older. These changes further increased female life
pectancy so that in 1970 a (white) woman at 40 could expect to live for
more years, whereas her 40-year-old counterpart in 1900 could antici-
e 29 more years.

These and other demographic changes have resulted in a popula-
n in which the median age increased from 22 years in 1900 to 30 years
1970, and the proportion of midlife women increased from 13% of the
pulation to 21%. By 1980 over 50% of midlife women were in the work
ce, a substantial increase from the 38% of 1950. Thus, the increased
ibility and prominence of midlife women results not only from nu-
rical changes but from role changes as well, making the health status
midlife women a significant issue for the whole society.

JOR HEALTH ISSUES FOR MIDLIFE WOMEN

Although mortality figures are at best a crude indication of the health
us of a population, they do provide a basis for comparison and
sent one aspect of the total picture. Tables 1 and 2 indicate the major
ses of death for midlife women. One can see that the major killers of
life women are not gynecological conditions. Mortality from cancer of
breast, cervix, and uterus is at the rate of 50.1 (per 100,000) for white
nen and 63 (per 100,000) for nonwhite women, whereas heart disease
cerebrovascular disease account for the largest number of deaths for
h white and nonwhite women (Table 1).

Looking at women divided according to white and nonwhite cate-
izations provides some very important information. It illustrates that
t disease, cerebrovascular diseases, and malignancies are major kill-

Table 1. Ten Leading Causes of Death for
Midlife Women[a,b]

Cause of death	Rate[c]
White women	
Malignant neoplasms	264.9
Heart disease	159.7
Cerebrovascular diseases	37.6
Cirrhosis	22.6
Accidents	22.0
Diabetes	14.1
Suicide	11.3
Influenza, pneumonia	10.1
Bronchitis, emphysema, asthma	8.5
Benign neoplasm	2.9
Nonwhite women	
Heart disease	324.1
Malignant neoplasms	301.0
Cerebrovascular diseases	97.3
Diabetes	42.0
Cirrhosis	39.4
Accidents	31.9
Influenza, pneumonia	20.0
Nephritis, nephrosis	15.5
Homicide	9.1
Septicemia	6.9

[a]Based on data from National Center for Health Statistics
(Dunn, 1981).
[b]Midlife defined as 45–55 years old for this table.
[c]Rates per 100,000.

ers of all women. The mortality rates for nonwhite women are greater
all categories, but the white/nonwhite designation does not tell us i
Native American woman has the same risks as a Hispanic woman
does not tell us how socioeconomic factors influence the data. F
quently it is assumed that a racial breakdown for health data is a sur
gate for socioeconomic influences, since many nonwhite persons
United States culture are relegated to lower socioeconomic status a
result of discriminatory practices. But making this assumption does
give much information concerning the risk factors for the middle-cl
black woman or the poor white woman, and it can serve to further
perpetuation of cultural stereotypes not based on fact.

Regarding the mortality studies in Table 1, what does it mean t
the mortality rate from suicide for white women is 11.3/100,000,
suicide is not listed in the 10 major killers of nonwhite women? '
higher rates for nonwhite women of heart disease and malignant r

Table 2. Causes of Death from Malignant Neoplasms for Midlife Women[a,b]

	45–49	50–54	55–59	60–64
east				
White	41.0	60.3	76.3	92.3
Nonwhite	43.5	59.1	72.2	82.4
rvix uteri				
White	6.7	7.3	8.6	10.4
Nonwhite	15.3	19.0	22.4	25.9
rpus uteri				
White	2.4	4.4	8.3	14.6
Nonwhite	4.0	7.2	13.7	24.2

[a]sed on data from National Center for Health Statistics (Dunn, 1981).
[b]tes per 100,000.

asms (cancers) may reflect greater stresses because of environmental fluences or, conversely, may reflect the poorer-quality health care ten available to persons in lower socioeconomic groups. Kidney dis-ses, nephritis and nephrosis, are major killers of nonwhite women but e not among the 10 major killers of white women.

Nonwhite women may have less access to preventive health/medi-l care or may encounter more toxins in the workplace, occupational zards with which poorer women are more likely to come into contact.

Other approaches used to determine the health status of a popula-n include looking at the use of health services, including physician sits and hospitalizations, and at how much illness interferes with daily tivities, the assumption being that one can infer the health status of e total group from this information. Although there are slight in-eases in use of health services associated with age for midlife women, e predominant differences, as throughout the life-span, are between en and women. Midlife women make 5.9 visits to physicians a year, % more than the 4.7 visits of midlife men (Givens, 1979), as well as ving an incidence of acute conditions 24% greater than men of the ne age. Midlife women's activities are restricted by illness 46% more n for midlife men, although this is 8% less than for women in gen-l.

There has been speculation that this type of information may reflect biases on the part of physicians, but this view has not been substan-ted by available data. In a rigorous analysis using National Ambulato-Medical Care Study (NAMCS) data, Verbrugge could find no exam-s where the differences in care could be attributed to physician bias erbrugge and Steiner, 1981). But it does not seem likely that only a logical or biomedical model is sufficient to explain these differences.

Other explanations for these differences take sociocultural aspects of women's roles into consideration, such as that it is more acceptable for women to report illness; that because of women's role responsibilities they can assume a sick role more easily than men; that women may indeed have more illness because their roles are more stressful; or that because of interviewing techniques of large surveys, women have greater probability than men of being interviewed directly but as a proxy for men, thus recalling greater illness for themselves and less for men (Nathanson, 1975; Verbrugge, 1976).

Finding the explanation for these sex differences in health experiences will provide significant information but will not directly approach the issue of whether care given to women is appropriate to their needs. Sex bias in health care may be impossible to measure because it is grounded in societal assumptions concerning women that are commonly held by providers, researchers, and often women themselves. Because of this it becomes difficult to evaluate the data that are available. How do we evaluate the fact that up to the present most research on heart disease, stress-related illness, or occupational health was done with male subjects and the results extrapolated to women? How do we evaluate the information that when men and women visit a physician or a clinic, women have fewer diagnostic tests and procedures done than men (Hadden, 1981)? Thus, although heart disease is a major killer of women, only 27% of women receive cardiograms compared to 41% of men. This may reflect sex bias or it may reflect physicians' perceptions of actual gender differences. It does not seem to reflect adequate assessment of the risk-factor profile. Assessment of health in midlife women becomes even more difficult because the effect of stereotypes about aging need to be added to the picture. Thus, the biases from age stereotypes as well as those of the medical model influence the way health care is planned and provided for midlife women. One result of this is that the literature presents a narrow view of midlife women's health, seeing menopause as the most important issue—a view that is often in conflict with what women themselves want or think.

In a random community survey of 120 midlife women and their physicians conducted by this author in 1981, no woman thought that menopause was a major health problem, but 21% of the physicians responded that menopause was the major health problem for midlife women. Moreover, 60% of the women replied that menopause was no concern to them, while 83% of the physicians thought it was a major concern to them (DeLorey, 1981). In follow-up discussions with some of the physicians, they consistently asked for any available information on midlife women, saying that the only information about midlife women they received in their medical training had been in pathophysiology ᵘurses, where menopause was discussed. There is clearly a need for ᵃajor changes in the existing structure of the medical education system.

Looking again at the leading causes of death in Table 1, we find that ᵒme are more relevant than others to a discussion of health for midlife ᵒomen. Heart disease and cerebrovascular disease are relevant because ᵉey account for a larger number of deaths as women age, and also ᵉcause many people are unaware of their importance to women. Can-r of the uterus, cervix, and breast are relevant because they are specifi-lly women's issues that begin to show their significance at midlife, ᵃrticularly breast cancer, the largest single cause of death for midlife ᵒomen.

Two other health issues of major importance to midlife women are ᵉnopause and occupational health. Menopause is important because it ᵃ a physiological transition that usually occurs at midlife. Occupational ᵉalth is important because 54% of midlife women are employed outside ᵉ home. Insufficient attention has been given to the health hazards of ᵉ workplace in general, and those that relate specifically to midlife ᵥe been ignored completely.

ᵉnopause

Menopause becomes a major issue for discussion in any considera-ᵒn of health and midlife women because it is experienced by most ᵒmen at midlife and because it overwhelmingly dominates the medical ᵉrature. In addition, there is a growing awareness that traditional ᵉas concerning the experience of menopause are not accurate and that ᵉerences are therefore made without adequate justification.

A major reason for inaccurate assessments of menopause is that ᵘch research concerning menopause and midlife is biased and frag-ᵉnted. It is biased because most studies are conducted with clinical ᵖulations; it is fragmented because many studies are done assuming ᵈy a biological, psychological, or sociocultural model of explanation ᵗh little integration of the models or awareness of how each relates to ᵉ other when attempting to explain the totality of the experience for ᵒmen.

Over the last 20 years menopause has gained increased recognition ᵃn acceptable area of scientific research, with the most dramatic in-ᵃase occurring in the last decade. Recognition has been stimulated by ᵥelopments in hormone research as well as the increasing numbers of ᵒmen experiencing menopause or postmenopausal stages of life. Al-ᵒugh behavioral and clinical aspects of menopause are studied, these ᵒ components are not related to each other or to the health care ᵒvided to midlife women.

With a few exceptions, research on menopause lacks clarity of de sign and methodological rigor. Definitions of menopause vary, for ex ample. Menopause usually refers to physiological aspects of change in the ovary, or cessation of the pituitary–ovarian feedback mechanism which in turn results in the cessation of menstruation. Climacterium usually refers to a sociocultural period of time of change occurring in th middle years of life. In many studies, menopause and climacterium ar used interchangeably (Dalton, 1976; Taich, 1978), with climacteriun often defined as the time period in which menopause occurs (Neu garten, 1963; Goodman, 1976; Utian, 1976). Frequently menopaus loosely refers to the time of the last menstruation (Neugarten, 196; McKinlay and Jefferys, 1974; Utian, 1976; Eskin, 1980) and is subdivide into premenopause, menopause, and postmenopause. These categorie are defined by the time elapsed since the most recent menstrual cycl (Thompson, 1973; McKinlay and Jefferys, 1974), as well as subjectiv response of women (Maoz, 1970). Even reports from conferences specif cally focused on menopause may fail to provide consistent or objectiv definitions of menopause (Ryan and Gibson, 1973; Beard, 1976; Cam; bell, 1976; van Keep, 1976).

The vagueness of definition not only prevents a clear understanc ing of the event, it precludes a definition of the true "population i risk." A standard definition of menopause would permit a clearer ui derstanding of the etiology of any problems, of the processes involve in the genesis of such problems, and of diagnosis and treatment issue

The fact that menopause occurs at the time in a woman's life whe other biological and social changes take place intensifies problems i volved in conducting research. Not only must the effects of menopau be separated from those of chronological aging, but the biological a pects of menopause need to be separated from the psychosocial to u derstand the role of each. Because menopause is both a biological and sociocultural event, this separation is even more difficult.

BIOLOGICAL ASPECTS OF MENOPAUSE. Although separating biolo ical and social factors is difficult, some aspects of menopause are consi ered as strictly biological. The biological changes are those directly i volved in alterations of the ovary and circulating estrogen supply. It not clear whether symptoms reported around the time of menopau are biological events of menopause, biological events of other process in the body (e.g., aging), or psychosocial events such as reactive depr sion to life events.

Estrogen. Because cessation of menstruation is a result of a dim ished, but not eliminated, supply of cyclical ovarian estrogen, there much controversy concerning estrogen's function in the me opausal/postmenopausal woman. A small number of researchers a

ractitioners consider menopause an estrogen deficiency disease and
ierefore suggest the use of estrogen as a therapeutic agent to alleviate
ymptoms associated with midlife. Discussion of the function of es-
ogen in the body and the use of estrogen replacement therapy must
cknowledge that different substances are considered. The first are en-
ogenous estrogens, natural steroids produced by the body. The others
re exogenous estrogens, which are either synthesized in the laboratory
r extracted from animals. There is no definitive evidence in the litera-
ire to indicate that exogenous estrogens have the same effect as those
strogens naturally produced by the body.

Treatment for the changes at midlife that get labeled as symptoms
f menopause varies according to how menopause is defined, how
ymptoms are evaluated, and how effective treatment is thought to be
Midwinter, 1976; Shoemaker, 1977). There are natural regimens for
iese "symptoms" that include exercise, nutritional changes, and vari-
us vitamin programs (Prensky, 1974; Seaman and Seaman, 1977; Siegal
id Michaud, 1980). Many women are prescribed tranquilizers, anti-
epressants, or antianxiety medications to alleviate problems, but the
iost prescribed and used treatment for menopause is exogenous es-
ogens. Three to four million women in the United States take ex-
zenous estrogens, with an estimated two to three million taking it for
iore than 3 months (Wolfe, 1977). The total number of prescriptions for
itrogen replacement increased by 35% from 1970 to 1975, but then
ecreased by 29% from 1975 to 1977. This decrease reversed a trend that
egan in the 1930s and increased dramatically in the 1960s. The reversal
iat began in 1975 may be associated with the publication of research
iggesting a causal link between endometrial cancer and estrogen use
Mack, Pike, Henderson, Pfeffer, Gerkins, Arthur, and Brown, 1976;
mith, 1975; Ziel and Finkle, 1975). Even with this decrease in total
rescriptions, a Food and Drug Administration Bulletin of 1976 con-
udes that estrogen is misused to an extent that cannot be explained
'ood and Drug Administration, 1976). Although there is general con-
:nsus that hot flushes, or flashes, and dryness of vaginal mucous mem-
:anes are the only symptoms altered by the administration of ex-
zenous estrogens, estrogen is often prescribed for "general well-
:ing" and just for "the menopause," with no clear criteria for prescrib-
ig it. Those practitioners who believe menopause is an "estrogen defi-
ency disease" suggest it be given to all menopausal women (Wilson,
161; Greenblatt, 1977; Lebich, 1976; Notelovitz, 1976; Wenderlein,
180), whereas other practitioners suggest using it sparingly and judi-
ously, specifically for hot flushes/flashes that are bothersome to the
dividual woman (Connell, 1977; Coope, 1976).

A number of unwanted effects of, and contraindications for, prescribing estrogen are recognized (Reitz, 1977; Seaman and Seaman 1977; Utian, 1976). Those receiving the most attention concern the car cinogeneity of estrogen replacement therapy. Cancer of the breast is on type of cancer linked with estrogens (Burch, 1971; Trichopoulos, 1972 Hoover, 1976; Lawson, Jick, Hunter, and Madsen, 1981). This hypoth esis linking estrogen with cancer of the breast is complex and not ye definitively demonstrated. The hypothesis suggests that the exposure c breast-duct epithelium to unopposed estrogen results in changes tha are precursors to cancer. Estrogens have been a causative factor of breas tumors in mammals (Cutts, 1964), and groups of women at high risk c breast cancer have higher plasma levels of estrogen (Henderson, an Canellos, 1980). Two major recent studies have indicated a greater ris of breast cancer with the use of menopausal estrogen, particularly a higher doses over long periods of time (Hoover, 1976; Ross, Paganin Hill, Gerkins, Mack, Pfeffer, Arthur, and Henderson, 1980; Lawsor Wick, Hunter, and Madsen, 1981). The study by Ross et al. indicates tha women who still had their ovaries and received estrogens had a 2.5-fol higher risk for breast cancer, and the study by Lawson et al. showed two-fold increase for women who use exogenous estrogen at midlife

Even though the relationship of estrogens and breast cancer is no receiving attention, most discussion and research on the carcinogenei of estrogens relate to cancer of the endometrium. Recent ep demiological research suggests that women taking estrogen over a per od of time have a greater risk of cancer of the endometrium (Smith, 197 Ziel and Finkle, 1975; Mack et al., 1976; Antunes, 1979). Though the has been disagreement as to the analytical procedures of the research f the mechanisms involved in the causality, there is agreement that son causal link exists between endometrial cancer and estrogen (Weis Szekely, and Austin, 1976; Mack et al., 1976; Proudfit, 1976). Some r search suggests that a causal link exists but only in women who a cancer-prone, and that the dangers of estrogen replacement theraf might be mitigated by prescribing cyclic estrogen with progesteror (Gambrell, 1976; Greenblatt, 1977).

In any studies linking cancer with estrogen use, the relationsh between large doses and long-term use is highlighted. This is partic larly relevant when we think of the women who are at midlife in tl United States in late 20th century. These are the women who receiv the synthetic estrogen diethylstilbestrol in the 1950s and 1960s as a pr tective intervention in what were defined as high-risk pregnancies, wl received the high-estrogen birth control pills in the 1960s, and/or wl received high doses of estrogen replacement therapy to keep the "feminine forever." The outcome of these estrogen interventions will difficult to determine because there are so many other factors that c confound the cause and progression of cancers.

Symptoms Attributed to Menopause. In discussing what are often des-
nated as the symptoms of menopause it is necessary to remember the
age in a woman's life when menopause occurs. It is a time of many
hysical changes that can influence both somatic and psychological ex-
eriences. A more realistic approach in assessing the health of midlife
omen would be to define the various signs of midlife, naming meno-
ause as one of them.

There is no accurate assessment of how many midlife women have
ymptoms of menopause, and of those women who do, to what extent.
his is because most studies relating to health and menopause are con-
icted using clinical groups of women and because few prospective
udies have been conducted.[1]

Information on the symptoms of menopause or how many women
perience them is lacking because there is no precise definition of the
ymptoms, because distinctions are not made between symptoms of
enopause and symptoms of other phenomena, and because re-
archers measure symptoms in different ways (Kaufert, 1981). Some
idies include such diverse experiences as insomnia, diarrhea, and
in-crawling as symptoms, whereas many researchers now believe that
ily two symptoms can be attributed to menopause: hot flashes and
yness of vaginal mucosa. In obtaining the data on symptoms, some
idies report clinical data while others report women's perceptions
er the fact. Estimations of the proportion of women who have "symp-
ms" of menopause reflect this lack of clarity in the research. These
timates range from 20% (Jern, 1973) to 37% (DeLorey, 1981) to 62%
ouncil of the Medical Women's Federation, 1933) and up to 80%
/ilson, 1962; Thompson, 1973; McKinlay and Jefferys, 1974; Weideger,
77). Most estimations of the proportion of women who see a physician
r menopausal symptoms report 50% or less (Weideger, 1977; Studd,
81; Evans, 1982).

There is no clear-cut evidence of a causal link between symptoms
sociated with menopause and a decrease of cyclical ovarian estrogen.
at is not to deny the existence of symptoms or to deny the experience
women who report them. But further research is needed from the
iological and experiential perspectives before the significance of these
mptoms can be evaluated. From the biological perspective, more in-

---

vo recent exceptions to this offer exciting prospects for future results and future re-
arch. Sonja McKinlay is conducting a prospective study on midlife women in the
nited States and expects to replicate the study with a Canadian cohort. Maryanne
olnalons-Nicolet and Elizabeth Markson are planning a prospective study on midlife
at will compare women in Switzerland, France, and the United States. These studies
ll provide more information on the midlife experience as well as highlight the factors
ost relevant to women's health in old age.

formation is needed on the clinical and epidemiological manifestation
of the symptoms and the women who experience them. From the expe
riential perspective, more information is needed concerning whic
women do and do not report symptoms, to determine antecedents tha
influence their health status, including their experience of menopause
at midlife.

PSYCHOSOCIAL ASPECTS OF MENOPAUSE. Menopause is a biologica
process that takes place within a particular social and cultural setting
Thus, the psychosocial aspects of menopause are as important a consic
eration as the biological aspects. Because of the symbolic representatio
of menopause, the social aspects produce profound changes in the wa
women at menopause view themselves and in turn are viewed b
society.

Menopause is discussed and evaluated as a social event in bot
professional and nonprofessional literature (Patrick, 1970; Crawfor
1973; Boston Women's Health Book Collective, 1976; Gray, 1976; Parle
1976; van Keep, 1976; Reitz, 1977; Bart, 1967; McCarter, 1982). The infl
ence of different cultural settings and different cultural backgrounds c
a woman's perception of menopause is well documented (Maoz, 197
McKinlay and Jefferys, 1974; van Keep, 1976; Griffin, 1978; Datan, 198
Frey, 1981) and is further evidence that a biological explanation is n
sufficient to explain the varied experiences of menopause.

Although there is evidence that class differences influence a won
an's perception of menopause (McKinlay and Jeffreys, 1974), as do
how a woman experiences her parental role (Bart, 1967), little is know
about other social factors. One interesting cross-cultural perspective
that of Marsha Flint, who has carried out anthropological studies
women of the Rajput caste in the Indian states of Rajasthan ar
Himachel Pradesh. These women had none of the symptoms Weste
women often associated with menopause. If they had not yet achieve
menopause they were looking forward to it, while those women wl
had already reached menopause were very positive about it.

Flint's explanation is that these Rajput women live in purdah ar
are not allowed in the company of men prior to menopause, when the
are released from these restrictions and allowed to publicly visit ar
socialize with men. The women view menopause as raising their statu
Flint contrasts the elevation of status in these Indian cultures with tl
changing roles of menopausal women in the United States, whose stat
declines as they age, and suggests that the rewards, or lack of them, c
influence women's experiences of menopause or midlife (Flint, 198.

Other recent research is exploring cross-cultural differenc
(Griffin, 1978; Datan, 1981) as well as sexuality and role norms (McC
ter, 1982).

Ieart Disease and Midlife Women

Much of the information concerning heart disease and midlife wom-
n assumes a connection with menopause, a connotation perpetuated
y a misinterpretation of the data, a denial of the multifactorial causes of
eart disease, and a lack of relevant research on women and heart
isease.

If menopause were responsible for increased heart-disease mor-
lity, then we would expect to see a sharp increase at the time of
1enopause, but instead the reality is that there is a gradual increase
ith age, with no acceleration at menopause (Ryan and Gibson, 1973;
auer, 1980). It is the *ratio* of deaths from heart disease between men and
omen that changes. For all ages, the female : male ratio for heart-dis-
1se fatalities is 2 : 36 for white women (1 : 47 for black women) but by 60
ears of age it becomes 1 : 71 for all groups. This change in the ratio
·flects the steadily increasing rate for women as well as a diminishing
f the acceleration of men's rates. The sharp difference in the
1ale : female ratios between blacks and whites should be noted. Black
1en and black women have higher death rates from heart disease
1roughout the life-span, but the ratio of black men to black women is
most half that of their white counterparts. There is yet no evidence
1at hormonal factors in black and white women differ, and if indeed
ormonal influences were protective for women against heart disease,
e would expect to see the ratios similar for black and white persons.
he role of estrogens in heart disease risk is not yet known.

It is more reasonable to assume that genetic, dietary, and life-style
ctors are more relevant to heart disease fatalities than menopause
atus. The linear increase with age may not be from aging factors or
ormonal changes but instead may reflect prolonged exposure to high
sk factors. In looking at heart disease, midlife women, and meno-
1use, we need to separate out those activities that confound each other
1ch as body size, smoking, and alcohol consumption, all of which are
·sociated with both an early menopause and cerebrovascular disease
Iill, 1979; Gordon, Kannell, Hjortland, and McNamara, 1978).

Coronary risk factors for women have received scant attention com-
1red to men. This is particularly striking for sociocultural factors. Re-
·nt work by Haynes and others in the Framingham Study indicate that
idlife women classified as high in Type-A behavior (emotional lability,
;ing worries, tension, and anger symptoms) have an increase in the
te of coronary heart disease compared to women who show less Type-
behavior. Employed women showed more Type-A behavior than
eir homemaker sisters and were similar to the Type-A men (Haynes,
·vine, Scotch, Feinlab, and Kannell, 1978); overall, only clerical work-

ers with family responsibilities actually had a higher coronary risk tha
homemakers.

Further epidemiological research is needed to explain male–femal
differences in cardiac mortality. But if the evidence is not yet available t
explain these differences, neither is it available to demonstrate tha
menopause is a cause of heart disease in midlife women.

Cancer and Midlife Women

Next to heart/cerebrovascular diseases, cancer is the leading kille
of midlife women. Cancers of the uterus, cervix, and breast account fc
approximately 40% of all female cancer deaths (see Table 2).

Cancer of the breast is responsible for 26% of all diagnosed cancer
and 19% of cancer mortality, or 30,000 deaths in the United State:
higher than for any other site in women. Although breast cancer mo.
tality has declined in past decades for women under 50 years of age, it :
on the rise for women over 50 (Tishler, 1978; Kopstein, 1972), with bot
incidence and mortality greater in black women.

The specific causes of breast cancer are unknown, and it is unlikel
that there is one single etiological factor. Instead, it appears to be depei
dent upon a number of factors, including age, familial history, enviror
ment, and exogenous hormones. A woman's risk of breast cancer ii
creases by 80% to 150% if her mother or sister has had breast cancer, b
it is not clear whether this increased risk is primarily inherited or is
reflection of common environmental experiences (Bain, Speizer, Rosne
Belanger, and Hennekens, 1981). The use of exogenous estrogens
midlife increases a woman's risk of breast cancer at least twofold (Ross
al., 1980; Lawson et al., 1981). Fibrocystic disease of the breast is anoth
factor thought to be associated with a higher risk of breast cancer, b
recent research questions this belief. It seems more likely that tho
other factors that put a woman at risk for breast cancer influence preca
cerous changes in the breast; these factors, rather than fibrocyst
changes, influence the risk status for breast cancer (Love, Gilman, ar
Silen, 1982).

The term breast cancer is in reality a general phrase used to designa
a heterogeneous group of cancers of the breast residing in a heter
geneous group of women. Thus, to think of the natural history of brea
cancer as a single phenomenon is fallacious (Fisher, Redmond, ai
Fisher 1978). This makes research on the progress of the disease ai
therapeutic interventions complex and often confusing. The complexi
in research can be addressed by doing prospective randomized clinic
trials in which, by design, women in different groups will be as simil
as possible, and any differences will therefore be from what is bei

valuated. The complexity in deciding upon treatment for individual
omen is made even more difficult by rapid changes of information
egarding diagnostic procedures and therapeutic decisions. Screening
rograms and breast self-examination are responsible for detecting the
ajority of breast tumors. The success of any screening program de-
ends on the stage of the lesions detected (Strax, 1978), but even this is
ow the subject of some controversy. Screening may not actually influ-
nce the survival rate by early detection. Instead, a tumor detected in a
creening program may just be diagnosed earlier in its natural history,
nd thus the longer survival time is an artifact of early detection. There
 also some consideration of another bias, in that slow-growing tumors
e more likely to be detected at screening while fast-growing tumors
ill be detected in the times between. Slow-growing tumors are less life-
reatening and respond to treatment better than fast-growing tumors
Henderson and Canellos, 1980).

Screening for breast cancer relies on three major components: clinical
amination (including palpation and inspection), mammography, and
ermography. Because of a high rate of false diagnoses and disagree-
ent on criteria of normalcy, thermography is not widely used at present
Moskowitz, Milbrath, Gartside, Zermeno, and Mandel, 1976). Mam-
ography is a form of X ray specifically designed for breast examinations.
s efficacy and safety have been challenged (Bailer 1976; Strax 1978), but
ith improvement in mammographic technique and the use of mam-
ography only for women over 50 years or in high-risk categories, the
ossible dangers are mitigated.

There are few remaining standards for the treatment of breast can-
r. Factors that must be considered in planning therapeutic interven-
on include the stage of the cancer at diagnosis, the natural history of
e tumor, and the type of tumor (Henderson and Canellos, 1980). In
e past, radical mastectomy (complete removal of the affected breast,
nderlying tissue, and lymph nodes) and chemotherapy were the major
eatments for breast cancer. The value of using such major interven-
ons on a routine basis is now questioned by some researchers and
actitioners on the grounds that the results are not any better than
her forms of treatment (Kohn, 1982). Alternative treatments for early
ages include primary irradiation after biopsy, lumpectomy (excision of
e tumor) with endocrine therapy, or combined chemotherapy for re-
rrence or advanced disease.

With the rapid changes in therapies as well as the resulting dis-
reements among practitioners, what is an individual woman to do
hen confronted with the possibility of breast cancer? Because it is a
mplex disease manifested differently in each woman, there is no one
rrect form of treatment. A woman must insist that her physician dis-

cuss all relevant options and their outcomes with her so that together they may make the decisions concerning her care. If her physician is reluctant, she should get a second opinion, now covered by most insurances. If she cannot get the information she needs, she can contact her nearest women's health center or consumer health information service

To the physician, breast cancer is seen as a life-threatening concern, but for the woman involved, it means not only confronting a life-threatening illness but the possible loss of a very significant part of her body with grief at this loss (Notman, 1979). It is therefore essential that a woman have full information so she can then make the most appropriate decisions for herself.

Cancer of the endometrium (*corpus uteri*) is not a major killer of women, but its relevance for midlife women has increased since a causal link between estrogen use and endometrial cancer has been proposed. Although some researchers suggest that the reported increase is an artifact of closer surveillance or lack of differentiation of cellular change (Campbell, 1976), most researchers indicate an increased risk of endometrial cancer from four- to eightfold with the use of exogenous estrogens (Weiss, Srekely, and Austin, 1976; Sartwell, 1976; Spengler, Clarke, Worlever, Newman, and Osborn, 1981).

Cervical cancer is not a major cause of death among United States women, accounting for only 3% of cancer deaths, and the mortality from it has been decreasing rapidly. Even though the mortality is decreasing there is wide disparity among groups, with black women three times more likely to die from cancer of the cervix than white women.

The availability and use of the Papanicolaou (Pap) test has often been credited with the declining mortality from cancer of the cervix. Recently, debate on this issue has centered around the fact that the decline may have started before Pap tests were routinely administered, that the decline exists where Pap tests are not done, and that increasing numbers of hysterectomies mask the epidemiological data since a woman cannot get cancer of the cervix if she has no uterus. Although debate on the issue continues, particularly concerning the costs of screening total population, even critics concede that screening according to high risk groups is appropriate (Kleinman, 1979). Women at high risk are those who have had sexual intercourse, particularly with early onset of sexual activity and multiple sexual partners (Canadian Task Force, 1976). Because screening programs can detect lesions before they have progressed, and because cervical cancer can be effectively treated when detected early enough, the most appropriate use of resources would be to screen those groups at high risk for cervical cancer and to educate women and physicians concerning the value of selective screening.

Occupational Health Issues for Midlife Women

If a paucity of information characterizes other aspects of health for midlife women, then it completely defines what we know about work and health and midlife women. Most of the attention to occupational health issues has been directed to young male workers and, to a lesser degree, to young female workers; typically, concern about females has centered around reproductive issues. Occupations that are predominantly female, such as clerical work and household work, have been consistently neglected in the determination of health hazards. Additionally, nontraditional occupations for women have been neglected in considering differential effects of health hazards on women. An important point for the group of women who are at midlife today is that these women 55–60 years old in the 1980s entered the work force in the 1940s, during World War II. These women are the Rosie the Riveters, who were exposed to all the hazards of the workplace usually considered relevant only to men.

Little research has been done on the hazards of the workplace that primarily affect women, and further research is needed to identify the epidemiology of work-related health conditions, rates of occupational illness, and occupational disabilities specific to midlife women.

A 1981 American Public Health Association report on older women and their health (Rathbone-McCuan and Dunn, 1981) suggests the following priorities for older women and occupational health:[2]

1. As more women enter craft-skill jobs and hazardous occupations that have yet to design equipment for women workers, the protective equipment needs of women must be investigated.
2. Working conditions such as ventilation inadequacies, excessive temperature ranges, and exposure to noise, dust, fume levels, and chemical substances should be investigated for their relationship to chronic diseases and related disabilities that have an impact on women.
3. Occupational stress and work-related crisis events should be examined in relation to the mental health of women as they age in a combined life-style of work and family.
4. The interrelationship of job satisfaction, economic status, job status, and future life-style decisions should be studied in the context of women's retirement planning and postretirement adaptations.

The priorities are quoted from the report, *The Surviving Majority: Older Women and Their Health,* with permission of the authors.

5. Studies of employee health services are needed to assess their relevance to the special needs of older women and to identify specific programs or modifications of services that will meet their health needs for prevention and early diagnosis and follow-up.

CONCLUSION

The American Public Health Association project on Older Women's Health Issues (1981) reported on social and physical health, aging, occupational health hazards, and research issues (Rathbone-McCuan and Dunn, 1981). The researchers reported that they were hindered by huge gaps in the information that they needed to make realistic assessments of the health of older women. This implies that the existing "medical model" health care system is inappropriate and ineffective to meet the health needs of older women. A new system with new perspectives is needed, one that considers all factors that relate to health. Because a person's life-style and past experiences are integral components of health status, it is crucial that health care include a life-style perspective. Events in women's lives do not follow a predetermined staircase pattern, as much of the biomedical literature assumes. Life-style factors such as a woman's work history, her reproductive history, or her nurturant responsibilities, as well as other role relationships, and the timing of each of these in her life cycle all need to be considered.

One cornerstone of the present medical system is the assumption that the gynecologist is the primary care provider for women. This is inappropriate as well as impractical, because gynecological health problems are not the major health problems or causes of death for women. Heart disease (*not* a gynecological problem) is the leading cause of death for women, accounting for 38% of all deaths (Kleinman, 1979). The fact that gynecology is a surgical specialty also argues against gynecologists being the primary providers for midlife women. In addition, it is conceptually and politically inappropriate to have gynecologists as the primary health providers for older women because it perpetuates the reductionist attitude of seeing women only as products of their reproductive organs and of prescribing surgery as the obvious solution of choice for many common health issues.

Furthermore, many gynecologists are out of step with women' genuine health needs. One indication of this lack of congruity between women and gynecologists is that almost all medical literature concerning midlife women focuses on menopause, whereas in reality menopause accounts for only 3% of physician visits made by midlife women (45 to 65 years old). Hypertension accounts for the largest number of visits 8.8%—almost three times as many visits as for menopause-related rea sons. Not surprisingly, gynecologists attribute the reasons for women's visits to menopausal reasons at a 64% higher rate than women themselves do (Cypress, 1980).

In a survey of medical literature it became clear that the information currently available to physicians perpetuates negative attitudes toward menopause and midlife women (DeLorey, 1981). Of over 30 textbooks concerning women, not one discusses midlife women without menopause as the predominant subject, and few even mention other aspects of health (Romney, 1975; Martin, 1978; Taylor, 1969; Wilson, 1979; Baden and Thornton, 1980). Less than one-third of the texts present menopause as a normal, nonpathological process (Beeson and McDermot, 1971; Jeffcoate, 1975; Novak, 1975; Romney, 1975; Martin, 1978; Parson and Sommers, 1978; Wilson, 1979; Baden and Thornton, 1980). By presenting menopause as negative and by focusing on menopause as the major midlife health issue, the authors perpetuate the reductionist perspective that women's reproductive organs are the central focus of their life and health.

If the existing system of health care is not appropriate for midlife women, what would an adequate health system include? Both as individuals and as a group, women need to be listened to and heard, and as a group they need to be given the opportunity to implement their ideas of good health care. Women need encouragement to seek and demand information concerning their own health, so that they themselves may make the decisions for, and have control of, their health and their bodies. In such a health care system prevention of disease would be stressed.

There already exists a strong movement of women of all ages concerned with health who are incorporating these ideas into actions. These women, part of the women's self-help health movement, are often associated with women-controlled health centers, and focus on menopause issues, midlife issues, and health for older women. This women's self-help movement goes beyond discussions of how or why the medical care system does not meet their needs; members view self-help as an action-oriented concept, with major goals being (a) to demystify health/medical care through sharing and translating medical literature, (b) to remedicalize health care for women, and (c) to empower women to reclaim control of their health and bodies through validation of their own experiences.

These goals are actualized through groups and centers that midlife women themselves control. These include such diverse groups as the Menopause Collective in the metropolitan Boston area, the Midlife and Older Women's Committee of the National Women's Health Network, the Older Women's League, and the Gray Panthers Health Project

Fund. It is from these older women's self-help groups, more than from medical sources, that valuable information has been generated and disseminated. This new information includes various ways to ameliorate hot flashes, why exercise continues to be important for women as they get older, and the continued importance of nutrition for older women. These groups also emphasize the need to separate normal aging from illness and the need to consider women's lives in totality.

Because the nature of the phenomena of midlife, women, and health make these difficult to study, the myths more than the realities of each have guided providers, policy-makers, and researchers. The implications of this lack of accurate information and perpetuation of stereotypes are far-reaching. The immediate implication is that midlife women cannot receive adequate and appropriate health care if every aspect of their health is seen as related to menopause. The long-term implication is that by the attribution of all symptoms or complaints of midlife to the diminution of ovarian estrogen, the possible consequences of these complaints and their relation to the aging process are ignored, perhaps to manifest themselves as chronic disease processes of old age that could have been alleviated with appropriate attention at midlife.

To provide appropriate health services for midlife women, both the structure of the existing services and the dearth of accurate information need to be addressed. To accomplish this we must do the following:

1. Establish priorities of health care that address women's priorities derived from their own experiences and that are based on the sociological and behavioral as well as the biomedical sciences
2. Establish an information base that considers the precursors of health at midlife. For example, one could focus on how nutrition and exercise throughout the life-span affect osteoporosis, rather than focus on medical intervention issues after the process has already begun.
3. Redefine research priorities so that nonclinical and prospective studies are conducted that give a more accurate assessment of midlife.
4. Present a more realistic, less pathological view of midlife women to health providers. This perspective is not readily available in the medical literature but is available in the literature from the behavioral sciences (Bart and Grossman, 1976; Parlee, 1976; Koeske, 1977; Bart, 1967; Notman, 1979; Rubin, 1979; Datan, 1981), as well as in the literature written by and for women (Boston Women's Health Book Collective, 1976; Clay, 1977; Reitz, 1977; Weideger, 1977; Sommers and Shields, 1980; Sand

Fe Health Education Project, 1980; Block, Davidson, and Grambs, 1981).

5. Support environments in which women can develop realistic expectations about midlife health issues. These environments already exist through many self-help groups and workshops conducted at women's health centers, and in other women's groups where women learn through sharing and validating their experiences with each other.

Midlife is an important stage of women's lives, but from the perpective of health issues, the domination of menopause has obscured our understanding of the totality of women's health experiences. Only when we look at all the facets of this rich experience can we begin to make valid statements and assessments relating to the health of midlife women. The task now is to hear what women themselves say of their xperiences of midlife, including menopause, so that both the social and iological significance of midlife can be seen as it really is, not as it is ssumed to be. Then, attention can be redirected to look at all the factors nfluencing women's health at midlife and women themselves will then ave accurate and appropriate information when they make choices bout their own health care.

REFERENCES

ntunes, C. M. F. Endometrial cancer and estrogen use. *New England Journal of Medicine*, 1979, *300*, 9–13.

aden, W. F., and Thornton, D. R. (Eds.). *Primary health care for obstetricians and gynecologists*. Baltimore: Williams and Wilkins, 1980.

ailer, J. V. Mammography: A contrary view. *Annals of Internal Medicine*, 1976, *84*, 77–84.

ain, C., Speizer, F. E., Rosner, B., Belanger, C., and Hennekens, C. H. Family history of breast cancer as a risk indicator for the diseases. *American Journal of Epidemiology*, 1981, *111*, 301–308.

art, P. *Depression in middle-aged women: Some sociocultural factors*. Doctoral dissertation, University of California at Los Angeles, 1967.

art, P., and Grossman, M. Menopause. *Women and Health*, 1976, *1*, 3–11.

eard, R. J. (Ed.). *The menopause: A guide to current research and practice*. Baltimore: University Park Press, 1976.

eeson, P. B., and McDermot, W. *Cecil-Loeb textbook of medicine*. Philadelphia: Saunders, 1971.

ock, M. R., Davidson, J. L., and Grambs, J. D. *Women over forty: Visions and realities*. New York: Springer, 1981.

oston Women's Health Book Collective. *Our bodies, ourselves*. New York: Simon & Schuster, 1976.

urch, J. C., and Byrd, B. F. Effects of long-term administration of estrogen on the occurrence of mammary cancer in women. *Annals of Surgery*, 1971, *174*, 414–418.

ureau of the Census. *A statistical portrait of women*. Current Population Reports, Special Studies: Series P-23 No. 58, Washington, D.C., 1975.

Campbell, S. (Ed.). *The management of the menopause and post-menopausal years.* Baltimore: University Park Press, 1976.

Canadian Task Force. Cervical cancer screening programs. *Canadian Medical Association Journal,* 1976, *114*, 1003–1033.

Clay, U. S. *Women: Menopause and middle age.* Pittsburgh: Know, Inc., 1977.

Connell, E. Estrogen: What to do until the results are in. In L. Rose (Ed.), *The menopause book.* New York: Hawthorn Books, 1977.

Coope, J. Double blind cross over study of estrogen replacement therapy. In S. Campbell (Ed.), *The management of the menopause and post-menopausal years.* Baltimore: University Park Press, 1976.

Council of the Medical Women's Federation. An investigation of the menopause in one thousand women. *Lancet,* 1933, *1*, 106.

Crawford, M., and Hooper, D. Menopausal aging. *The Family* 1973, *7*, 464–482.

Cutts, J. H., and Noble, R. L. Estrone-induced mammary tumors in the rat. *Cancer Research,* 1964, *24*, 1116–1123.

Cypress, B. K. *Office visits by women.* Vital and Health Statistics: Series 13; No. 45 (DHEW Publication No. (PHS) 80-1796). Hyattsville, Md.: 1980.

Dalton, K. Menopause: A clinician's view. *Royal Society of Health Journal,* 1976, *96*, 75–81.

Datan, N. *A time to reap.* Baltimore: Johns Hopkins University Press, 1981.

DeLorey, C. *Health care for midlife women.* Unpublished doctoral dissertation, Harvard University, 1981.

Department of Commerce. *Historical statistics of the United States* (DHEW Publication No. 004-024-00120-9), Washington, D.C.: U.S. Government Printing Office, 1975.

Dunn, L. National Center for Health Statistics, personal communication, December 1981.

Eskin, B. A. *The menopause: Comprehensive management.* New York: Masson, 1980.

Evans, B. *Life change.* London: Pan Books, 1982.

Fisher, B., Redmond, C., and Fisher, E. R. Clinical trials and the surgical treatment of breast cancer. *Surgical Clinics of North America,* 1978, *58*, 723–735.

Flint, M. Male and female menopause: A cultural put-on. In A. M. Voda, M. Dinnerstein and S. R. O'Donnell (Eds.), *Changing perspectives on menopause.* Austin: University of Texas Press, 1982.

Food and Drug Administration. *FDA drug bulletin.* February/March 1976.

Frey, A. K. Middle-aged women's experience and perceptions of menopause. *Women and Health,* 1981, *6*, 25–36.

Gambrell, R. D. Estrogens, progestogens and endometrial cancer. In P. A. Van Keep, R. F. Greenblatt, and M. Albeaux-Fernet (Eds.), *Consensus of menopause research.* Baltimore: University Park Press, 1976.

Givens, J. D. *Current estimates from the health interview survey.* Vital and Health Statistics Series 10, No. 130 (DHEW Publication No. (PHS) 80-1551). Hyattsville, Md.: U.S. Government Printing Office, 1979.

Goodman, M. *Menopause: A pilot study.* University of Hawaii Women's Studies Program, Working Paper Series, 1976, *1*, 1–23.

Gordon, T., Kannell, W. B., Hjortland, M. C., and McNamara, P. M. Menopause and coronary heart disease. *Journal of the American Medical Association,* 1978, *89*, 157–161.

Gray, R. H. The menopause—Epidemiological and demographic consideration. In R. Beard (Ed.), *The menopause.* Baltimore: University Park Press, 1976.

Greenblatt, R. B. Estrogens and endometrial cancer—Gross exaggeration or fact? *Geriatric* 1977, *32*, 60–72.

Griffin, J. A cross-cultural investigation of behavioral changes at menopause. In K. O'Connor-Blumhagen and W. D. Johnson (Eds.), *Women's studies: An interdisciplinary collection.* Westport, Conn.: Greenwood Press, 1978.

Hadden, W. C. *Basic data on health care needs of adults ages 25–74 years, United States*

1971–1975. Vital and Health Statistics: Series 11, No. 218 (DHEW Publication No. (PHS) 81-1668). Hyattsville, Md.: U.S. Government Printing Office, 1981.

Haynes, S. G., Levine, S., Scotch, N., Feinlab, M., and Kannell, W. B. The relationship of psychosocial factors to coronary heart disease in the Framingham study. *American Journal of Epidemiology*, 1978, *107*, 384–401.

Henderson, I. C., and Canellos, G. P. Cancer of the breast: The past decade. *New England Journal of Medicine*, 1980, *302*, 17–30.

Hill, J. *Menopause and cardiovascular disease.* Paper presented at the Interdisciplinary Research Conference on Menopause, Tucson, 1979.

Hoover, R. Menopausal estrogens and breast cancer. *New England Journal of Medicine*, 1976, *295*, 401–405.

Jeffcoate, N. *Principles of gynecology.* Boston: Butterworths, 1975.

Kern, H. *Hormone therapy of the menopause and aging.* Springfield, Ill.: Charles C Thomas, 1973.

Kaufert, P. Symptom reporting at the menopause. *Social Science and Medicine*, 1981, *151*, 173–184.

Kleinmann, J. C. Death rates from cervical cancer by health service area 1968–72. *Statistical Notes for Health Planners*, No. 8, August 1979 (DHEW Publication No. (PHS) 79-1237). Washington: U.S. Government Printing Office, 1979.

Koeske, R. K. *Theoretical perspectives on menstrual cycle research.* Paper presented at the Menstrual Cycle Conference, Chicago, 1977.

Kohn, J. Treating breast cancer conservatively: Dissension, contention continue. *Journal of the American Medical Association*, 1982, *248*, 1793–1802.

Kopstein, A. N. Breast cancer death rates by health service area, 1968–72. *Statistical Notes for Health Planners*, No. 30, July 1978 (DHEW Publication No. (PHS) 78-1250). Washington: U.S. Government Printing Office, 1972.

Lawson, D. H., Jick, H., Hunter, J., and Madsen, S. Exogenous estrogens and breast cancer. *American Journal of Epidemiology*, 1981, *114*, 710–713.

Lebich, P. E. Effects and side effects of estrogen therapy. In D. A. Van Keep, R. B. Gesenblatt, and M. Albeaux-Fernet (Eds.), *Consensus of menopause research.* Baltimore: University Park Press, 1976.

Love, S. M., Gilman, R. S., and Silen, W. Fibrocystic "disease" of the breast—A non-disease? *New England Journal of Medicine*, 1982, *307*, 1010–1014.

Mack, T. M., Pike, M. C., Henderson, B. E., Pfeffer, R. I., Gerkins, V. R., Arthur, M., and Brown, S. E. Estrogens and endometrial cancer in a retirement community. *New England Journal of Medicine*, 1976, *294*, 1262–1267.

Maoz, B. Female attitudes to menopause. *Social Psychiatry*, 1970, *5*, 35–40.

Martin, L. L. *Health care of women.* Philadelphia: Lippincott, 1978.

McCarter, S. S. Physical changes related to menopause. In S. L. Tyler and G. M. Woodall (Eds.), *Female health and gynecology across the lifespan.* Bowie, Md.: Robert J. Brady, 1982.

McKinlay, S. M., and Jefferys, M. The menopausal syndrome. *British Journal of Preventive and Social Medicine*, 1974, *28*, 108–115.

McKinlay, S., Jefferys, M., and Thompson, B. An investigation of the age at menopause. *Journal of Biosocial Science*, 1971, *4*, 161–173.

Midwinter, A., Contra-indications to estrogen therapy and management of the menopausal syndrome in these cases. In S. Campbell (Ed.), *The management of the menopausal and post-menopausal years.* Baltimore: University Park Press, 1976.

Mishler, E. G., Amarasingham, L. R., Hauser, S., Liem, R., Osherson, S. D., and Waxler, N. E. *Social contexts of health, illness, and patient care.* New York: Cambridge University Press, 1981.

Moskovitz, M., Milbrath, J., Gertside, P., Zermeno, A., and Mandel, D. Lack of efficacy of thermography as a screening tool for minimal and Stage I cancer. *New England Journal of Medicine*, 1976, *295*, 249–252.

Nathanson, A. Illness and the feminine role: A theoretical review. *Social Science and Medicine*, 1975, *9*, 57–62.

Neugarten, B. L. Women's attitudes toward the menopause. *Vita Humanae*, 1963, *6*, 140–146.

Notelovitz, M. The effect of long term estrogen replacement therapy on glucose and lipid metabolism in post-menopausal women. *South African Medical Journal*, 1976, *50*, 2001–2003.

Notman, M. Midlife concerns of women: Implications of the menopause. *American Journal of Psychiatry*, 1979, *136*, 1270–1274.

Novak, E. R. *Novak's text book of gynecology*. Baltimore: Williams and Wilkins, 1975.

Parlee, M. B. Social factors in the psychology of menstruation, birth, and menopause. *Primary Care*, 1976, *3*, 477–490.

Parson, L., and Sommers, S. C. *Gynecology*. Philadelphia: Saunders, 1978.

Patrick, M. L. *A study of middle-aged women and menopause*. Unpublished doctoral dissertation, University of California at Los Angeles, 1970.

Prensky, J. *Healing yourself*. New York: Bantam, 1974.

Proudfit, C. D. Estrogens and menopause. *Journal of the American Medical Association*, 1976, *236*, 939–940.

Rathbone-McCuan, E., and Dunn, T. *The surviving majority: Older women and their health* (APHA Project No. 440032). Washington, D.C.: American Public Health Association, 1981.

Reitz, R. *Menopause: A positive approach*. Radnor, Pa.: Chilton, 1977.

Romney, S. *Gynecology and obstetrics: The health care of women*. New York: McGraw-Hill, 1975.

Ross, R. K., Paganini-Hill, A., Gerkins, O. R., Mack, T. M., Pfeffer, R. I., Arthur, M., and Henderson, B. E. A case-control study of menopausal estrogen therapy and breast cancer. *Journal of the American Medical Association*, 1980, *243*, 1635–1638.

Rubin, L. B. *Women of a certain age: The midlife search for self*. New York: Harper & Row, 1979.

Ryan, K. J., and Givson, D. C. *Menopause and aging* (DHEW Publication No. (NIH) 73-319). Washington: U.S. Government Printing Office, 1973.

Santa Fe Health Education Project. *Menopause: A self care manual*. Santa Fe, N. Mex.: Santa Fe Health Education Project, 1980.

Sartwell, P. Estrogen replacement theory and endometrial carcinoma: Epidemiologic evidence. *Clinical Obstetrics and Gynecology*, 1976, *19*, 817–823.

Sauer, H. I. *Geographic patterns in the risk of dying and associated factors, ages 35–74, United States, 1968–1972*. Vital and Health Statistics: Series 3: No. 18 (DHHS Publication No. (PHS) 80-1402). Hyattsville, Md.: U.S. Government Printing Office, 1980.

Seaman, B., and Seaman, G. *Women and the crisis in sex hormones*. New York: Rawson Associates, 1977.

Shoemaker, S. Estrogen treatment of post-menopausal women: Benefits and risks. *Journal of the American Medical Association*, 1977, *238*, 1524–1530.

Siegal, D., and Michaud, A. Exercise at menopause. *WomanWise*, 1980, *3*, 7.

Smith, D. Association of exogenous estrogen and endometrial cancer. *New England Journal of Medicine*, 1975, *293*, 1164–1167.

Sommers, T., and Shields, L. Older women and health care. In *Gray paper no. 3*. Oakland, Calif.: Older Women's League, 1980.

Spengler, R. F., Clarke, E. A., Worlever, D. A., Newman, A. M., and Osborn, R. Exogenous estrogens and endometrial cancer: A case-control study and assessment of potential biases. *American Journal of Epidemiology*, 1981, *114*, 497–506.

ᴋax, P. Evaluation of screening programs for the early diagnosis of breast cancer. *Surgical Clinics of North America*, 1978, *58*, 667–679.

ᴜdd, J. W. W. *The menopause*. London: Guideway, 1981.

ᴚich, A. *Social implications of menopause*. Paper presented at the American Women in Psychology Conference, Pittsburgh, 1978.

ᴀylor, E. S. *Essentials of gynecology*. Philadelphia: Lea and Febiger, 1969.

ᴚompson, B. Menopausal age and symptomatology in a general practice. *Journal of Biosocial Sciences*, 1973, *71*, 1973.

ᴚhler, S. L. Breast disorders. In M. T. Notman and C. C. Nadelson (Eds.), *The woman patient*. New York: Plenum Press, 1978.

ᴚichopoulos, D. Menopause and breast cancer risk. *Journal of the National Cancer Institute*, 1972, *48*, 605–613.

ᴚian, W. H. The scientific basis for post-menopausal estrogen therapy: The management of specific symptoms and rationale for long-term replacement. In R. J. Beard (Ed.), *The menopause*. Baltimore: University Park Press, 1976.

ᴚn Keep, P. A., Greenblatt, R. B., and Albeauz-Fernet, M. (Eds.). *Consensus on menopause research*. Baltimore: University Park Press, 1976.

ᴚrbrugge, L. M. Females and illness: Recent trends in sex differences in the United States. *Journal of Health and Social Behavior*, 1976, *17*, 387–403.

ᴚrbrugge, L. M., and Steiner, R. P. Physician treatment of men and women patients: Sex bias or appropriate care? *Medical Care*, 1981, *19*, 609–632.

ᴚeideger, P. *Menstruation and menopause*. New York: Dell, 1977.

ᴚeiss, N. S., Szekely, D. R., and Austin, D. F. Increasing incidence of endometrial cancer in the United States. *New England Journal of Medicine*, 1976, *294*, 1259–1262.

ᴚenderlein, J. M. Psychotherapeutic effects of estrogen substitution during the climacteric period. In N. Pasetto, R. Paoletti, and J. L. Ambrus (Eds.), *The menopause and postmenopause*. Baltimore: University Park Press, 1980.

ᴚilson, J. *Obstetrics and gynecology*. St. Louis: C. V. Mosby, 1979.

ᴚilson, R. A. *Feminine forever*. New York: M. Evans, 1961.

ᴚilson, R. J. Roles of estrogen and progesterone in breast and genital cancer. *Journal of the American Medical Association*, 1962, *82*, 327–331.

ᴚolfe, S. M. Affidavit of Sidney M. Wolf, M.D., United States District Court for the District of Delaware: *Pharmaceutical Manufacturers Association* vs. *Food and Drug Administration*, September 22, 1977.

ᴚomen's Bureau. *Mature women workers*. Washington, D.C.: U.S. Department of Labor, 1976.

ᴚel, H. K., and Finkle, W. D. Increased risk of endometrial carcinoma among users of conjugated estrogens. *New England Journal of Medicine*, 1975, *293*, 1167–1170.

Chapter 13

Reproductive Issues, Including Menopause

MARY BROWN PARLEE

Scientific and clinical knowledge about the psychology of female reproduction has expanded rapidly over the past 15 years. Not only is there more research on the psychology of menstruation, pregnancy, birth, and menopause, it is better: more grounded in empirical data and more reflective of the complexity of the phenomena.[1]

A good deal of credit for this progress belongs to feminist researchers, scholars, and health care workers, both inside and outside academia and traditional health care institutions. Beginning with the groundbreaking *Our Bodies, Ourselves* (Bosten Women's Health Book Collective, 1973), these investigators reexamined and reevaluated literature on female health and reproduction, identifying implicit assumptions in the traditional work and pointing at gaps in knowledge where further research was needed. Such critiques—analyses of underlying assumptions and their implications for research—have played a central role in advances in research on the psychology of female reproduction, particularly in research on the psychology of menstruation (Dan, Graham, and Beecher, 1981; Komnenich, McSweeney, Noack, and Elder, 1981; Friedman, 1982; Golub, in press).

Despite significant progress in psychological research on menstruation and menarche, research and thinking about the psychology of menopause does not appear to have progressed as far (Voda, Dinnerstein, and O'Donnell, 1982). Why is that? Why should the psychological

MARY BROWN PARLEE • Center for the Study of Women and Society, Graduate School and University Center, City University of New York, 33 West 42nd Street, New York, New York 10036. This work was supported in part by a grant from the Ford Foundation to the Center for the Study of Women and Society, Graduate School and University Center, City University of New York.

aspects of menopause have proved so much more intractable to concep
tual and empirical analysis than have other stages of the female re
productive life cycle?

Part of the answer may be that menopause is psychologically signif
icant in different domains of experience and behavior from those of th
menstrual cycle or pregnancy, and that psychological researchers, in
cluding feminists, have been working with assumptions that do no
usually lead them to explore these domains fruitfully.[2] These assump
tions may be resistant to change, furthermore, because they reflect an
are embedded in an important set of social processes that not only shap
the experience and actions of women in midlife but also serve to main
tain the stable functioning of society as a whole. Catherine DeLore
(Chapter 12, this volume) discusses some of these significant social pro
cesses related to menopause—among them, how middle-aged wome
interact with health care systems. Other potentially fruitful domains fo
menopause research will also be suggested as the following line of rea
soning is developed.

In brief, I would like to suggest that feminist critiques of research o
the psychology of menopause point to the importance of what will b
called here a *psychological* rather than a *biological* perspective. This di
tinction does not coincide with one between social/psychological an
biological *causation*. Such critiques have not so far led to programmat
research, however, because of a further general problem pervading so
entific thinking about the psychology of female reproduction, a proble
that the topic of menopause represents in a particular acute form. Th
problem is that the language and concepts of psychological research o
female reproduction tend to mirror the language and thought of socie
as a whole, and these linguistic/conceptual patterns are an integral pa
of a set of important social processes whose equilibrium depends upo
them. To change scientific thinking and research about the psycholog
of female reproduction, then, means that researchers would need
step outside everyday ways of thinking, a bootstrap operation that
perhaps never completely possible.[3] If this operation were successfu

---

[2]As will become apparent, my analysis in no way resembles, in content, in tone, or,
think, in rigor, Judith Posner's disparaging commentary on the caricature she presents
feminist research on menopause (Posner, 1979). While I agree with her observation th
"the relationship of political ideology to research into human behavior" is crucial, I do n
think conceptual clarity on the issues is likely to emerge from the "straw man" s
constructs and then labels "the feminist position."

[3]As research on the psychology of female reproduction has improved (including that
menopause and the climacterium), investigators increasingly point to the importance
studying biological–psychological–social *interactions* (e.g., van Keep and Humphre
1976). The problem is that no one does it or, seemingly, can point to a body of exempla
research. It is issues that still may be blocking the development of those appropriate ne
paradigms to which the present chapter is addressed.

urthermore, it would inevitably raise questions about—perhaps posing hallenges to—the social processes in which the usual patterns of hought are embedded.

If this analysis is correct, then it follows that research on the psychology of female reproduction will be successful (1) to the extent that veryday ways of thinking about the phenomenon are compatible with uitful paradigms for empirical research and/or (2) to the degree to rhich alteration of these ways of thinking can be absorbed without isruption of the social processes of which they are a part. I think one eason psychological research on menopause has not developed satisactorily is that scientific concepts based on everyday thinking are highly nappropriate: They incorporate assumptions about the usefulness of a iological perspective in studying domains of behavior and experience or which adoption of a psychological perspective would probably be seful. For a variety of reasons, two of which will be discussed in detail, nis mismatch between the research perspective adopted and the do—main of psychological phenomena being investigated is greater for nenopause than for other events in the female reproductive life cycle. his argument will now be elaborated in greater detail.

In Chapter 12, DeLorey rightly points to the fragmented and biased ature of previous research on menopause and to the lack of a conceptual nodel integrating biological, psychological, and sociocultural processes. eLorey and others have, further, identified several key assumptions nderlying traditional psychological research on menopause. Their analses, together with the related research supporting them, appear to onverge on the following four points: (1) Judging from self-reports, nenopause and the symptoms traditionally thought to be associated with do not seem to be dominant or universal features of the experience and ehavior of middle-aged women in the United States (Neugarten, Wood, raines, and Loomis, 1963; Neugarten and Kraines, 1965; Greene, 1976; olit and LaRocco, 1980; Townsend and Carbone, 1980). (2) Women's xperience and behavior are affected by midlife changes in their social •les as well as those of others with whom they are emotionally in—olved—husband, children, parents, friends (Ballinger, 1975; Flint, 1975; art and Grossman, 1976; van Keep and Kellerhals, 1976; Barnett and aruch, 1978; Nadelson, Polonsky, and Mathews, 1979; Severne, 1979; reene and Cooke, 1980). (3) The psychological significance of meno—ause as an event in a continuing process (the climacterium) is difficult to sentangle from the psychological significance of more general age-lated physiological changes (Ballinger, 1976; Goodman, Stewart, and ilbert, 1977). (4) Menopause is often invoked by physicians and by ypeople as an implicit or explicit explanation for symptoms or behaviors ising from other causes (Donovan, 1951; Osofsky and Seidenberg, 1970; senberg, 1979; Weissman, 1979; Cowan, in press). These four claims,

arising largely from feminist analyses of traditional research, seem suffi-
ciently obvious and well documented by now to serve as assumptons, as
starting points for further research. That investigators have tended to
reiterate these points rather than use them as the basis for new research
suggests that additional, still implicit assumptions must be operating that
impair the development of programmatic research and theory.

Elsewhere I have suggested that researchers interested in the psychological aspects of female reproductive processes tend to approach the
problem in one of two ways (Parlee, 1981, 1982). If they approach the
study of psychological phenomena from a *biological* perspective, their
conceptual starting point is the *biological process* (menstrual cycle, pregnancy, menopause). The psychological question asked from this perspective is: What are the psychological consequences of these particular
biological changes?

This is a reasonable way to study biological influences on behavior
and experience. Its success depends upon the investigator's being able
to identify those psychological phenomena that are in fact fairly directly
influenced by underlying biological changes, with minimal individual
differences arising from current social influences and/or personality
structure. In research on the psychology of the menstrual cycle, for
example, phenomena related to basic sensory processes appear to be a
domain of psychological functioning for which a biological perspective is
fruitful (Baker, 1975; Parlee, 1982). Similarly, in psychological research
on menopause, it may well be the case that psychological phenomena
related to and including hot flashes are best studied from a biological
perspective (Nelson, 1979).

On the other hand, researchers can also adopt a *psychological* perspective in studying the psychology of female reproduction. From this
perspective, the conceptual starting point is *psychological change over time*.
The research question is: What is the nature of the processes—biological, social, and psychological—that produce psychological changes?

In the study of the psychology of women at midlife, researchers are
adopting what is here called a psychological perspective when they
hypothesize and examine the ways in which changes in social roles
might cause psychological changes in middle-aged women (Barnett and
Baruch, 1978). Such psychological changes might or might not also be
influenced by the biological changes of the climacterium. From a psychological perspective, then, researchers can in principle take into account multiple, covarying causal processes of different kinds (biological,
social, psychological). As with the biological perspective, the success of
research conducted from a psychological perspective depends upon the
investigator's being able to find an appropriate fit between the kind of
psychological phenomenon being studied and the kind(s) of causal pro-

ess(es) by which it is influenced. This is very difficult to do, particularly
then the psychological phenomenon under investigation (changes in
epression, for example) may be subject to different causal influences
perating at the same time and also to primary causation by one kind of
rocess (biological changes) at one time and another kind of process
ole loss) at another.

In addition to the inherent difficulty of the subject matter, psycho-
gical research on female reproduction in general, and on menopause
particular, is made more difficult by the way in which everyday lan-
uage and thought highlight some features of the phenomenon and
task others. According to stereotypes popular in much of the United
tates, certain aspects of women's behavior under particular conditions
nd to be causally attributed to their reproductive biology. As Randi
oeske has pointed out and demonstrated (Koeske, 1981; Koeske and
oeske, 1975), premenstrual changes in physiology are often taken to be
ie cause for negative, out-of-role behavior for women (e.g., anger,
;gression). Stereotypes about a "premenstrual tension syndrome," re-
ardless of the extent to which they are descriptively accurate, can thus
:rve as a cohesive explanatory framework, assimilating within it ac-
ons and experiences that might also have nonbiological causes.

For the present argument, it is important to note that *everyday*
ought and language tend to impute a causal role to female reproductive biology
major transition points in the social life cycle. It is also at such points that
eviancy from role expectations might be predicted by sociologists to
igger social labeling and other social processes that either produce
nformity or isolate the deviant individual as mad (sick) or bad (Scheff,
166). The phrase "postpartum depression," for example, serves to
ghlight and isolate a physiological event (birth) as the implicit cause of
.e psychological phenomenon to be explained (depression). "New
other depression," of course, would be an equally accurate description
 the concurrent biological, psychological, and social events. A woman
ho is depressed after the birth of a child, however, departs from the
neral social expectation that motherhood is usually a pleasurable and
lfilling role. Deviancy theory would predict that when such behavior
reatens the smooth functioning of an important social institution (in
is case, the family), the deviant individual is labeled and becomes a
cus of social processes (or social interactions shaped by roles within
stitutions) that serve to protect the integrity of society as a whole
emert, 1964).

Thus, the new mother who is depressed is described as suffering
)m "postpartum depression." Her behavior will be tolerated because
 her "illness" until she is ready to take up her nondepressing role as
other. In extreme cases, doctors may prescribe drugs for her or recom-

mend hospitalization to cure her "postpartum depression." Social changes that might make the role of mother less depressing are not considered, since the assumption (incorporated in the label) is that the individual woman is suffering psychological problems as a result of changes in her postpartum reproductive biology. Some postpartum depressions may, in fact, as the label implies, have fairly clear and direct biological causes. The important point for the present argument, however, is that the labeling and social processes mobilized in response to it make no effort to discriminate women with such biologically caused postpartum depression from those whose depression arises from role changes and thus, if understood and acted upon, might represent a threat to the stability of social roles within the family.

As with other labeling phenomena studied by deviancy theorists, it is particularly striking that the social responses to potential deviance are usually initiated and carried out by decent, well-meaning, caring people. The husband, family, friends, and doctors of the depressed mother are not conspiring to disregard or mask the real sources of her depression by making causal attributions to reproductive biology. They genuinely want to help. The fact is, however, that ordinary language and thought focus attention exclusively on biology, and these thought patterns are deeply implicated in both social roles and institutions and in the psychology of individuals in them. The acquisition of culture by the individual through language makes it unlikely that he or she will focus on (think about) the presence and properties of phenomena that are unnamed in everyday language and thought (Scribner and Cole, 1974) or that different names and meanings will be given to those that are named.

Researchers as well as laypeople have found it difficult to break away from an everyday explanatory framework that attributes postpartum psychological changes to reproductive biology. One consequence of this has been an inability to develop a cumulative body of psychological research and theory on the postpartum period (Parlee, 1978). Everyday thought has encouraged a biological perspective in the research when a psychological perspective seems also to be appropriate and necessary if scientific progress is to be made.

Labeling and thinking about certain psychological phenomena as "menopausal" has had much the same effect, both in life and in research. The word's reference to biological changes highlights their potential causal significance and implicitly masks concomitant changes in social roles and in age-related psychological development. It is applied to women at a transition point in the social life cycle when several major roles are likely to be changing, either because they have run their natural course or because of general physical changes of the aging process.

While it is not clear what the role expectations for a "menopausal woman" are, it is fairly clear that, as deviance theory would predict, labeling her in this way has consequences for the way others treat her, and perhaps also for the way she regards herself and her possibilities in life. The biological label may thus serve to reduce the likelihood that she and others will examine her experiences in light of possible social and psychological causes.

The problem of linguistic/conceptual bias toward exclusively biological causes is much more acute with menopause, however, than with any of the other major stages of the female reproductive life cycle, One reason is that a much broader range of psychological phenomena are causally attributed to the menopause than to either the recurring changes of the menstrual cycle or to pregnancy, birth, and postpartum. Stereotypes about the "menopausal woman" not only encompass emotional and perhaps cognitive changes but also seem to carry with them a subtle pejorative reference to her inconsequential social status and perhaps also to her physical appearance. Research concepts arising from everyday language and thought, then, seem implicitly to assimilate multiple domains and levels of psychological functioning within the single explanatory framework of changes in reproductive biology. This seems implausible on the face of it, and no body of research has been accumulated to date that would suggest that this biological perspective alone will prove adequate.

There is a second, related reason why research based on concepts from everyday language and thought is more problematic for menopause than for other phases of the reproductive life cycle, It is that the time scales of the psychological, social, and biological changes are not coincident in the way they are for the menstrual cycle and for pregnancy and birth. The biological changes of pregnancy, for example, are temporally concomitant with the psychological changes. Regardless of whether one adopts a psychological or a biological perspective in psychological research on pregnancy, it makes sense to examine biological influences on all the psychological processes occurring over the given time period.

In psychological research on menopause, however, the situation is different. If one adopts a biological perspective, the task is to identify the domain(s) of psychological functioning that are causally influenced by biological changes occurring over a time period defined in terms of biological markers. If one adopts a psychological perspective, the task is to identify a relatively limited domain of psychological functioning that changes over a given time period (defined by psychological markers) and then to ask what biological, psychological, and social processes might account for these changes. Many of the areas of psychological functioning that one might want to explore in women in midlife occu over a different time scale—longer, shorter, or at a different time al together—from physiological changes of the climacterium (including menopause). For example, one might be interested in changes in de pression or self-esteem in women at midlife. Such changes could occu in conjunction with major changes in social roles, with menopause as discrete event marking the end of fertility, with difficulty in separatin from children or parents, with the physical changes of the climacteric with repeated social encounters with those disdainful of "menopausa women." One needs to discover the major causal influences on clearl defined psychological changes through psychological research. But obviously need not be assumed at the start that the psychologica changes of interest will be concomitant in time with the psychologica changes of the climacteric and menopause.

As psychologists interested in women at midlife, we need to ident fy those psychological issues and processes we think are of greater sig nificance or interest according to whatever criteria we choose to use. M hunch is that from this psychological perspective, the significant psy chological issues at midlife are not greatly affected by physiologica changes of the climacterium. Most psychologists are probably more in terested in specific aspects of psychological changes and development i personality and behavior over the course of the middle years than in th more limited class of psychological events that present evidence sug gests is fairly directly caused by the climacterium (Nadelson *et al.*, 197 Notman, 1979).

The conclusions from feminist research and critique (outline above) all point to the same inference. The ongoing changes in behavic and experience occurring in midlife women are not very closely relate to the climacteric or to menopause. Yet too often researchers intereste in midlife have continued to focus on menopause as the conceptu starting point for the research, attempting to assimilate within its pote tial explanatory domain relatively large arenas of behavior extendir over long periods of time. It is of course difficult to avoid in research th patterns of language and thought in the culture that have conflate middle age and menopause. But it can and must be done if scientif psychological research and theory are to proceed beyond critiques.

The fragmented, noncumulative state of the psychological literatu on menopause continues unambiguously to suggest that a biological pe spective is not appropriate, except in research on the psychological n ture and consequences of hot flashes and flushes (Nelson, 1979; Fel man, Postlethwaite, and Glenn, 1976). If researchers interested specific psychological changes occurring in women in the middle yea consistently adopt a psychological perspective, they may well find th enopause plays little or no causal role (Barnett and Baruch, 1978; Notan, 1979; Wood, 1979). The time has surely come when investigators udying middle-aged women can respond to the implicit or explicit ery "But what about menopause?" with "What *about* menopause?" nd let it go at that. The stereotypes imputing causal significance to enopause need be granted no scientific standing. The burden of proof n now be placed on those who want to argue that menopause is ychologically significant in such-and-such (and let them specify) doains of behavior and experience.

In fact, I think menopause may be psychologically significant in at ıst the following two domains: (1) It may be the stimulus for applica·n of a social label (stigma) that triggers social interactions having gative consequences for women. DeLorey describes some that occur one very important social institution, the health-care system. It is ear, however, that it is the application of the label and not the phys-ogical event that is psychologically significant. Women who are or ıght to be menopausal may be treated in certain ways (and we need to ıow what these are), regardless of their actual biological status. (2) enopause may be psychologically significant as one marker of the ssation of fertility, an event that seems likely to have different mean-ɜs for different women. It is important, however, to note here, too, ıt menopause is only one event that may trigger psychological con-ɛn with and resolution of issues related to fertility. Some women may ɑl with such issues when they have a hysterectomy, others when they ɛ diagnosed by a physician as infertile.

In both of these potential areas of research, it is the psychological ɔcesses and issues that are the main focus. Menopause plays a role, t not the direct causal role implied in the biological perspective. Con-tently adopting a psychological perspective in research on midlife ɔmen, then, may even enable us to learn more about the genuine ychological significance of menopause—and a great deal more about ychological changes in midlife.

FERENCES

linger, C. B. Psychiatric morbidity and the menopause; screening of general population sample. *British Medical Journal*, 1975, *2*, 344–346.
ıinger, C. B. Subjective sleep disturbance at the menopause. *Journal of Psychosomatic Research*, 1976, *20*, 509–513.
ɪnett, R. C., and Baruch, G. K. Women in the middle years: A critique of research and theory. *Psychology of Women Quarterly*, 1978, *3*, 187–197.
t, P. B., and Grossman, M. Menopause. *Women and Health*, 1976, *1*, 3–11.

Boston Women's Health Book Collective. *Our bodies, ourselves.* New York: Simon & Schu
ter, 1973.

Cowan, G. Medical perceptions of menopausal symptoms. *Psychology of Women Quarterl*
in press.

Dan, A. J., Graham, E. A., and Beecher, C. P. (Eds.). *The menstrual cycle (Vol. 1): A synthes*
of interdisciplinary research. New York: Springer, 1981.

Donovan, J. C. Menopausal syndrome: A study of case histories. *American Journal*
Obstetrics and Gynecology, 1951, *62,* 1281–1286.

Eisenberg, J. M. Sociologic influences on decision-making by clinicians. *Annals of Interr*
Medicine, 1979, *90,* 957–964.

Feldman, J. M., Postlethwaite, R. W., and Glenn, J. F. Hot flashes and sweats in men wi
testicular insufficiency. *Archives of Internal Medicine,* 1976, *136,* 606–608.

Flint, M. The menopause: Reward or punishment? *Psychosomatics,* 1975, *16,* 161–163.

Friedman, R. C. (Ed.). *Behavior and the menstrual cycle.* New York: Marcell Dekker, 198

Golub, S. (Ed.). *Menarche.* Boston: Heath, in press.

Goodman, M. J., Stewart, C. J., and Gilbert, F., Jr. Patterns of menopause: A study
certain medical and physiological variables among Caucasian and Japanese wom
living in Hawaii. *Journal of Gerontology,* 1977, *32,* 291–98.

Greene, J. G. A factor analytic study of climacteric symptoms. *Journal of Psychosoma*
Research, 1976, *20,* 425–430.

Greene, J. G., and Cooke, D. J. Life stress and symptons at the climacterium. *British Jourr*
of Psychiatry, 1980, *136,* 486–491.

Koeske, R. D. Theoretical perspectives for menstrual cycle research. In A. J. Dan, E.
Graham, and C. P. Beecher (Eds.), *The menstrual cycle (Vol. 1): A synthesis of int*
disciplinary research. New York: Springer, 1981.

Koeske, R. D., and Koeske, G. F. An attributional approach to moods and the menstr
cycle. *Journal of Personality and Social Psychology,* 1975, *31,* 473–478.

Komnenich, P., McSweeney, M., Noack, J. A., and Elder, S. N. (Eds.). *The menstrual cyc*
(Vol. 2): Research and implications for women's health. New York: Springer, 1981.

Lemert, E. M. Social structure, social control, and deviation. In M. B. Clinard (Ed.), *Ano*
and deviant behavior. New York: Free Press of Glencoe, 1964.

Nadelson, C. C., Polonsky, D. C., and Mathews, M. A. Marriage and midlife: The imp
of social change. *Journal of Clinical Psychiatry,* 1979, *40,* 292–298.

Nelson, S. B. Flooding, flashing, and flushing: Emotional repercussions. *Arizona Medic*
1979, *36,* 675–678.

Neugarten, B. L., and Kraines, R. J. "Menopausal symptoms" in women of various ag
Psychosomatic Medicine, 1965, *27,* 266–273.

Neugarten, B. L., Wood, V., Kraines, R. J., and Loomis, B. Women's attitudes toward
menopause. *Vita Humana,* 1963, *6,* 140–151.

Notman, M. Midlife concerns of women: Implications of the menopause. *American Jour*
of Psychiatry, 1979, *136,* 1270–1274.

Osofsky, H. J., and Seidenberg, R. Is female menopausal depression inevitable? *Obstet*
and Gynecology, 1970, *36,* 611–615.

Parlee, M. B. Psychological aspects of menstruation, childbirth, and menopause. In J.
Sherman and F. L. Denmark (Eds.), *The psychology of women: Future directions of*
search. New York: Psychological Dimensions, 1978.

Parlee, M. B. Gaps in behavioral research on the menstrual cycle. In P. Komnenich,
McSweeney, J. A. Noack, and S. N. Elder (Eds.), *The menstrual cycle, (Vol. 2): Rese*
and implications for women's health. New York: Springer, 1981.

Parlee, M. B. The psychology of the menstrual cycle: Biological and psychological persp
tives. In R. C. Friedman (Ed.), *Behavior and the menstrual cycle.* New York: Ma
Dekker, 1982.

lit, D. F., and LaRocco. Social and psychological correlates of menopausal symptoms. *Psychosomatic Medicine*, 1980, *42*, 335–345.

sner, J. It's all in your head: Feminist and medical models of menopause (strange bedfellows). *Sex Roles*, 1979, *5*, 179–190.

heff, T. J. *Being mentally ill: A sociological theory*. Chicago: Aldine, 1966.

ribner, S., and Cole, M. *Culture and thought*. New York: Wiley, 1974.

verne, L. Psycho-social aspects of the menopause. In A. A. Haspels and H. Musaph (Eds.), *Psychosomatics in peri-menopause*. Baltimore: University Park Press, 1979.

wnsend, J. M., and Carbone, C. L. Menopausal syndrome: Illness or social role—A transcultural analysis. *Culture, Medicine, and Psychiatry*, 1980, *4*, 229–248.

n Keep, P. A., and Humphrey, M. Psycho-social aspects of the climacteric. In P. A. van Keep, R. B. Greenblatt, and M. Albeaux-Femet (Eds.), *Consensus on menopause research*. Baltimore: University Park Press, 1976.

n Keep, P. A., and Kellerhals, J. M. The ageing women: About the influence of some social and cultural factors on the changes in attitude and behavior that occur during and after the menopause. *Acta Obstetricia et Gynecologica Scandinavica, Supplement*, 1976, *51*, 19–27.

eissman, M. M. The myth of involutional melancholia. *Journal of the American Medical Association*, 1979, *242*, 742–744.

ood, C. Menopausal myths. *Medical Journal of Australia*, 1979, *1*, 496–499.

The Midlife Woman as Student

Nancy K. Schlossberg

learning explosion is under way in this country. According to a study
>nducted by the College Board's Future Directions for a Learning Soci-
y, "half of all Americans 25 years and older (over 60 million adults)
arned one or more topics in the past year" (Aslanian and Brickell,
'80, p. 43). Women constituted over half (52%) of this group of learn-
s. The definition of *learning* used in the college board study was broad,
icompassing informal and independent learning activities as well as
ganized, formal instruction. Hence, the estimated participation rate is
iusually high.

Other estimates of adult participation in learning are more modest.
>r example, the National Center for Education Statistics (NCES) reports
at in 1978 over 18 million people participated in adult education, de-
ied as "courses and organized educational activities other than those
ken by full-time students in programs leading toward a high school
ploma or an academic degree and in occupational programs of six
onths or more duration" (Dearman and Plisko, 1980, p. 230). Thus, of
e age-25-and-over population, about 12% were involved in adult edu-
tion. Of these 18 million participants, 36% were 25–34 years old, 34%
ere 35–54 years old, and 2.4% were age 65 and older. Women outnum-
red men in all age groups among adult-education participants, con-
tuting 57% of the total. Their predominance was particularly evident
the older groups: They account for 61% of the 55–64-year-olds and
% of the age-65-and-older group of adult education participants.

Because of recent definitional changes, reliable trends are difficult to
lculate from NCES data for 1978. Earlier statistics show, however, that

ncy K. Schlossberg • Department of Education, University of Maryland, College
k, Maryland 20742.

between 1969 and 1975, the number of adults particpating in continuing education activities increased by 30.8%, while the total adult population increased by only 12.6%. This growth in the number of adult education participants was much greater among women (an annual average of 6.4%) than among men (an annual average of 1.9%), though it was smallest for women between 35 and 54 years old (2.5% annually) and largest for women aged 55 and over (7.6% annually) (Entine, 1978, p 156). The proportion of the population aged 17 and older who partici- pate in adult education seems to have stabilized at about 12.5% since 1975, but the actual number has continued to increase as the adult popu lation has increased. Moreover, "the size of the adult population is projected to grow further throughout the 1980's, suggesting that if the participation rate remains constant, the number of adult education par ticipants will continue to grow" (Dearman and Plisko, 1980, p. 231)

The number of adults enrolling in the *collegiate* sector has increased even more dramatically. Indeed, according to an article by Magarrel (1981), "institutions concerned about maintaining their enrollment lev els are looking to the older groups to offset, at least partially, a decline in the population of 18-year-olds during the 1980s" (p. 3). Although the number of students aged 35 and older attending the nation's college and universities increased by 36.8% between 1975 and 1979, only a smal proportion of the total adult population aged 35 and older were attend ing higher education institutions. To summarize, "over 18 million adult participated in . . . formal education . . . in 1978 . . . [while] over 13 million adults did not participate" (Charner, 1981).

Granting that more adults are becoming involved in formal educa tion programs, what else do we know about who they are, besides the fact that more are women? We know that relative to the general adu population, adult education participants tended to be well educated, t have high incomes, to live in the suburbs rather than the central city c rural areas, and to hold high-status jobs; underrepresented are the blue collar and farm workers, the unemployed blacks and Hispanics (Dear man and Plisko, 1980, p. 232).

We know that of those women participating in higher education the majority still "have more marginal status and stand on more ten uous educational ground than men" (Randour, Strasburg, and Lipman Blumen, 1981, p. 33). They are still concentrated in female-intensiv fields whose status and market value is low, they are less well-repre sented at each higher degree level, and they are more likely than men be enrolled in public institutions and to attend college on a part-tim basis. Randour *et al* deplore the increasing tendency of women to ente community colleges, which have been shown negatively to affect degre aspirations and persistance (see Astin, 1975; Karabel, 1972). Thus, won en have not yet achieved parity with men in higher education. Despite these reservations, the authors agree that older women have made rapid strides in recent years.

This theme is sounded again in a recent release from the Project on the Status and Education of Women: "Re-entry women—women over 25 who have interrupted their education for at least a few years and are now entering or re-entering postsecondary institutions—comprise the largest potential source of students, and their participation in higher education is expected to increase for some time to come" (Hall and Gleaves, 1981, p. 1).

In short, statistics show and observers agree that increasing numbers of adult women engage in learning activities and pursue formal education, although the number of nonparticipants far exceeds the number of participants. This background provides the context for the remainder of this chapter, which is based on a series of questions: (1) Is there such an entity as the adult learner? (2) What factors motivate women to become learners? (3) What are the barriers hindering women from pursuing education? (4) What can be said of the learning experience itself for those women pursuing education? The following sections address these questions.

THE ADULT LEARNER: SOME ASSUMPTIONS

Is there such an entity as "the adult learner"? As evidenced by the growing number of articles and books on the subject, adult learners have special needs and capacities that distinguish them from traditional-aged students. At the same time, the group is very diverse. Adult learners are a heterogeneous group, just as younger learners are. Some are bright, others dull; some are knowledgeable, other ignorant; some are energetic, others apathetic; some are anxious, others self-confident.

Either position gives rise to certain difficulties. To say that the adult learner is a distinctive category feeds into the agism of our society and evokes other stereotypes that bear little relation to reality. For instance, many minority women (and other special populations) are hesitant to enroll in reentry and continuing education programs because they have a "gilded cage" image of such programs, seeing them as aimed primarily at "bored, middle-class, middle-aged housewives" (Hall and Gleaves, 1981, p. 5). Similarly, adult and continuing education is often denigrated on the grounds that it consists chiefly of such courses as basket weaving and flower arranging. Even if one avoids these oversimplifications, making age the central variable still carries some dangers. One is apt to overlook other important characteristics of the adult learner or, worse, to conclude that some people are simply too old to learn.

On the other hand, denying the existence of adult learners as a distinct category may well lead to overlooking some of the special needs of that population, needs that should be addressed by policy-makers and educators.

In brief, age may be a salient but not the central defining variable. Given these caveats, we will examine two issues: (1) the relationship between age and learning capacity and (2) the categorization of midlife women.

The Relationship of Age to Learning Capacity

Though few people in this day and age would subscribe to the notion that "you can't teach an old dog new tricks," the conventional wisdom seems to be that intellectual functioning slows down with age. For instance, Cattell (1963) differentiated *fluid intelligence* (the ability to process information rapidly in problem solving) from *crystallized intelligence* (stored information such as vocabulary and general knowledge). The former seems to decline with age, whereas the latter seems to remain stable and even to improve (Gallagher, Thompson, and Levy, 1980, p. 23). While brain cells are continually being destroyed as a person ages, there are more than enough active brain cells to ensure that the intellectual functioning of most men and women will remain adequate until they die, except in cases of illness where, for instance, the circulatory supply to the brain is disturbed (Ramey, 1981).

Reviewing issues connected with the study of adult intelligence, Willis and Baltes (1980) conclude: "Chronological age per se accounts for a relatively modest amount of the variance observed in intellectual aging during late adulthood up to the 60s or early 70s" (p. 263). According to Willis and Baltes, one must take into account three sets of influences on intellectual functioning.

> *Age-graded influences:*—those biological and environmental determinants that are correlated with chronological age; "their occurrence, timing, and duration are fairly similar for all individuals of a given set of aging cohorts" (p. 267).
> *History-graded influences*—those biological and environmental events correlated with historical change: "Their degree of generality and predictability varies. Some of them, however, are fairly normative in that they apply to most members of a given set of aging cohorts in similar ways" (p. 267). For instance, people who grew up during the Great Depression may differ in consistent ways from people

who grew up in the post-World War II era of economic expansion, and these differences may be reflected in their cognitive functioning. Similarly, intergenerational differences in labor force participation or family life may result in intergenerational differences in intellectual development.

Nonnormative critical life events—those events in the life of the individual that are relatively idiosyncratic: e.g., usual opportunities for learning, illness, unemployment, bereavement. Such events may affect intellectual development directly (as in the case of disease that results in brain damage) or indirectly, through stress.

Willis and Baltes maintain that, if investigators are to arrive at an understanding of intellectual development over the life-span, they must give greater attention in their research designs to history-graded influences and nonnormative critical life events.

Learning capacity may improve rather than decrease over time in certain situations. Kohn (1980) and his associates identified more than 50 job dimensions or occupational conditions, 12 of which were found to have significant positive effects on psychological functioning, after all other pertinent factors were statistically controlled. The most important of these dimensions is *substantive complexity*, defined as "the degree to which the work, in its very substance, requires thought and independent judgment. Substantively complex work by its very nature requires making many decisions that must take into account ill-defined or apparently conflicting contingencies. . . . The index of substantive complexity that we have generally employed is based on the degree of complexity of the person's work with things, with data, and with people" (Kohn, 1980, p. 197). Kohn further asserts that substantive complexity is a central structural characteristic of the work experience; that it is related to a wide range of psychological factors including job satisfaction, occupational commitment, self-direction, self-esteem, authoritarian conservatism, and intellectual flexibility; and that the causal relation is reciprocal—that is, one's psychological functioning affects the substantive complexity of the work one does, and the substantive complexity of the work one does affects one's psychological functioning. Looking in particular at intellectual flexibility, as indicated by performance and behavior on tests and during interviews, Kohn states:

> If two men of equivalent intellectual flexibility were to start their careers in jobs different in substantive complexity, the man in the more complex job would be likely to outstrip the other in further intellectual growth. This, in time, might lead to his attaining jobs of greater complexity, further affecting his intellectual growth. Meantime, the man in the less complex job would develop intellectually at a slower pace, perhaps not at all, and in the extreme

case might even decline in his intellectual functioning. As a result, small differences in the substantive complexity of early jobs might lead to increasing differences in intellectual development. (Kohn, 1980, p. 203)

Moreover, similar results emerged from a study of 269 employed married women. Those women whose work was substantively complex and, in addition, nonroutinized (i.e., involved a variety of unpredictable tasks) demonstrated greater intellectual flexibility than those women performing relatively simple, routine work (Miller, Schooler, Kohn, and Miller, 1979, p. 80).

How do these findings apply to the topic of midlife women and education? Women who have been continuously exposed to stimulating and complex environments that exercise their problem-solving abilities may be more intellectually flexible—and thus more likely to benefit from learning activities—than those women who work in environments where they perform only routine and repetitive tasks. Although the research of Kohn and his associates has been limited to employed adults, one could argue that many women who do not hold outside jobs nonetheless perform work—in the home and in the community—of considerable substantive complexity. Further, those women who do play occupational, as well as conjugal and maternal, roles may live substantively complex lives even if their jobs are relatively low-level.

In brief, age is not the sole, or even the primary, determinant of learning capacity. History-graded influences, nonnormative critical life events, and the substantive complexity of the environment must also be considered in assessing the individual's learning capacity. These points deserve emphasis because many midlife women (and men as well) are victims of the age stereotypes that pervade our society. Because they feel they have slowed down intellectually, they may be fearful of committing themselves to educational activities. The evidence cited here indicates that such fears are probably groundless.

Categorizing Midlife Women

Two ways to classify women as students are in terms of cognitive development (Perry, 1970) and in terms of role involvement (Campbell, Wilson, and Harrison, 1980; Lowenthal, Thurnher, and Chiriboga, 1975). Both these classificatory schemes seem particularly well-suited to studying the midlife women as learner because they touch on aspects of her life and personality that are directly connected with her response to education, and they may be useful for planning curricula and advising midlife students.

COGNITIVE DEVELOPMENT. Perry's model of cognitive development (1970) grew out of his empirical work with several cohorts of Harvard undergraduates, who were studied longitudinally from their freshman to their senior years. In interviews at the end of each year, the students were asked a broad general question about what had "stood out" for them during the year and then were questioned in more detail. Their responses were found to reflect attitudes about the nature of knowledge and thinking, the function of educational institutions and teachers, the responsibility of the learner, and so forth. Perry defined a set of hierarchical stages, which are as follows:

Basic Duality. The world is seen in terms of such polarities as good–bad, right–wrong. Knowledge is absolute, and Authority (the teacher) has the Right Answer, which will duly be revealed to the hardworking and obedient student.

Multiplicity Prelegitimate. Differences of opinion exist, but they are attributable to confusion on the part of the teacher or are an exercise set by the teacher so that students can find the Right Answer for themselves.

Multiplicity. Uncertainty and differences of opinion are acceptable in some areas where the Right Answer simply has not been discovered yet. At the extreme, the student believes that "anyone has a right to his own opinion" and that all opinions have equal validity.

Relativism. All knowledge and values, including those of Authority, are contextual and relativistic.

Commitment. Although absolute certainty is impossible, some kind of personal commitment or affirmation is needed. The student makes such a commitment. As this commitment develops, the student affirms his or her own identity.

Not all students progress through the stages easily and smoothly to attain the highest level. Most difficult for both traditional-aged and adult students is the shift from Multiplicity to Relativism, which involves "discarding the view that knowledge is a quantitative accretion of discrete rightness, including the kind of discrete rightness in which everyone has a right to his own opinion, and adopting a conception of knowledge as the qualitative assessment of contextual observations and relationships" (Weathersby and Tarule, 1980, p. 34). In addition, Perry's model resembles Kohlberg's (1970) theory of moral development and Loevinger's (1976) theory of ego development in that all three view development as progression from the simple to the complex, from an external orientation (where the individual is dependent on authority or on the judgment of others) to an inner orientation (where the individual takes responsibility for the consequences of his or her own actions), from absolutism and dogmatism to increasing tolerance for ambiguity and uncertainty, from a tendency to perceive those outside one's own immediate group in stereotypic terms to increasing awareness of individual differences and greater empathy with others, and "from a strong self focus to a posture of conformity to the group and then to a mature focus on mutual interdependence on others. The individual is truly autonomous and inner-directed when she arrives at the point of acknowledging her interdependence on others in her life" (Knefelkamp, Widick, and Stroad, 1976, p. 16).

Perry's model is useful because of its direct applicability to understanding adult learners. It is more useful to know whether a learner is a dualist or a relativist rather than whether he or she is age 20, 40, or 60. Teaching and curriculum development should be geared to the individual's style of learning and not the individual's chronological age.

ROLE INVOLVEMENT. Some attention needs to be given to the midlife woman student's involvement in other roles and activities as one way of understanding her attitudes toward and response to education. The role-involvement typology most directly related to adult learners was developed in a study of age-25-and-over undergraduates at the University of Texas in 1979 (Campbell et al., 1980). On the basis of time spent in various activities (e.g., working at a paying job, doing schoolwork, doing things with the family), these adult students were classified into five types:

Type 1. These were full-time students who were not employed and who spent more than 40 hours a week with their families and had little free time. This group was largely women (75%), most of whom had at least one child at home.

Type 2. This category comprised full-time students who were not employed and who had few family responsibilities and a considerable amount of free time. Forty-two percent were women. Over half of the total group were single or divorced.

Type 3. These were part-time students who were employed full time, spent little time with their families, and had considerable free time. Again, women constituted a little under half of this group (47%).

Type 4. In this group were full-time students who were not employed and who, despite their family ties, spent little time in family or social/recreational activities but a great deal of time (an average of over 60 hours a week) on schoolwork and had little free time. About half of this group (42%) were women; about a third of the total group had at least one child at home.

Type 5. This type were students who were employed full time, had signed up for one or two courses, spent a great deal of time in family activities, and had very little free time. Forty-nine percent were women; 49% had one child.

Campbell and his associates found that the five types of adult learn ers differed "on a number of background characteristics, on the degree of difficulty they had in deciding to return to school, and on the kind of problems they had after enrollment. . . . Members of one type were as likely as members of another to have difficulties adjusting to student life; however, the reasons for these difficulties varied by type" (Campbell *et al.*, 1980, p. 85).

This discussion of role involvement points out that there is no single category of midlife women. Women have many kinds of role involvement. To some degree, those involvements will determine whether a particular midlife women will decide to pursue education at all. The next section examines in more detail the various "push" and "pull" factors that may motivate the midlife woman to return to school.

MOTIVATION FOR LEARNING

Reviewing the literature on motivation for learning, Cross (1981) distinguishes those investigators who deal with types of learners from those who deal with clusters of learning motives. A broad perspective on learning motives is offered by Kuhlen (1963), who suggests that adult behavior in general is impelled by two "meta-motives": The first is a positive drive for expansion and growth; the second is a self-protective drive, based on anxiety and insecurity, to compensate for perceived inadequacies. Obviously, both motives may be present in the pursuit of education; that is, adult learners may be motivated by a desire to achieve in their careers, to improve their social skills and interpersonal relations, or simply to expand their knowledge of the world; or they may be "pushed" by the fear that, without further education, they will lose their jobs, their friends, or their cognitive powers.

Like Kuhlen, White (1976) believes that people have a lifelong drive for competence, a need to expand, explore, and achieve mastery over the world and over themsleves. As they grow older, they continually try out new coping mechanisms that will facilitate "successful transaction with the environment." Empirical support for this view comes from a study of the wives of coal miners (Giesen and Datan, 1980), women between the ages of 47 and 62 who had fewer resources than most women in this age group. Contradicting the stereotype of older women as "dependent, passive, incompetent, and generally unable to deal with the problems and crises of life" (p. 57), this study found that most of the women interviewed gave evidence of being able to "interact effectively with the environment" and "to cope with and solve problems" (p. 60). Moreover, most of them felt they had gained in competence and were better able to handle life than they had been at a younger age. Similarly, a study of women who lead complex lives found that those who were satisfied with their multiple roles also showed gains in competence and in sense of well-being (Baruch and Barnett, 1980).

Obviously, there are many possible approaches to the question of what motivates midlife women to pursue learning. In the remainder of this section, two recent contributions to the literature will be presented. The first, by Aslanian and Brickell (1980), see life changes as providing the impetus for adult learning. The second, while not dealing directly with adult education, is nonetheless highly suggestive; it is Marjorie Fiske's (1980) view of changes in value commitments over time.

Life Changes

Aslanian and Brickell (1980) attribute the learning explosion currently under way in the United States to the aging of the population; the greater labor force participation of women; the growth in the proportions of part-time workers and of professional, managerial, and service workers and the concomitant decline in the proportions of laborers, factory operatives, and craft workers; and the increase in leisure time. More adults are seeking and will continue to seek learning opportunities as a means of facilitating their adaptation to these transitions.

Aslanian and Brickell define a *transition* as a "change in status . . . that makes learning necessary. The adult needs to become competent at something that he or she could not do before in order to succeed in the new status" (pp. 38–39). It should be noted that learning can be informal and self-directed; it need not involve formal, organized instruction. The authors further distinguish between a transition and a *trigger*, defined as the specific life event that precipitates "the decision to learn at that point in time" (p. 39). The trigger is not necessarily related either to the transition or to the topic studied. For instance, an unemployed woman who is suddenly widowed may enroll in a medical technology course in order to become qualified for a job. The transition is the change of status from nonworker to worker; the triggering event is the husband's death.

Finally, Aslanian and Brickell identify seven life areas into which both transitions and triggers may be classified: career, family, health religion, citizenship, art, and leisure. Within this theoretical framework they examine the data collected through personal and telephone interviews with a national sample of approximately 1500 subjects who were 25 years of age or older. Among the most notable findings to emerge from this survey were the following:

1. Close to half the sample indicated that they were engaged in

some kind of learning activity at the time of the survey or had been so engaged during the previous year.

2. Over four in five of the learners (83%) said that they were motivated to learn by some transition in their lives; only 17% were learning simply for the sake of learning.

3. Of those who said that some life transition had motivated them, 56% cited career transitions, 16% cited family transitions, and 13% cited leisure transitions.

4. Sex differences in reasons for learning were evident: 71% of the men, but only 42% of the women, mentioned career transition. Twice as many women (21%) as men (10%) mentioned family transitions. Women were also more likely than men to mention transitions in the areas of leisure, health, religion, art, and citizenship. In short, women show greater variation in their reasons for learning.

Looking more closely at the various life areas, career transitions—he top-ranked reasons for both men and women—include moving into a new job, adapting to a changing job, and advancing in a career. Specific triggers included such events as technological or organizational changes demanding the acquisition of new skills, an offer of advancement, job termination, and retirement. The triggering event for many women who engage in learning for career-related reasons often lies in family life: The youngest child enters school or leaves home, the couple is divorced or separated, the husband dies.

In the area of family life, many women pursue education to learn how to can food, how to prepare special cuisines, how to make household repairs, how to sew. Other transitions in this area include adapting to shifts in family income or changes in the health of a family member. Family-centered events that may trigger learning activities include marriage, pregnancy, children's progress through school, divorce, residential moves, the retirement or death of a family member, and changes in family income.

Transitions in the area of leisure involved acquiring "skills in sports, crafts, hobbies, and social activities, for the sole purpose of making constructive use of free time" (Aslanian and Brickell, 1980, p. 77). Triggers for these changes always occurred in some other areas: For instance, retirement from a job, a reduction in the work week, or a child's entering kindergarten may all lead to an increase in the leisure time of an adult; similarly, a residential move or a divorce may lead to a change in one's social circle and thus to the development of new interests. Closely related to leisure are changes in artistic life that prompt the adult to take piano lessons (for instance) or to take a course in art appreciation. Transitions in the area of personal health take two forms: recovering from illness or injury and maintaining physical fitness. Transitions in religious life include religious conversions; transitions in citizenship including becoming a citizen and becoming a volunteer worker.

Clearly, career transitions are the primary reasons behind learning for both sexes, while changes in family life are much more likely to be triggers for women (52%) than for men (20%). Aslanian and Brickell suggest, "To know an adult's life schedule is to know an adult's learning schedule" (p. 61).

Changes in Commitments

A look at changing commitments—or what gives meaning to one's life—throws some additional light on why many midlife women pursue education. According to Fiske (1980), the individual's value hierarchy does not remain constant over the life-span; rather, major changes or reorientations in commitment may occur. As she grows older, the woman may become increasingly concerned with mastery, competence, and dominance. Even if such a value shift does not take place, she may find that her interpersonal and altruistic commitments can no longer be fulfilled by family life. In either case, she may be motivated to pursue education as a means of giving expression to her value commitments.

BARRIERS TO LEARNING

What of the other side of the coin? With the various life and commitment changes that may be pushing her to pursue education, what factors prevent the midlife woman from reentering an educational program? Cross (1981) identifies three types of barriers:

> Situational—those barriers "arising from one's situation in life at a given time" (p. 98): e.g., lack of time, lack of funds.
> Institutional—"all those practices and procedures that exclude or discourage . . . participation" (p. 98): e.g., financial aid policies, scheduling of classes.
> Dispositional—those barriers "related to attitudes and self-perceptions about oneself as a learner" (p. 98): e.g., lack of confidence in academic ability, lack of energy, fear of being too old to begin.

Carp, Peterson, and Roelfs (1974) surveyed "potential learners" (i.e., those who indicated that they had a desire to learn but that they were not currently engaged in any kind of organized educational program) to find out the relative importance of various barriers (Table 1) which will be discussed in the following section.

Table 1. Perceived Barriers to Learning[a]

Barriers	Percent of potential learners[b]
Situational barriers	
Cost, including tuition, books, child care, etc.	53[c]
Not enough time	46
Home responsibilities	32
Job responsibilities	28
No child care	11
No transportation	8
No place to study or practice	7
Friends or family don't like the idea	3
Institutional barriers	
Don't want to go to school full time	35
Amount of time required to complete program	21
Courses aren't scheduled when I can attend	16
No information about offerings	16
Strict attendance requirements	15
Courses I want don't seem to be available	12
Too much red tape in getting enrolled	10
Don't meet requirements to begin program	6
No way to get credit or a degree	5
Dispositional barriers	
Afraid that I'm too old to begin	17
Low grades in past, not confident of my ability	12
Don't enjoy studying	9
Not enough energy and stamina	9
Tired of school, tired of classrooms	6
Don't know what to learn or what it would lead to	5
Hesitate to seem too ambitious	3

Source: Cross, 1981, p. 99. Adapted from Carp, Peterson, and Roelfs, 1974, p. 46.
[b]Potential learners are those who indicated a desire to learn but who are not currently engaged in organized instruction.
[c]Respondents were asked to check all items that applied.

Situational Barriers

Situational barriers—especially costs and lack of time—are mentioned most frequently as impediments to learning in most studies (Table 1). The situational barriers vary somewhat by subgroup: For instance, low-income adults most frequently identify costs as a major barrier, whereas young mothers are more inclined than other groups to mention lack of child care.

The costs of education include not only direct costs (such as tuition and books) but also indirect costs (foregone income, child care, transportation). Given these high costs, it is not surprising that one finds socioeconomic class differences with respect to participation in adult education. For instance, persons with annual incomes of under $10,000 constituted 30% of the U. S. population but only 17% of adult education participants. Conversely, 60% of those persons enrolled in adult education, but only 44% of the U.S. population aged 17 and over, come from families with incomes of $15,000 or more (Dearman and Plisko, 1980, p. 244). Clearly, the affluent find it easier to pay for education. But there is more to it than that.

According to Boaz (1978), about one-third of all blacks enrolled in adult education are supported by public funds, and about one-third of all white males are supported by their employers; "this leaves white females the only population subgroup presented in NCES data in which a majority of learners (66 percent) are supporting educational costs from their own or family funds" (Boaz, 1978, p. 73). This no doubt explains why more women than men say that the cost of education constitutes a barrier for them. Another problem may be that women feel guilty about spending money on themselves; education may seem like an indulgence (Cross, 1981, p. 101).

Other frequently mentioned situational barriers include lack of time (mentioned by 46% of the potential learners in the Carp *et al.*, 1974 survey), home responsibilities (32%), and job responsibilities (28%). Obviously, these items overlap to some extent—that is, the individual with home or job responsibilities often does not have enough time to pursue education, especially the woman with children. Ages of the children, rather than the number of children, seems to be the decisive factor in limiting education (Westervelt, 1975).

As was reported earlier, participation in adult education has increased much more among women than among men, but the rate of increase between 1969 and 1975 was smallest among women in the 35–54 age group. Soldo (1980) suggests one possible reason for their lower rate: For women, middle age may be "a time of maximum responsibility" (p. 1). Middle-aged women are often caught in a "dependency squeeze" caused by the "competing pressures of employment, . . . children, home life *and* older relatives" (p. 1), especially aging parents who require care. As the life-span has lengthened, and as four-generation families have become more common, midlife women often find themselves having to provide care not only for grandchildren but also for older relatives. To demonstrate more clearly the impact of these responsibilities, Soldo divided middle-aged women into two age groups: the 40–49-year-olds and the 50–59-year-olds. Only 7% of the younger group, but 55% of the older group, were providing care for an older relative. By age 60, nearly 1 million women are involved in kin care. Moreover, given the exorbitant cost of nursing care, women in upper income brackets are just as likely to be faced with these responsibilities as are low-income women.

The seriousness of this problem was brought home to me by the situation of a client, a 42-year-old woman who had just been elected to the city council. At about the same time, her husband's mother broke her hip and was incapacitated to the extent of requiring constant nursing care. Because there were four children in the family, three of them in college, money was an issue, even though the family was relatively well off in absolute terms. Moreover, the husband strenuously objected to the idea of placing his mother in a nursing home. Thus, my client was caught in a no-win situation: She was the only one who could stay home to care for the older woman, so she was expected to resign her membership on the city council.

This case illustrates several points: (a) The middle-aged wife is the family member who is expected to care for children, grandchildren, and aging relatives. (b) The woman is more likely than the man to require care as she ages. (c) Thus, the women—especially the married woman in her middle years—is less likely to be able to take advantage of learning opportunties.

Other situational constraints include lack of a private place in which to study, a particular problem for married women with children. Moreover, transportation to and from the educational institution may be difficult unless the institution is relatively close to home, which may account in part for the overrepresentation of adult women in community colleges; these tend to be more geographically accessible than other types of institutions.

Institutional Barriers

Numerous reports have proposed recommendations designed to reduce or eliminate the institutional barriers that women encounter as they seek education. These categories include admissions practices, financial aid practices, institutional regulations, curriculum planning and student personnel services, and faculty and staff attitudes.

Examples of barriers in the form of admissions practices include the imposition of higher standards (high school grade-average, aptitude test scores) for female applicants than for male applicants; age restrictions many graduate schools will not accept applicants who are over 35 or 40 years of age, a practice that discriminates against women, who are more likely to delay their education than are men; and regulations governing the transferability of credit (many institutions do not accept credits after a certain number of years have lapsed or limit the junior-college credits that can be transferred).

Most financial aid is targeted to full-time students. Thus, midlife women (and others) who must attend school part time because of job or family responsibilities are denied access to such funds. Women may also find themselves ineligible for financial assistance because they are married or pregnant and because they are concentrated in "soft" fields— e.g., education, arts, and humanities—which receive less support than the sciences and engineering. Moreover, even when women do receive grants, the amounts are typically smaller than the amounts awarded to men, even when their income levels are the same. The lack of aid to pay for child care constitutes another financial barrier for adult women.

Among the institutional regulations that seem to work a particular hardship on women are time limits on certain kinds of certificate and degree programs that make full-time study a necessity.

In the area of curriculum planning and student personnel services, the location and scheduling of classes may constitute a formidable barrier for many adult women, especially those who have to travel some distance if they are to attend classes. Similarly, adult women may find it hard to make full use of such academic resources as libraries, laboratories, and computer centers, or of such student services as administrative offices, health centers, and counseling centers.

Finally, faculty and staff attitudes, including subtle forms of sex and age discrimination, may discourage midlife women from pursuing education. The lack of female role models among faculty and administrators is another aspect of the institutional environment that has received much attention as a possible deterrent to potential learners among adult women.

These and other institutional barriers are regularly addressed in reports from the Project on the Status and Education of Women. For instance, Hall and Gleaves (1981) examine the needs of special populations of reentry women (including minority women, single parents, displaced homemakers, older women, and disabled women) and offer a series of recommendations covering the categories discussed above, as well as recruitment and basic skills programs.

As the traditional-aged college population continues to shrink, it seems likely that higher education institutions will make greater efforts to attract "nontraditional" students, including midlife women, and that many of the institutional barriers discussed above will be eliminated.

Dispositional Factors

As Table 1 indicates, dispositional factors were less frequently perceived to be a barrier to education than were situational and institutional factors, although 17% of the potential learners indicated they were fraid they were too old to learn, and 12% said they had made low rades in the past and lacked confidence in their academic ability. It hould be pointed out, however, that "potential learners" were defined y their desire to learn; many adults may lack this desire because of ispositional factors. Moreover, even those people who have a desire to arn may not be able to recognize the psychological characteristics that revent them from pursuing education. Thus, it seems probable that ispositional factors constitute more of a barrier to learning than the gures in the table suggest.

For instance, many older people, influenced by the age stereotypes revalent in American society, may tacitly accept the assumption that arning ability declines with age and thus may not even consider enroll- ig in an educational program. Others may feel anxious about compet- ig with younger students but may be unwilling to express their nxiety.

Similarly, because of internalized sex-role stereotypes, many wom- 1 may not see education as a viable option. Lipman-Blumen (1972) has ointed out that our society socializes women to "vicarious achieve- ient" (i.e., through the men in their lives) rather than "direct achieve- ient." While norms have changed somewhat in recent years and while ounger women are likely to reject the "vicarious achievement ethic," it ay still influence the thinking and behavior of many middle-aged omen, especially those from low socioeconomic backgrounds where ollege-going is not a tradition.

Hall and Gleaves (1981) cite a number of other dispositional factors at are particularly likely to prevent minority women and other "spe- al populations" from pursuing education. First, as was mentioned irlier, these women may have a "gilded cage" image of reentry and ntinuing education programs, seeing them as directed at affluent hite women with ample leisure time. Second, they may fear that such urses will not be related "to their employment, community, and cul- ral needs" and "will serve to divorce them from their own cultural ickground" (pp. 5–6). Third, they may suffer from a "fear of 'chilly aters,'" feeling that they will be the only ones from their particular opulation to enroll in a given program.

Other dispositional factors listed in Table 1 as barriers to the pursuit education seem more idiosyncratic. Thus, some people indicated sim- y that they did not enjoy studying or that they were tired of school.

IE FINAL EQUATION

Having considered some of the motivations for and barriers to irning, we are still left with the question of why some midlife women

Table 2. Motivators and Barriers

Motivators
  Life changes occurring primarily in the areas of career and family
  Changes in value commitments
  Desire for mastery/competence and a need to fulfill interpersonal and altruistic
    commitments outside the home
Barriers
  Situational factors, including economic contraints and multiple family responsibilities
    such as the care of aging relatives
  Institutional factors that work a particular hardship on midlife women, such as
    various kinds of discrimination against part-time students
  Dispositional factors that may in part represent the internalization of societal norms
    regarding sex and age

---

choose to pursue education and others do not. To arrive at some kind of final equation that will help to explain this difference, one has to balance the various factors discussed above. Table 2 outlines the motivators and barriers that can simultaneously push and pull an individual to return to school.

As was pointed out earlier, participants in adult education tend to be relatively well educated already. For instance, in 1978 they were almost twice as likely as adults in the total population to have at least some college experience (57% vs. 30%; Dearman and Plisko, 1980, p. 242). What accounts for the greater tendency of the well educated to seek more education? Cross (1978) suggests three hypotheses by way of explanation.

> First, the more people experience [education] the more they like it—either for its intrinsic or extrinsic rewards. A second hypothesis is that those who have been successful in the fairly narrow demands of the educational system stay in it longer and also wish to return to the scene of their earlier success. A third hypothesis is that human beings are basically curious and enjoy learning, but that the "haves" possess the information and wherewithal to pursue learning that interests them, whereas the "have nots" are handicapped and thwarted in attaining what all people basically desire. . . . [Thus,] those with high motivation, high past success, good information networks, and adequate funds get more and more education while those already dragging in the educational race fall farther and farther behind. (Cross, 1978, p. 12)

But is this gloomy conclusion justified? Are certain groups destined to remain have-nots insofar as education (and its rewards) are concerned? Recent data on freshmen enrollments suggest that this is not necessarily the case: In the fall of 1980, close to half of all full-time freshmen entering the nation's colleges and universities indicated that their parents had not gone beyond the high school level; thus, they were first-generation college students (Astin, King, and Richardson, 198

oreover, as the statistics cited earlier show, adult women account for
i increasing proportion of both part- and full-time enrollments in regu-
r college courses, as well as making up the majority of adult education
rticipants; the implication is that a large number who for some reason
d not enter or complete postsecondary education at traditional college
e are now catching up. Finally, the proportions of minority women
ho go on to college or participate in adult education have increased
mewhat over the last decade or so and are projected to continue to
crease in the decades ahead (Fisher-Thompson and Kuhn, 1981).
us, many former have-nots are becoming haves, at least insofar as
ucation is concerned. Although progress is indicated, the number of
turning women is still a relatively small proportion of the potential
ol.

IE EXPERIENCE OF EDUCATION

So far, the discussion has dealt with the bare fact of participation in
ucation. But what of the actual experience? Once the adult woman
s made the decision and actually entered a formal education program,
hat happens then?

Campbell *et al.* (1980), studying the adjustment process for adults
5 years and older) returning to school as undergraduates at the Uni-
rsity of Texas, take an ecological approach in assessing the educa-
nal experience: "The focus is on the degree of fit between the charac-
ristics of the individual student and the properties of the student's
vironment. Psychological adjustment is conceived in terms of per-
n–environment fit" (p. 1). The authors first identified four stages in
e return to school (represented diagramatically in Figure 1).

Balance. The person is in a state of equilibrium, "neither enrolled in
hool nor actively considering a return to school," but employed full
ne, taking care of the home and raising children, or whatever. "The
erall degree of person–environment fit may range, however, from
ry good to poor" (p. 4).

Conflict. The equilibrium is threatened, and the person actively con-
mplates returning to school. The motivating forces may be personal
g., need for intellectual stimulation) or environmental (e.g., job re-
irements, need for a second income in the family). Other forces act as
rriers to the return (e.g., lack of confidence in academic ability, finan-
l constraints, family opposition). "Thus, individuals considering re-
rollment are typically in a state of conflict" (p. 4).

Transition. The person makes a commitment to enroll in school, "a
jor decision having impact on all realms of the person's life
d . . . therefore, potentially a highly stressful period" (p. 5).

I. Balance	II. Conflict	III. Transition	IV. Outcome (New Balance)
	Environmental Forces Toward and Against Return to School	Environmental Mediators of Psychosocial Adjustments	Good P–E Fit
State of Person– Environment Balance	State of Indecision	Decision to Return	Potentially Stressful Situation
	Personal Forces toward and against Return to School	Personal Mediators of Psychosocial Adjustment	Poor P–E Fit

Figure 1. Four-stage process model of psychosocial adjustment of returning adult students. Sour... Campbell, Wilson, and Hanson (1980, p. 5).

Outcome. The person achieves a new state of equilibrium incorpora... ing the return to school. Again, the person–environment fit may rang... from very good to poor.

Next, Campbell and his associates categorized the 440 adult stu... dents in their sample into five groups, on the basis of time spent i... various activities (e.g., paid employment, school work, family life). (Th... five types were discussed earlier, in the section entitled Role Involv... ment). To assess the person–environment fit in both the balance and th... outcome stage, they used an Index of Well-Being (Campbell, Convers... and Rogers, 1976), an instrument predicated on the assumption that...

> the optimum "fit" occurs . . . when (1) the particular combination of social settings provides multiple opportunities for fulfilling a wide range of personal needs; (2) the person is accommodating to the demands of each social setting; (3) in negotiating the environment to meet these needs and social demands, the individual is experiencing a degree of challenge that stimulated personal growth but is not overwhelming; and (4) in addition to satisfying personal needs the person is progressing toward fulfillment of higher-order needs. (Campbell *et al.*, 1980, p. 134)

Some of the major findings to emerge from this particular stu... provide a useful summary for the entire discussion of midlife wome... and education:

1. Most adults returned to school because they were dissatisfie... with their lives and regarded education as a way to a better life. T... majority had definite career-related goals in mind: "They want traini... that will help them develop a career, advance in a current career,... change to a better career" (p. 89).

2. Two-thirds of these adults had wanted to enroll sooner than th... actually did but were impeded by institutional barriers (chiefly a univ...

ity requirement that students get special permission to enroll for fewer
than 12 credit hours and the lack of evening courses) or situational
barriers (family and job responsibilities).

3. Their greatest apprehensions prior to returning to school were
connected with lack of funds, multiple responsibilities, academic performance, the impact of the return on their families, and their own ability
to adjust. "A lack of information about what to expect after enrollment
seems to have contributed to the conflict" (p. 81).

4. Most found that their life-style was disrupted considerably by
returning to school.

5. Background characteristics such as age and sex bore little relation
to ease or difficulty of adjustment.

6. Adjustment was most difficult for those who were coping with
other major life changes (e.g., a divorce, a job change), those who had
been anxious about the return, those whose life-styles were changed
most drastically, and those with heavy family responsibilities (e.g., single parents).

7. Of the adult students saying they needed campus services, those
who experienced the most adjustment difficulty were least likely to
make use of such services. The implication is that "those students who
used campus resources when problems arose were able to reduce the
overall levels of stress and difficulty associated with the transition process" (p. 83).

8. For most students, the person–environment fit was better, and
the sense of well-being greater, 4 months after enrollment than prior to
enrollment.

9. All five types of students experience some difficulty in adjusting
the return to school, but the sources of the difficulty differed by type:

a. Type 1 students (mostly married women with children) had
"the greatest difficulty deciding to return to school; they were
the most apprehensive, yet they were also looking forward to
school more than the other types" (p. 85), and the chief source
of their difficulty was balancing the demands of school and
family.

b. Type 2 students most closely resembled traditional-aged students in that few were either married or employed. They had a
fairly easy time adjusting to the return to school. Their difficulties stemmed chiefly from "adjusting to a lowered standard of
living and maintaining an adequate social life" (p. 86).

c. Type 3 students (most unmarried adults employed full time
and attending school part time) had considerable difficulty
adjusting because of financial and academic problems; many
dropped out after one semester.

d. Type 4 students (mostly full-time students who were married but spent little time with their families and devoted a great deal of time to their studies) experienced few academic problems but nonetheless reported "high levels of difficulty and stress during the adjustment period," probably because they "were not able to fulfill important social needs" (p. 87).

e. Type 5 students (mostly married, employed full time, and enrolled in only one or two courses) indicated that returning to school did not change their life-style but nonetheless experienced some stress, chiefly because "they had trouble fitting school in their already busy lives" (p. 87).

In summary, ease of adjustment and sense of well-being seemed to depend on the student's particular situation following enrollment. Competing demands on time were a greater source of stress than were academic demands *per se*.

CONCLUSION AND RECOMMENDATIONS

In the foregoing discussion, a series of questions related to midlife women and education have been raised. To the overriding question: What use does the midlife woman make of education? What value does it have for her? My answer must be: It all depends. It depends on the woman's particular situation, on her level of cognitive development, her role involvements, the motives that drive her, and the barriers that impede her. Although one can, for convenience, differentiate adult learners from traditional-age learners, one cannot talk about the "midlife woman" without doing violence to reality. To some women, midlife is a period of greater freedom and opportunity; to others, it is a period of greater constraint and responsibility. To the former group, education may be a vehicle for growth and renewal; to the latter, it might simply constitute an added burden.

Even though the number of adult learners—particularly women—has increased dramatically, it is important to remember that a far greater number do not participate in formal learning activities. Projections indicate that by the year 2010 there will be 36 million women between the ages of 45 and 64 in this nation. Will most of them be so preoccupied with their roles as workers and caretakers that they will be unable to utilize education?

Earlier, situational, institutional, and dispositional factors that impede midlife women's participation in education were outlined. The following two recommendations would help remove all three sets of barriers.

1. *Postsecondary educational institutions should initiate policies more responsive to the needs of adult students.* These policies would include (a) granting credit for life experiences that have been appropriately evaluated; (b) giving financial aid to part-time as well as full-time students; (c) establishing internships (paid and unpaid) that will give adult students a chance to explore a new field before making a full commitment to it; (d) revision of schedules; (e) revision of admissions procedures (Charner, 1981, p. 2).

2. *Regional Adult Counseling Centers should be established, to serve both as model centers and as resources for satellite centers throughout the region.* These centers would offer a comprehensive array of services, including individual and group counseling, career planning, skills training, and special-interest workshops. Satellite centers might offer only some of these services, referring clients to the regional center for other services as necessary. Despite the proliferation of counseling centers serving adults of both sexes, such services are not universally available. So far, there is no systematic delivery system to assure that the ordinary adult woman in any given community will have somewhere to go for help in uncovering educational and other options.

Until we have social policies that offer opportunities for education throughout life and provide help in caring for children or aging relatives, many midlife women will continue to be excluded from the learning opportunities now enjoyed by only a few of this age group.

REFERENCES

Aslanian, C. B., and Brickell, H. M. *American in transition: Life changes as reasons for adult learning.* New York: College Entrance Examination Board, 1980.
Astin, A. W. *Preventing students from dropping out.* San Francisco: Jossey-Bass, 1975.
Astin, A. W., King, M. R., and Richardson, G. T. *The American freshman: National norms for fall 1980.* Los Angeles: Cooperative Institutional Research Program, 1981.
Baruch, G. K., and Barnett, R. C. On the well-being of adult women. In L. A. Bond and J. C. Rosen (Eds.), *Competence and coping during adulthood.* Hanover, N.H.: University Press of New England, 1980.
Boaz, R. L. *Participation in adult education: Final report, 1975.* Washington, D.C.: National Center for Education Statistics, 1978.
Campbell, A., Converse, P., and Rodgers, W. *The quality of American life.* New York: Russell Sage Foundation, 1976.
Campbell, M. D., Wilson, L. G., and Hanson, G. R. *The invisible minority: A study of adult university students.* (Final report submitted to the Hogg Foundation for Mental Health). Austin: Office of the Dean of Students, University of Texas, 1980.
Carp, A., Peterson, R. E., and Roelfs, P. J. Adult learning: Interests and experiences. in K. P. Cross, J. R. Valley, and Associates, *Planning non-traditional programs.* San Francisco: Jossey-Bass, 1974.
Cattell, R. B. Theory of fluid and crystallized intelligence: A critical experiment. *Journal of Educational Psychology,* 1963, *54,* 1–22.

Charner, I. Motivating adult learning through planned change. *National Center for Educa* *tional Brokering Bulletin*, 1981, 6 (7), 1.

Cross, K. P. A critical review of state and national studies of the needs and interests o adult learners. In C. B. Stalford (Ed.), *Conference report: Adult learning needs and th demand for lifelong learning.* Washington, D. C.: National Institute of Education, U.S Department of Health, Education and Welfare, 1978.

Cross, K. P. *Adults as learners.* San Francisco: Jossey-Bass, 1981.

Dearman, N. B., and Plisko, V. W. *The condition of education, 1980 edition.* Washington National Center for Education, 1980.

Entine, A. D. The role of continuing education. In *Women in mid-life: Security and fulfillmen Part I.* A compendium of papers submitted to the Select Committee on Aging, U.S House of Representatives, 95th Congress. Comm. Pub. No. 95–107, 1978.

Fisher-Thompson, J., and Kuhn, J. A. *Re-entry women: Relevant statistics.* Washington D.C.: Project on the Status and Education of Women, Association of American Co leges, 1981.

Fiske, M. Changing hierarchies of commitment in adulthood. In N. J. Smelser and E. H Erikson (Eds.), *Themes of work and love in adulthood.* Cambridge, Mass.: Harvard Un versity Press, 1980.

Gallagher, D., Thompson, L. W., and Levy, S. M. Clinical psychological assessment (older adults. In L. W. Poon (Ed.), *Aging in the 1980's: Psychological issues.* Washingto D. C.: American Psychological Association, 1980.

Giesen, C. B., and Datan, N. The competent older woman. In N. Datan and N. Lohman (Eds.), *Transitions in aging.* New York: Academic Press, 1980.

Gutmann, D. C. The cross-cultural perspective: Notes toward a comparative psychology (aging. In J. E. Birren and K. W. Schaie (Eds.), *Handbook of the psychology of aging.* Ne York: Van Nostrand Reinhold, 1977.

Hall, R. B., and Gleaves, F. D. *Re-entry women: Special programs for special population* Washington, D.C.: Project on the Status and Education of Women, Association (American Colleges, 1981.

Karabel, J. Community colleges and social stratification. *Harvard Educational Review*, 197 42, 521–562.

Knefelkamp, L. L., Widick, C. C., and Stroad, B. Cognitive-developmental theory: guide to counseling women. *Counseling Psychologist*, 1976, 6, 15–19.

Kohlberg, L. Stages of moral development as a basis for moral education. In C. Beck and Sullivan (Eds.), *Moral education.* Canada: University of Toronto, 1970.

Kohn, M. L. Job complexity and adult personality. In N. J. Smelser and E. H. Eriks((Eds.), *Themes of work and love in adulthood.* Cambridge, Mass.: Harvard Universi Press, 1980.

Kuhlen, R. G. Motivational changes during the adult years. In R. G. Kuhlen (Ed.), *Psych logical backgrounds of adult education.* Chicago: Center for the Study of Liberal Educatic for Adults, 1963.

Lipman-Blumen, J. How ideology shapes women's lives. *Scientific American*, 1972, 22 34–42.

Loevinger, J. *Ego development: Conceptions and theories.* San Francisco: Jossey-Bass, 197

Lowenthal, M. F., Thurnher, M., and Chiriboga, D. *Four stages of life: A comparative study men and women facing transitions.* San Francisco: Jossey-Bass, 1975.

Magarrell, J. The enrollment boom among older Americans: 1 in 3 college students is nc over 25 years old. *Chronicle of Higher Education*, May 4, 1981, p. 3.

Miller, J., Schooler, C., Kohn, M. E., and Miller, K. A. Women and work: The psycholo; cal effects of occupational conditions. *American Journal of Sociology*, 1979, 85, 66–S rry, W. G. *Forms of intellectual and ethical development in the college years.* New York: Holt, Rinehart & Winston, 1970.

mey, E. *Anatomy—Destiny: Is burn-out inevitable?* Paper presented at the 6th Annual Conference of Helpers of Adults, University of Maryland, May 1981.

ndour, M. L., Strasburg, G., & Lipman-Blumen, J. *Women in higher education: Trends in enrollments and degrees earned.* Unpublished manuscript, 1981.

do, B. *The dependency squeeze on middle-aged women.* Paper presented to the Secretary's Committee on the Rights and Responsibilities of Women, Department of Health, Education and Welfare. Washington, D.C.: Center for Population Research, Georgetown University, 1980.

eathersby, R. P., and Tarule, J. M. *Adult development: Implications for higher education* (AAHE-ERIC Higher Education Research Report No. 4). Washington, D.C.: American Association for Higher Education, 1980.

estervelt, E. M. *Barriers to women's participation in postsecondary education: A review of research and commentary as of 1973–1974.* Washington, D. C.: National Center for Education Statistics, 1975.

ite, R. Strategies of adaptation: An attempt at systematic description. In R. Moos (Ed.), *Human adaptation: Coping with life crises.* Lexington, Mass.: Heath, 1976.

llis, S. L., and Baltes, P. B. Intelligence in adulthood and aging: Contemporary issues. In L. W. Poon (Ed.), *Aging in the 1980's: Psychological issues.* Washington, D.C.: American Psychological Association, 1980.

'he Anxiety of the Unknown—Choice, Risk, Responsibility

'herapeutic Issues for Today's Adult Women

OSALIND C. BARNETT

ithin the last several years we have seen a plethora of research find-
ξs and demographic data describing current social changes, especially
they affect women. The changes that have received greatest attention
:lude the lengthening life-span, the widespread movement of women
o the labor force, the rising divorce rate, and steadily growing infla-
n. These massive changes in our social environment have undoubted-
affected women's views of themselves and their life satisfaction. Yet
plicit work on exploring the implications of these widely discussed
:ial shifts on the psychological experiences of women and on the
ues they bring into therapy has not kept pace. Several recent reviews
aracek and Johnson, 1980; McMahon, 1980) focus on the process of
:rapy—the form, not the content. Other overviews deal with the psy-
atric aspects of particular and frequent presenting problems, such as
ortion, sexual dysfunctions, eating disorders (see, for example, Not-
n and Nadelson, 1978). These efforts, however, rarely address the
pact that the sweeping changes in the social and political definitions
women's roles have had on the issues with which adult women are
ppling, especially in their middle years.

Research in such diverse fields as life-span developmental psychol-
y and social gerontology has illuminated such relevant topics as (1)
ividual adjustment to a longer life-span and, in particular, to in-

ALIND C. BARNETT • Wellesley College Center for Research on Women, Wellesley,
sachusetts 02181.

tergenerational relationships over the life-span (Hagestad, 1981; Hage
stad, Smyer, and Stierman, 1982); (2) the psychological well-being o
women in the middle years as it relates to women's employment an
family statuses (Barnett and Baruch, 1981); and (3) the influence of sc
cial-historical events on individual adjustment (Elder, 1979; Hareven
1976; Pearlin, 1975).

The Social Context

This chapter is an attempt to articulate several pressing therapeuti
issues for mature women in the 1980s that grow out of this new socia
context and to view them against the backdrop provided by pertiner
research findings. These issues reflect women's growing realization tha
they need to shape their lives actively, to take risks, and to be respons
ble for their own happiness. Underlying these issues are the dual cor
cerns over establishing one's sense of femininity and of sexuality in
time when old prescriptions are shattered and newer ones are not yet
place.

My comments pertain predominantly to middle-class Caucasia
women and to the concerns they are bringing into therapy. These cor
cerns are not necessarily new; however, they have a new urgency ar
intensity that calls for special attention from therapists.

For mature women, the last decade has been one of radical depa
tures. The steady stream of demographic statistics makes it absolute
clear that the life patterns of today's women differ dramatically from tl
pattern that their mothers followed and for which they were socialize
Compared to their mothers, today's women are far better educated, a
more often in the paid labor force for their entire adult lives, are marr
ing later or not marrying at all, are having fewer children later or none
all, and are dissolving bad marriages rather than preserving them '
least until the children are grown up." As a percentage of the fem
population, women who live out over the long term the idealized l
pattern of being married and at home with children are now a minori

Awareness that the old norms no longer apply is only the first st
in accepting that diversity and normlessness are the new norms. Und
standably, yet sadly, full acceptance of alternative life patterns
"right," "fitting," or "fulfilling" lags, creating a psychological gap. I
many women, this gap results in anxiety, depression, and painful so
searching, particularly as they approach the middle years.

For a long time educated women have acknowledged intellectua
that freedom to choose one's life pattern is essential. Awareness
demographic shifts, of the need to prepare for future goals, is reflect
in the growing numbers of women completing higher education a

ommitting themselves to continuous employment. For many women, owever, these alternative patterns have been experienced as largely relevant for defining their core identities and for fulfilling themselves women. While intellectually championing the importance of non-aditional roles, most middle-class women have difficulty embracing em as means of satisfying their basic personal needs. This difficulty ows in part out of their upbringing and is sustained by the realization what their mothers' lives have been and what their own expectations erefore are. With the demise of the old norms and the new emphasis alternative life patterns comes the need to reevaluate nontraditional les for their capacity to fulfill basic needs. And conscious reevaluation alternative life patterns raises the issue of choice.

AKING CHOICES

Resistant to planning ahead, reared to believe that the future will be ken care of by the man of their dreams, women are now grappling ith the need to plan for themselves and to take responsibility for their vn lives. These needs are very anxiety-producing, raising concerns out essential femininity, responsibility for oneself, relations to one's other. Hard-hit by the demands of the changing social situation are men in their 30s and 40s. These women have been reared by mothers bodying the Feminine Mystique and have absorbed the expectation at at midlife they too would be in a similarly stable family situation.

Many women struggling with these issues enter therapy. For some re is still conflict, even when knowing consciously that they value ir independence and their time alone, that they do not want to be rried, that they do not want children, that the ideal relationship for m is one that is free of long-term commitments. Conflict arises be-se their feelings don't quite match their conscious beliefs. They ago-e over whether they are emotionally ready to live out the new "pat-ns" they may have chosen or that may seem desirable. They both w what they want and aren't sure whether they want it. How do I w these things? Am I perhaps still rebelling against my mother? Was erhaps caught up in the politicization of women's issues and am still ner-waving? Conflict leads to questioning. How can I want such a ferent life pattern from the one my mother chose and the one I am posed to "want"?

Departures from known patterns also have consequences for the ental generation. Mothers watch as their daughters mature under ial conditions with which they have a difficult time identifying. The ninine Mystique mother never had to deal consciously with the array hoices confronting her daughter. She may not understand or be able

to support her daughter who postpones marriage to finish a degree
chooses to have an abortion rather than drop out of school, brings some
one in to care for her young children so that she may resume work, or
divorces her husband when her children are still young. Under these
pressures, mothers may feel useless, incompetent, and rejected as mod
els. Hence, they may retreat, criticize, or in other ways fail to acknow
edge their daughters' choices, thus inadvertently adding to their daugh
ters' anxiety about the "rightness" of the life choices they are making
The potential for a sense of betrayal on both sides is great, fueling th
daughter's concern over being someone her mother can approve of o
the one hand, and, on the other, generating tension over inadequaci
in knowing how to parent an adult daughter whose life bears so littl
resemblance to her own.

The following vignette illustrates how a mother's behavior can un
wittingly add to her daughter's anxiety.

Alice, a 34-year-old married professional woman, has an infant daughter.
She continued to work actively until the day before her daughter was born
and returned to work shortly thereafter. She managed her new role by arranging to work from her home office part of the time, and she hired a live-in
maid to assist with the baby. Her colleagues and professional women friends
had made similar arrangements and were supportive of the pattern she had
worked out. However, Alice had a nagging sense that her choices would not
be approved of by her mother, and this realization increased her uncertainty
about the "rightness" of the life-style she was developing. Her uncertainty
and anxiety predated the birth of her child. She is from a large traditional
family and is the first child and grandchild to have completed a professional
degree. As a woman and as a member of this family she was an anomaly;
none of her close relatives had life experiences that were, in critical ways, at
all similar to hers. Within her own family she first began to feel a lack of
understanding and a distance during her college years, when it became clear
to her that she wanted to pursue advanced training. Her parents had fully
supported her in completing a college education. However, graduate school
was another thing. They had never known anyone who had gone to graduate school and certainly never expected their daughter to make that choice.

The difference between what they had expected for her and her actual
choices began to mount. She did not get married when all her friends did.
She explained to her parents that she wasn't ready to marry because she had
not decided what to do with her life. They had a difficult time understanding
what she meant.

She completed her program and got married. She decided to postpone
having children until her career was established. Again, her parents, who
had expected her to marry and start a family years before, were unable to
comprehend. They never openly confronted her on these issues, but they
made their disappointments known largely by not asking personal questions
and never inquiring about her professional life. Alice knew that they were
having trouble understanding the life choices she was making. Nevertheless,
her mother's inability, or lack of effort, to understand served as a constant
reminder of her own uncertainty about the new pattern she was following. In

therapy she related the following incident, which reflected the various strains in her relationship with her mother: Her parents came to visit her when the baby was just a few weeks old. Alice brought the baby over so that her mother could hold her. Her mother was delighted and took the baby in her arms. After just a few seconds, she turned to Alice and said, "No, you take her; after all you don't get to hold her too often."

This interchange underscored the attempts these two women were making to connect with one another as well as the tension, implicit criticism, and consequent anxiety generated by these attempts.

The remainder of this chapter focuses on several sources of anxiety today's women—specifically, concerns over being feminine and being ⁣xual—and how therapists can understand the related issues of choice, ⁣k, and responsibility. Women caught in these struggles come into ⁣erapy with questions such as the following: Why am I not married? ⁣hat is wrong with me? What will happen to me if I never marry, if I get ⁣vorced? What will my life be like if I never have a child? How can I ⁣ssibly have a child when my professional life is so unsettled?

The intensity of affect around these concerns—all of which touch on ⁣finitions of femininity—gives striking evidence of the hold traditional ⁣as about femininity have on the psyches of today's women. There is ⁣acute intrapsychic struggle being waged within many women pa⁣nts (and nonpatients) over these issues, and the struggle takes several ⁣ms.

Among never-married women, for example, many who enjoy their ⁣-style wonder whether their ability to enjoy life without a permanent ⁣rtner reflects a personality deficit. And they fear that the happiness ⁣y now enjoy will be short-lived—that the price of deviating from ⁣ial and maternal norms will have to be paid eventually. Those who ⁣ anguished about not being in a permanent relationship feel rejected, ⁣ssed by, "out of synch." They experience themselves as deviant, ⁣feminine, essentially unlovable—and the proof lies in their unmarried ⁣te. Women approaching 40 who are childless—whether married or ⁣t—wrestle painfully with feelings of being incomplete, of being less ⁣n a whole female.

Rarely do women patients experience these life dilemmas as ⁣ices. Why then did I use the word *choice* in the title of this chapter? ⁣arly, the word needs some clarification. Hard as it may be for many ⁣men to acknowledge their part in creating the dilemmas in which ⁣y find themselves, they inevitably did make choices—consciously or ⁣consciously—and understanding that they did so is crucial to any ⁣olution.

One recently married 37-year-old women patient was acutely de⁣ssed over the realization that her husband refused to have a child. ⁣ entered the marriage knowing his feelings, but wanting so much to

be married that she discounted his resolve. Two years later, painfull
aware of her approaching 40th birthday, she again raised the issue
From her husband's point of view there was nothing to discuss. H
understood how she felt, but he had been perfectly clear about hi
feelings at the outset and they had not changed.

She was desperate. She yearned to have a child, to care for a baby
to nurture, to fulfill her own expectations, yet she did not want t
divorce her husband. On balance, her life was happier than it had bee
before she married, and realistically the possibility of establishing ar
other relationship and having a child was negligible. Her initial depres
sion was accompanied by feelings of being incomplete and of blamin
her husband for impeding the fulfillment of her femininity.

Treatment centered around disentangling her sense of her ow
femininity from that of being a mother, and accepting responsibility fc
the marital choice she had made. As her anger at her husband diss
pated, she was able to recognize that prior to her marriage, she was
vivacious, independent, outgoing woman with lots of friends wh
while lonely at times, was not burdened by a sense of her inadequacy i
a female. As a single woman she had no assumptions about the nece
sary conditions for fulfilling herself as a woman and was able to "put c
hold" all the expectations and social pressures that surfaced after h
marriage. However, being married, the only role for which her ear
rearing prepared her, carried with it emotionally charged prescription
She was now in a position to have a child, thereby "completing" h
femininity and fulfilling what she perceived as her mother's expect
tions for her.

In therapy she worked through the various meanings she had i
tached to having a child and realized that her feelings about herself ar
her relationship with her mother were essentially independent
whether she had a child or not. Certainly her sense of loss was real; sl
was not going to be a mother, and she came to accept that she mig
always experience some pain around that loss. But the life she h
chosen offered many opportunities for her to meet other needs, and h
fulfillment depended on developing and enjoying those opportunitie

Taking Risks

As with any choice, there are costs as well as benefits. One cost
the anxiety of the unknown, of being on a path untraveled by on
mother or maybe by anyone else in one's immediate circle. (The rarity
role models for "deviant" life patterns will undoubtedly be less an iss
for tomorrow's mature women.) This anxiety is often associated with

eed for affirmation. And one's mother is the primary person from whom that affirmation is sought.

For patients, the abstract knowledge that mature women can lead ighly rewarding lives in alternative patterns is reassuring but inadeuate. The road to the end point of full acceptance is often very difficult, s is illustrated by the following case:

> The issues of choice, risk, and responsibility came together for a 40-year-old patient who, after years of a stagnant marriage, acknowledged that she was miserable. Ostensibly things were going well. She had two preteenage sons and a husband who earned a good living. Unlike the situation in her own family while she was growing up, her husband did not drink, there were no brawls, there were no disagreements or arguments, calm reigned, albeit at the cost to her of subordinating the fun-loving, vibrant parts of her personality. Like her mother, she conformed to the depressive life-style dictated by her husband's moodiness. Unlike her mother, she could not blame her misfortune on her husband's drinking. In fact, she could not begin to explain to her mother why she felt so miserable; her mother would never have understood. The religious/moral/social beliefs that kept her mother in a terrible marriage also kept her from any understanding of her daughter's desire to break out of her marriage and to live her own life. She stayed away from her mother in part because she accused herself of the same selfish motives she was sure her mother would accuse her of: Bob makes no demands, he is so easygoing, why can't you go along? What is wrong with you? Is what you want important enough to destroy your family?
>
> Underneath all these accusations was the fear that her mother would accuse her of not being feminine—not supportive, self-denying, patient, undemanding—an accusation with which she tormented herself. But times and attitudes had changed, and being a socially aware woman, she knew she had to get out of her marriage; she had to do what she had wished her mother had done. And she did. It took her three years of procrastinating, of changing lawyers, of not making her needs clear. During this period, she learned how to stand up for herself at work, how to ask her friends for what she needed; she reached out to her mother, was rebuffed, and recovered. She learned that her mother's limitations made it impossible for her to be the mother she wanted—to affirm her decision to divorce and to appreciate her as a worthwhile person. She learned that her own growing sense of her worth was what counted, and she took responsibility for cultivating her self-esteem. She began to feel confident enough to accept herself as a female and as a divorced woman. With her newly grounded sense of self, she tackled the divorce process with conviction, completing in a few months what otherwise would have taken years.

Ironically, the greater the departure from her mother's model, the eater a daughter's need for affirmation and the harder it may be to tain. Interestingly, findings from recent research (Barnett and Baruch, 32) lend support to this formulation. This study was designed to exore the relationship between psychological well-being and varying tterns of work and family status among women 35 to 55. The women in the study (N = 238) were in one of four family statuses: never-mar ried, married with children, married without children, and divorce with children. For most of the women, a close relationship to thei mothers was associated with high self-esteem and a sense of psycholog cal well being (Baruch and Barnett, 1983). For the divorced womer however, all of whom were employed and had children, a negativ association was found. That is, the closer they were to their mothers, th lower was their sense of well-being. One interpretation of this finding i that the mothers of divorced women may not be able to shed the negative views about divorce; they may not know how to mother daughter who has done something they were reared to believe wa "wrong," "shameful," or "immoral." By extension they may feel the they have failed as mothers and may take on the shame that they assoc ate with their daughter's divorce. Thus, for the divorced daughter closeness to their mothers may result in exacerbating the very anxie that motivated the desire for closeness.

Further evidence supporting this conjecture comes from a descri tive study of recently divorced middle-aged parents (mean age, 48 years for the women). A focus of the study was on the intergeneration impact of the divorce experience. The researchers (Hagestad et al., 198 report that about one-fourth of the women who had parents living at tl time of the marital disruption never discussed their marital situatic with their parents, typically because they expected disapproval or la of understanding. One woman said, "I am ashamed to say it, but at fif I am still afraid of what my mother thinks—she intimidates me. I w divorced almost a year before I told her." And a few of the peop interviewed admitted that the "divorce had been delayed because of t anticipated negative reactions from parents."

The process of accepting oneself as a complete and acceptab female in an atypical life pattern is itself experienced with anxiety. F acceptance involves taking the risk of presenting oneself both private and publicly as, for example, a divorced woman, a successful nev married professional, or a voluntarily childless married career woma The successful career woman who refuses an opportunity that wou make her more visible professionally may be acting out her anxiety o making clear her choice of a life pattern radically different from t idealized one that she assumed she would be following. Such a pub statement would make impossible future retreat into the safety of tl which is known.

Fortunately, the risks involved are most often greater in prosp than they are in actuality. For women who are struggling with achievi maternal approval, images of a powerful, threatening, difficult-to-ple mother, reminiscent of childhood perceptions of larger-than-life-p

nts, still abound. And in these times of change, it is tempting for
aughters to attribute the lack of maternal approval they feel to life
attern differences. Old images die hard. They do not allow for changes
nothers may have made in the course of their own lives or in response
o witnessing their daughter's experiments with new patterns.

When appropriate, I ask mature women patients to bring their
nothers with them into therapy. Typically they react with dread. Com-
etent, successful women are terrified at the prospect of talking openly
vith their mothers. Most often, this initial resistance is overcome and
ne mother in invited. Almost always she accepts. Initially the session is
nse—the daughter is on guard for signs that her mother really doesn't
alue her; the mother is defensive. As the session progresses, it becomes
ear to the mother that she is a very significant person in her daughter's
fe and that is why she was asked to be part of the therapy. Thus
assured, mothers relax and participate. Outcomes vary, of course, but
t the very least, old images are shaken up or destroyed. The "rigid,
emanding mother" is often just as eager to be accepted by her daughter
s the daughter is to be accepted by her mother.

The basic lesson is that opting for one life pattern over another in
rder to gain maternal approval is a strategy that is doomed to fail.
Iany adult patients struggle to free themselves of the need for approval
om their mothers. Many are engaged in a reexamination of their goals
light of what they see as their own values, not merely extensions of
hat they perceive their mothers want for them. This process takes on
ecial poignancy today because of the assumed relationship between
e goals women choose and their need to see themselves as "femi-
ine." Not long ago there was a certain consensus and therefore comfort
r women in the knowledge that they would follow their mothers'
ath—they would marry and have children—thereby automatically es-
blishing their femininity.

Now it is more difficult. There is no longer a reasonable certainty
at women will take this path, nor that, given the choice, they will find
at it meets the needs many adult women are expressing. However,
sues highly relevant to the content of therapy with today's women
ise from serious questioning about relinquishing marriage and/or
otherhood. As women contemplate alternative life patterns, the ques-
on of how one defines oneself as feminine becomes salient.

HE QUESTION OF FEMININITY

We all need to see ourselves as being like others of our sex (Kagan,
964; Kohlberg, 1966); that is, women need to see themselves as being
minine. Historically, this was accomplished by marrying and rearing

children. Thus, a woman was reassured that she was feminine because she was caring for a husband and children—following her mother's model and engaged in the same nurturing activities as her female peers Reliance on this once widely available and accepted behavioral resolution of an essentially psychological issue is no longer viable.

Many women in nontraditional as well as traditional patterns reject the view of femininity as a status ascribed only to those who have married and have had children. Rather, they view femininity as a status to be attained. Thus, they ask: Does a woman need to be in a long-term relationship with a man to prove to herself or others that she is truly feminine? Can a woman feel completely feminine if she devotes her energies to her career? How does her definition of herself as a female relate to her sense of herself as a sexual being? The sense of loneliness and the questioning of choices expressed in therapy by women who have alternative life patterns often masks the underlying fear that the price of these choices goes beyond feeling "out of sync." The price, they fear, may be living with perpetual doubt about their adequacy a females.

How does one go about achieving femininity? Is it possible? How will I ever know if I'll feel complete as a woman? This anxiety-laden self-questioning process is rendered more painful because it is being conducted on an individual basis. In the absence of social consensus women have to arrive at idiosyncratic definitions of femininity.

I envision a future in which individuals will separate definitions of feminity from behavioral prescriptions; where a woman's femininity will not be called into question, by herself or by others, because she choose not to marry or not to have children. I would like to see girls and boy reared in an environment in which adult women are portrayed as complete and feminine, independent of their marital and parental roles However, the psychological reality for today's women is that these two are entangled. In fact, the persistent scrutiny, the external and internal doubts about the independence of femininity and life pattern constitute a major obstacle to achieving separation of the two.

The goal of feeling comfortable with oneself as a female apart from one's life choices is far from trivial. How can therapists be helpful to women caught in the struggle to attain it? One answer comes from a unexpected source. Years ago, Harvard sociologist Alex Inkeles addressed the question "What is sociology?" (Inkeles, 1964). He approached this question in several ways. One intriguing approach was to define sociology as "what sociologists do." By analogy, femininity may not best be defined directly. Rather, femininity can be thought of as what females are or describe themselves as, including feelings, traits attitudes. This approach can be useful if the temptation is resisted t urn it into another quest for what is typically "feminine," and then to efine *that* as what females "ought" to do or be. If we as females can ccept our own feelings, traits, and attitudes as feminine by definition, ve can resist our need to obtain external approval. Such acceptance vould also help us disarm social criticism.

CKNOWLEDGING ONE'S SEXUALITY

A related issue, that of acknowledging and actualizing one's sexu-ity, is particularly problematic for today's women. Growing awareness f their own sexual needs often creates monumental problems for wom-n in nontraditional life patterns, as well as for married women. In the urrent climate, mature women "know" they have sexual needs, yet arning what those sexual needs are and how to fulfill them, and grow-g to accept oneself as a "sexual being," requires a revolution in inking.

The first lesson most adult women learned as children was not to ink about sex at all. Good girls didn't. Then, during their late teen ears, sexual standards loosened dramatically. The sexual revolution fected women differently, depending in large part on when in their evelopment they experienced its impact. For many women, experi-enting with sexuality was just that; they felt their behavior was wrong," more like play-acting than learning how to create a mutually tisfying sexual relationship. Most women brought to their early sexual ncounters the lesson of their youth—that sexual performance meant eeting their partner's needs. Following this prescription affirmed a oman as nurturant, supportive, caring, and loving. These qualities ere supposed to assure her satisfaction, but they obviously could not cause her needs were not addressed. As sexual taboos loosened, omen became aware that they were not alone in their frustration and at dissatisfaction, anger, and resentment grew out of culturally sanc-oned denial of their own sexual needs. Now adult women are discover-g their own sexuality. Along with this discovery is the need to engage eir partners in fulfilling their needs. These efforts are often initiated infully, shyly, with great difficulty, and with women not knowing w to ask, anxious over having expectations and needs, and fearing at their needs will be condemned as illegitimate and will therefore not met.

The presence of a marital sexual partner does not and certainly has t automatically provided for the satisfaction of women's sexual needs; e absence of a marital partner, however, creates additional problems r today's women. The nonmarried woman who tries to have her sexu-needs met has few choices: She can defy old prohibitions and permit herself to become sexually involved with one or more men with whom she is not in a committed relationship. In this action she is supported by current social mores, yet her internal struggle goes on. Seeing herself through her mother's eyes, she feels guilty over being promiscuous, over feeling like a whore. These feelings are part of her heritage. Again, women grapple individually with this issue and there is no easy solution. A classic case of this struggle is the sophisticated divorced woman involved romantically with a married man. Loving him, she is caught between two sexual moralities. She agonizes over how to remain in this fulfilling, yet clearly limited relationship; she is already overinvested and dreams a monogamous dream, yet she knows the relationship will never meet those needs. And her basic sexual-moral feeling is that she has to be loyal to him, to a married man who is being unfaithful. The reality of the situation does not elude her, yet neither does it point clearly to a way out. She sees the irrationality of her predicament, yet she can't make the emotional leap. Monogamous sexual feelings are part-and-parcel of her makeup—the psychological gap is still too wide.

Of course, not all women can or want to work out their sexual needs with a man. Some prefer to take care of their needs themselves; learning to nurture and pleasure themselves puts them safely in charge of their sexuality. Again, overcoming guilt is a necessary step before this course becomes viable. Other women turn to female partners. And these alternatives are not mutually exclusive. Whatever route one takes reflects an affirmation of one's sexuality and an acknowledgment that sexual needs are not to be denied. This is a mammoth undertaking, particularly for midlife women, one fraught with anxiety, self-doubt, recrimination, and enormous fear of the consequences.

The Role of the Therapist

The therapist alert to the centrality of these issues can help separate them from the manifest context in which they are raised. Thus, a presenting problem—for example, the sense of failure experienced around an impending divorce—can be hypothesized as arising in large part from the threat a woman experiences to her sense of femininity. What does her divorce imply about her femininity? How can she establish a sense of femininity when she is no longer in a marital relationship? In addressing these basic questions we can help our women patients redefine femininity as an inherent attitude, not an achieved status. Their essential femininity is then not threatened by divorce. Once this issue is dealt with, the risks inherent in contemplating a nontraditional life pattern are greatly reduced.

The position that femininity is independent of one's life pattern is
pported by several research findings. Of all the "choices" today's
omen are contemplating, the one that calls up the issue of femininity
ost acutely is that of choosing not to have children. Women who make
at choice are open to being stigmatized as unfeminine, i.e., selfish,
amature, irresponsible, unnatural. To explore the personality traits of
oluntarily childless women, psychologist Judith Teicholtz (1978) com-
ared a group of 38 married women who had decided never to bear
aildren (the age range was 23 to 38; the mean age was 30 years) to a
oup of 32 unmarried women who planned to have children (the age
nge was 24 to 37; the mean age was 28 years). While hers was not a
ndom sample and the findings must therefore be taken only as sug-
estive, she found no significant differences between the two groups of
omen on measures of adjustment, social responsibility, maturity, and
ost important—femininity. These two groups of women described
emselves in essentially identical ways on several measures assessing
conscious or unconscious" feminine identity.

In their interview study, based on a random sample of somewhat
der women, 35 to 55, Barnett and Baruch (1981) obtained similar find-
gs. Using the Bem Sex Role Inventory (Bem, 1974), a measure of self-
ncept that asks women to rate themselves on adjectives widely con-
dered to reflect femininity and masculinity, the mean femininity scores
r women in four family statuses—never-married, married with chil-
en, married without children, and divorced with children—were vir-
ally indistinguishable. The range on this instrument is 1 to 10, and the
eans for the four family status groups all clustered tightly around 5.7,
ith the highest being 5.9 and the lowest 5.6!

It might be argued that the women Teicholz studied were young
ad still had the option of changing their minds and therefore did not
ave to deal with the impact on their femininity of actually not having
aildren. The women in the Barnett and Baruch study described above,
owever, were almost all past the point in their lives when having
aildren was an open issue.

A second finding from the same study may be useful to therapists
orking with divorced women patients. Divorced women, it is widely
lieved, suffer a loss of self-esteem related to their sense of failure as
omen and wives. The divorced women in the study were all employed
others and had been divorced for an average of 7 years. On the indices
well-being, these women scored very high. As a group, they had high
vels of self-esteem and did not report many symptoms of anxiety or
pression. Knowing that divorced mothers who are employed and
ao have been divorced for several years feel as positive about them-

selves as do their married counterparts ought to help therapists in supporting their women patients who are struggling with divorce and cannot imagine how they can put together a satisfying postdivorce life.

Such research findings can be particularly helpful to women agonizing over the risk to their "femininity" of making deviant choices. These findings are also useful for therapists who do not have enough personal experience with women in these various alternative patterns to draw upon. And many of us are dealing personally with these issues and may have a difficult time separating our concerns from those of our patients.

Most women who come into therapy with these concerns are acutely depressed and cannot imagine a personal future free of the anxiety they are currently experiencing. Commonly heard are such painful formulations as these: What will I do to fill the emptiness of my life? How can I possibly come home every night to a childless home? Knowing that women typically can move beyond these crises, create meaningful lives and have a firm sense of their own femininity can help therapists, and in turn their patients, to develop a life-span perspective, focusing more on the resolution of the crises than on the crises *per se*.

BEING RESPONSIBLE

Perceiving that one needs to make choices, and confronting the risks involved in so doing, inevitably raises the question of responsibility. Traditionally, women did what they were "supposed" to do; they did not have to take responsibility for their lives. Happiness was marrying the right man and having children of whom you could be proud. Misery was having an alcoholic husband, or one who was an insufficient provider, or having children who were a disappointment. Whatever the outcome, women were passive victims of life's circumstances.

It is much harder today for women to avoid seeing themselves as responsible for the way their lives turn out. However, many adult women are ill prepared for feeling in control, for being able to take appropriate pride in choices that work out well and for assuming personal blame for those that do not. Not too long ago, even when economic necessity did not force a woman into the labor market, she could claim that she was working for her family—the college tuition bill was more than her husband could handle, the children needed money for extras. These claims were attractive because they lent social approval to her choice and left her free of personal responsibility. With their consciousnesses newly raised, adult women can no longer "get away" with such rationalizations. Moreover, such decisions as not to marry or not to have children do not easily lend themselves to self-sacrificial explanations.

Women also experience anxiety over the fear that the choices they re making are the "wrong" choices. A major psychological obstacle to 1aking active choices is fear of taking responsibility for how one's life urns out. The women who puts off having children so that she does not 2opardize her career advancement may find that being vice-president of he company is not as rewarding as she thought it would be. And there 5 no one to blame. For the woman who took a new path and failed, it 1ay be especially hard to hear "I told you so," particularly if this mes-age comes from one's mother.

The vocabulary of right and wrong choices seems highly inap-ropriate. When the marriage that seemed so right 15 years ago is so rrong today, the notion of right and wrong needs scrutiny. The test of vhether a decision is right cannot be how things turn out years later. 'oo much is in flux. Perhaps what is right needs to be defined in terms f what conforms best to one's truest feelings as one knows them at the me. This is not a comfortable definition. Traditional definitions of mo-ality (the old familiar standbys—security, stability, commitment, loy-lty, faithfulness) alone are not enough to sustain us. A hard look re-eals that these old definitions of what is right didn't sustain us anyway, nly we weren't willing to take a hard look. We weren't willing to uestion our faith in prescriptions.

While it is difficult to see oneself as actively choosing a life pattern or which one has no precedents and that has been and may still be tigmatized, there are substantial psychological gains to be had for so oing. Recent findings support the speculation that knowing yourself ell enough to know what life pattern you want, and being in that attern, contributes to feelings of well-being (Hoffman, 1976). If you are nonemployed mother and prefer to be employed, your self-esteem is ower compared to your counterparts who prefer to be homemakers. eing in a pattern because someone else wants you to be in that pattern, r because you are afraid of what others might think if you were to make change, turns out to exact a high price in a woman's feelings about erself. While such a woman may experience the comfort of not taking ole command of her life and of avoiding responsibility, there are no oticeable long-term rewards for that strategy.

In fact, recent data (Baruch, Barnett, and Rivers, 1983) indicate that elings of well-being for a woman in the middle years are associated ith her preferring to be in whatever life pattern she is in. Never-1arried women who prefer to be single are higher in well-being than ever-married women who wish they were married. Employed women ho would choose to remain employed even if they had enough money • live comfortably are higher in well-being than employed women who ould rather be homemakers, and so on. Clearly, it is difficult to dis-nguish preference from adaptation and denial. Perhaps never-married women "really" prefer to be married but are denying that preference. Our interpretation, based on additional findings from the same study, is that denial is not an adequate explanation, although adaptation—increasing the goodness of fit of self and role—may be. Indeed, it appears as if the never-married women at the midpoint in their adult lives have organized a life-style that is rich and meaningful and in which the absence of marriage is not significant.

But as independent adult women we need to learn that there are no guarantees; in a sense, we are all involved in experiments in which we cannot predict the outcomes. All we can do is make honest choices, learn to take whatever consequences follow from those choices, and deal with the outcomes. Since the old formulas for women have failed miserably, newer ideas about finding a life pattern that fits one's realistic appraisal of what one needs is a better long-term bet. But it is still only a bet.

References

Barnett, R. C., and Baruch, G. K. *Role strain, number of roles and psychological well-being.* Working paper of the Wellesley College Center for Research on Women, 1981.

Barnett, R. C., and Baruch, G. K. *On the psychological well-being of women in the mid-years.* Working paper of the Wellesley College Center for Research on Women, 1982.

Baruch, G. K., Barnett, R. C., & Rivers, C. *Lifeprints: New patterns of love and work for today's women.* New York: McGraw-Hill, 1983.

Bem, S. L. The measurement of psychological androgyny. *Journal of Consulting and Clinical Psychology,* 1974, 42, 155–162.

Elder, G. H. Historical change in life patterns and personality. In P. Baltes and O. G. Brim Jr. (Eds.), *Life-span development and behavior* (Vol. 2). New York: Academic Press, 1979.

Hagestad, G. O. Problems and promises in the social psychology of intergeneration relations. In R. W. Fogel, E. Hatfield, S. Kiesler, and J. March (Eds.), *Stability and change in the family.* New York: Academic Press, 1981.

Hagestad, G., Smyer, M., and Stierman, K. Parent–child relations in adulthood: The impact of divorce in middle age. In R. Cohen, S. Weissman, and B. Cohler (Eds.), *Parenthood as an adult experience.* New York: Guilford Press, 1982.

Hareven, T. K. The last stage: Adulthood and old age. *Daedalus,* 1976, 105, 13–27.

Hoffman, L. M. Effects of maternal employment on the child: A review of the research. In A. G. Kaplan and J. P. Bean (Eds.), *Beyond sex role stereotypes: Readings toward a psychology of androgyny.* Boston: Little, Brown, 1976.

Inkeles, A. *What is sociology?* Englewood Cliffs, N.J.: Prentice-Hall, 1964.

Kagan, J. Acquisition and significance of sex typing and sex role identification. In M. Hoffman and L. W. Hoffman (Eds.), *Review of child development research* (Vol. 1). New York: Russell Sage, 1964.

Kohlberg, L. A cognitive-developmental analysis of children's sex-role concepts and attitudes. In E. Maccoby (Ed.), *The development of sex differences.* Stanford, Calif.: Stanford University Press, 1966.

Marecek, J., and Johnson, M. Gender and the process of therapy. In A. M. Brodsky and T. Hare-Mustin (Eds.), *Women and psychotherapy.* New York: Guilford Press, 1980.

McMahon, S. L. Women in marital transition. In A. M. Brodsky and R. T. Hare-Mustin (Eds.), *Women in psychotherapy*. New York: Guilford Press, 1980.

Notman, M. T., and Nadelson, C. C. The woman patient. In M. Notman and C. C. Nadelson (Eds.), *The woman patient*, Vol. 1. New York: Plenum, 1978.

Pearlin, L. Sex roles and depression. In N. Datan and L. H. Ginsberg (Eds.), *Life-span developmental psychology: Normative life crises*. New York: Academic Press, 1975.

Veicholtz, J. *Psychological correlates of voluntary childlessness in married women*. Paper presented at the meeting of the Eastern Psychological Association, Washington, D.C., 1978.

Chapter 16

Reflections and Perspectives on Therapeutic Issues for Today's Adult Women'

Malkah T. Notman

Women in their middle years are at varying points in their own life cycles. One women at 40 may be a grandmother, another may be having her first child. Women's lives are also not linear—that is, they do not progress in a predictable sequence; many roles, positions, and psychological states may occur in varying sequences. Although women are affected by their reproductive timetable, this is not the only major framework, and the interrelated components of biology, culture, and psychology have an enormous impact. Therefore, women who are in their "middle years" will bring a variety of therapeutic issues to attention. There is some similarity, however, in the threads that run through many of these issues, particularly if one focuses on the midlife aspects of the problems presented. In confronting the finiteness of life as one comes to perceive it in midlife, an assessment is made of where one is and where one might like to be. Choices that were made, choices that still can be made, and their consequences are considered and evaluated. For women these sometimes concern decisions about having children, sometimes about careers, marriages.

In the past few years, many women have come for consultation and help with problems about these choices, whatever paths they have taken. Barnett has written about some of the central concerns that today's adult women are confronting and that they have been bringing to therapists. She has attempted to suggest the impact of recent major

Malkah T. Notman • Tufts University, Boston, Massachusetts 02146.

social changes in women's roles on these issues. The emphasis on the need to take risks, the importance of assuming responsibility for one's own life, and the importance of choice are crucial. But choice exists on many levels and it is a complex issue with many dimensions, related both to external reality and to internal reality. A few of these complex issues will be addressed and then some clinical examples described that have a bearing on choices and their implications.

Although we are all struck with the enormous impact of social change on women's roles, it is sometimes impossible to separate those problems that are related to these social changes from those that seem to be "old wine in new bottles." For example, the particular manifestations of generational conflicts and value shifts in our current historical period reflect not only new possibilities for women's lives but also some of the inevitable consequences of generational discontinuity, competition, and conflict, as well as identifications.

There is also some question as to how far-reaching the changes in opportunities for women have been (see Alington and Troll, Chapter 7) There is no question as to the availability of reproductive control, at least for middle-class Caucasian women, and therefore, of opportunities for limiting family size, clearly a far-reaching social phenomenon with lasting consequences. The increase in the life-span also means that commitments, such as marital commitments, and expectations of the content of one's life are different. A life can have a number of sequential periods. Some women today talk about their lives as if they have conscious expectations of phases, one to be occupied by marriage and child-rearing, another in which aloneness may not be chosen but may nevertheless have to be confronted. Longevity also means that marital commitments of fidelity and exclusivity, which were intended to last a shorter lifetime than now exists, may be strained as partners develop with the increasing years (Bernard, 1978). These issues are also brought to therapists, sometimes precipitated by the role changes of one or the other partner. They are sometimes presented as questions or disappointments, sometimes as newly awakened wishes that are conflicted.

There is also confusion as to which phases should precede which, whether childbearing and child-rearing should precede establishment of a career, whether this sequence should be the reverse, or whether both can take place concomitantly with some new integration of work and family at a later phase. These questions are also brought into therapy. The possibility of even considering an approach involving a series of life phases is based on the new expectation of many productive and healthy years.

In other spheres, however, the actual impact of social changes does not seem quite as clear. Given the enormous increase of women in the work force, their advancement into positions of high status, economic achievement, and authority has lagged far behind (Scott, 1982). Informal experience and contact with a number of women also indicate that although they may function with varying degrees of freedom at work, once they leave work and return home to their families and friends, their expectations of how they "should" be and what is expected of them are very different and much more conventional, and they speak about leading "schizophrenic" lives.

There are limitations of choice, then, which derive from the realities of particular work conditons and social options. Limitations of choice also are internal; for some women, the determing realities, the exigencies of the demands others make on them, and the limits of their situation may make options much less free in reality than they appear to be.

Most women who are aspiring to carrers do indeed have life potentials that are very different from the expectations that their mothers confronted. There is considerable disparity between the choices made by women today and the lives of their mothers. Dr. Barnett (Chapter 15, this volume) portrays the mother as the inhibiting, awe-inspiring, and feared person whom the daughter may be afraid to confront and who may limit her movement in new directions; Barnett points out that some of this image may be the daugher's internal perception and not actually correct. Situations where the daughters expect maternal disapproval certainly are common. Many women do express their own conflicts in terms of fearing their mother's disapproval. Sometimes this appears to be similar to an issue defined in an old way by psychoanalytic theory, as due to oedipal competitive anxieties—that is, anxiety at doing better than one's mother. This may be an internal concern, remaining from old unresolved conflicts, as well as externally reenforced. Competition with one's mother and the desire to exceed her achievements are often fraught with guilt even when success is not measured in terms of personal career achievement but in other dimensions. Applegarth (1976) describes a syndrome in which daughters fulfill a narcissistic role for the mother. They fulfill the mother's ambitions, and the mother sees them as part of herself. A gifted girl, then, may refuse, consciously or unconciously, to use her gifts, as a means of establishing separateness for herself or for the purposes of rebellion and revenge. This possibility needs to be considered in relation to difficulties and inhibitions that women have in moving ahead in work. This dynamic may complicate what is consciously perceived as a choice, or a lack of one.

People teaching at an advanced level, or working with women who are striving for demanding careers, have also begun to see a reversal in the traditional picture, namely, to see women pressured by parents, including mothers, to move ahead. This may not be motivated by quite the same narcissistic gratification as that of the mothers to whom Applegarth refers. A mother simply may wish that her daughter not miss opportunities that she herself was unable to fulfill, without seeing her as a narcissistic extension of herself. However, this pressure can nevertheless create problems relating to achievement for the daughter. It may be expressed as the reverse of Barnett's example of the mother who cannot understand why a woman might prefer to have an abortion and finish school. The mother sometimes would prefer for the daughter to finish school, while the daughter—for her own reasons, as we have indicated—may choose not to have the abortion.

Many women need approval from others, and their mothers figure importantly in this. However, it is also interesting to observe movement and change take place in the mother, since we are concerned with the spectrum of adult women in midlife. A woman in her mid-20s or in her 30s today may have a mother in her mid-50s. This woman is also in midlife and may have confronted life situations or internal changes that have also made for adaptations of her own.

A clinical example illustrates this.

> Mrs. E was 55 and had had no previous work experience when she went to work in a large firm. First she was a relatively unskilled file clerk, but she eventually became a managing secretary of a whole unit. She described her life over the past 10 years. She had had three daughters, was married to a fairly conventional man who was a skilled worked, and lived in a tightly knit neighborhood where she was very much part of the community of women— a devout churchgoer, a supporter of all school activities, and a dependable friend, mother, and wife. As her daughters grew older, she felt distant from them. She could not understand their preferences in clothes, such as choosing what seemed to her to be unconventional or too seductive or too "loud" kinds of dresses or pants. One of them was allied with a political group that took a stand against racial bais, a stand that was much more overt than the family's position had been. Another had been active in the antiwar protest movement. Then, unexpectedly, Mr. E was killed in a work-related accident. Mrs. E was overwhelmed, felt helpless, lost, bewildered for a time. She relied for a while on the support of her family but then realized that both for her own well-being and for financial reasons she would have to seek paid work. She had few marketable skills, so she went to secretarial school and then into the inner city to take the best of the jobs that were available to her. There she met a whole different group of women. She began to wear pants to work, particularly in the winter. She cut her hair, since she could not take the time for visits to the beauty parlor. She found she had to cut corners in housekeeping, was less interested in some of the homemaking activities she had shared with her friends earlier. In contact with people from very different backgrounds, she found her attitude changing. She said that although she missed her husband a great deal and felt very lonely, the activities that she found she needed most help with were those that involved physical strength. She found new friends and discovered she could do by herself most of the household things for which she had previously relied on her husband.

She had begun to date but really did not feel optimistic about finding some-body that she might marry; she realized she valued some aspects of her independence and freedom. To her amazement, she found that she began to share more of her daughters' attitudes. Her understanding of their positions and beliefs increased, as did the closeness of their relationship. At the same time, her shared activities with her friends diminished of necessity, and although she felt warm toward them, there was less time to do things with them as her own patterns changed.

This is an example of a woman whose own circumstances brought bout both more understanding through a change in life-style that be-ame closer to that of her daughters. (These changes can happen also by ie effects of interactions between people, not only by force of life rcumstances.)

Other mothers, of course, may remain disapproving. For many omen, however, the extent to which they are fearful of their mother's pinions, or the opinions of others close to them, represents their own nflicts about choices and decisions. Their own ambivalence may be rojected outward, so it is the other person who is seen as disapproving, ther than oneself who is in conflict.

A choice may thus involve internal discrepancies and potential con-ct, not only a risk in a new uncharted direction, perhaps with less rotection than in the past. It also contains the potential for confusion id disappointment when one feels one has done the right thing but has t experienced fulfillment. To recognize these internal issues brings eater possibilities for resolution.

A number of women currently come for help because they have ne what seems to be the "right" thing, in contemporary terms, yet do t feel it has worked well enough. They have worked hard, earned omotions, higher degrees, job advancements, positions with consid-able status and sometimes with considerable financial rewards. Nev-theless, they feel some sense of incompleteness or lack of fulfillment.

At times, the conflict has to do with "femininity" and with child-aring. Women who have initially made the decision not to have chil-en fear that they may regret it and may then decide to have children. owever, there may be a different issue, a conflict involving what one s intellectually chosen to do yet feels emotionally is unresolved. For ample, a woman who has internal conflicts about achievement and ccess may not feel comfortable in a successful position. There may be onflict between internalized expectations and current roles, which is rived not only from the way one's mother grew up and the conse-ent expectations but from problems reconciling the costs and benefits their choices. Some of these women are not aware of their internal nflict but develop symptoms, feel depressed, or are puzzled about eir dissatisfaction.

There are complicated determinants of most choices. Sometimes the conscious reason is not entirely consistent with some of the less conscious functions of a choice. For example, one may make a choice toward academic success and fulfillment and find that the process carrie with it the need to be competitive and aggressive. This not only raise issues of femininity, as Barnett indicates, but stirs up conflicts about aggression itself.

There has been a good deal of restriction placed upon girls in both their sexual and aggressive expression (Nadelson, Notman, Miller & Zilbach, 1982). Women may have particular conflicts around aggression that often produce problems with achievement. Men have difficultie concerning aggression that may be expressed in relation to work; however, they can have a somewhat different constellation in that in the rest of men's lives, aggressive expression is not so limited.

A woman's triumph may feel like surpassing and showing up her mother as weak, stupid, and "only a woman." The "unfeminine" aspect of being aggressive and competitive has been mentioned. It touches more on the larger issue of self-esteem, not just femininity.

The concept of *femininity* has been very confused. One may use the term descriptively, normatively, and in a variety of other ways. Barnet finds a woman's own concept of femininity closely connected with her feeling about her reproductive or marital status, and that is indeed often the way women see it. If one considers femininity in relation to self esteem, a woman who does not feel "feminine," in whatever terms she defines it, has a lower opinion of herself than one who does, since feminine is what women are "supposed" to be. Thus, problems ca develop in the discrepancies or contradictions between one's own view of oneself and the ideal. If an individual receives sufficient support for competence and mastery, she is likely to have less concern as to whether or not she is feminine, even if unmarried or not a mother.

For some women, however, a career itself may be defined inevitable as a masculine activity, rather than be assessed in terms of its fulfillment. The extent to which this is true despite conscious decisions to the contrary is sometimes astounding.

A woman premedical student, who had come to an interest in medicine after exploring a variety of other jobs and fields, and therefore felt she was making a mature and reasoned choice, found herself unable complete the last two courses of her premedical requirements. After many starts and failures, she stopped and decided to look more deeply into the conflicts that must be contained in this behavior. She realized that she was consciously committed to the values and choice of a career in medicine, but when she came to the threshold of the commitment thinking of the number of hours involved in the training and in t

ork, she could only see a man doing this and not a woman. Further-
ore, she felt that she could not bring herself to exceed the accomplish-
ents of her mother without paralyzing guilt. Her mother was moder-
tely supportive of her studies, but she herself could not at this point
esolve her ambivalence and accept the support. It took a good deal of
orting out of her past attitudes and expectations from her current ones
efore she could proceed.

Another woman, an accomplished professional, had been for sever-
years in a fairly stable, not very demanding job. She decided that she
as bored by this and would prefer another job that was becoming
vailable, which had as part of its appeal the fact that there was a clear
ossibility of advancement and even a position of some prominence.
he became extremely anxious. When this was explored she said, "It
els like I'm going public with my ambition." This competent woman
ad been able to function well with her apparently successful career
ntil a new situation brought what seemed a more open acknowledg-
ent of a competitive and aggressive aspect that she had not previously
ealt with directly. She was then forced to confront the fact that she
ted as if she felt that ambition was a "bad thing."

To reurn to the question of the definition of femininity as related to
ildbearing, this relationship was assumed for a long period, and as
arnett emphasizes, the potential separation of the two issues needs to
 made. However, the wish for a child is not always accompanied by a
ish for a traditional or a conventional life-style. It is a very complex
ish and involves not only narcissistic aspects, such as perpetuating
eself, but also the wish to care for another human being, or some
entification with one's mother, which need not be a complete identifi-
tion with one's mother's life-style. The woman who decides against
ildbearing or finds herself in a position where she is unlikely to have
ildren must confront a real loss if this has been an important goal for
er. Although it is possible to find fulfillment in other directions, the
ss and its meaning for that individual cannot be ignored.

In the same way, the woman who does not marry may find certain
eedoms, but she may also face loneliness, which makes her vulnerable
 depression. This is not only because of the consequences of choosing
 deviant path. The time limits on reproduction—that is, the limited
me during which women may bear children—are important in the
hole context of women's lives. Anxiety may result if a woman has not
d children, finds herself growing older, and feels the opportunity is
ssing her by.

Women live their reproductive lives in a more time-related frame-
ork than men. Menarche is an abrupt beginning of reproductive po-
ntial, and menopause is a relatively clear-cut ending, even though it

has a less abrupt quality. In addition, the monthly reminder of the menstrual periods constitutes an "inner clock," which many women feel is very much a part of their self-concept. These limitations may heighten awareness and significance of the passage of time, the changes that come with aging, and the limits of what can be accomplished in other directions. Choices about children thus become pressing in a different way from that for men, although many other choices and developmental experiences are unrelated to the reproductive timetable.

A recurrent theme in Barnett's chapter concerns the benefits of freeing oneself from old patterns, unfulfilling relationships, and need for support. The importance of developing the sense of self and of independence is stressed. Although these are indeed very important and differ from traditional goals for women and traditional components of femininity, it would be a mistake then to equate maturity with aloneness or to equate maturity and autonomy with nonrelatedness. Affirmation comes in the context of relationships, whether traditional, therapeutic, or other. Women sometimes need help in restructuring their relationships rather than in leaving them; their strengths also lie in the capacity to adapt, to compromise, to help others to change so that one's own needs as well as other people's needs are more adequately met. Not only independence but assertions and fulfillment within relationships are important and also take some knowledge of what one wants and courage to go after it.

Similar problems exist in sorting out the attitudes of *others* (including parents) toward steps that take a woman into a more unconventional position from one's *own* feelings of regret, loss, or failure—feelings that may be projected onto critical outsiders.

It is particularly crucial in dealing with patients to separate one's own concerns and values from those of the patient. For a therapist, the agenda must be to try to understand the patient's goals rather than to judge the patient's situation in terms of one's goals. A clinical example illustrates this. Mrs. A came for a consultation because of increasing marital difficulties. These were of long standing. She was married to an engineer with a predominantly unresponsive personality with many compulsive defenses. He was, however, reliable and companionable even though his range of affect seemed rather limited. They had two children who were adolescents. She recognized the limitations of her marriage and had gone back to school to a program that would permit her to develop her work in a new direction. She had been in therapy and her therapist, sensing the inadequacy of the marriage, had strongly supported her leaving her husband. Mrs. A felt that she really was not prepared to make that decision. She discovered that the therapist had recently been divorced, and then felt uncomfortable discussing her own ambivalence with this therapist. She wondered whether, because the herapist had found this solution effective for herself, she was proposing strongly for her patient without taking fully into account the patient's own balance of dependency, attachment, and discontent.

This important problem can be expressed in many directions; for example, the therapist may have a bias in favor of marriage, of divorce, of the value of childbearing, or other issues. It is important to maintain as much clarity as possible as to which choices are appropriate for the patient. Certainly, there are fewer automatic answers today; the automatic attempt to establish self-esteem and femininity by marriage and childbearing was very unsuccessful for many women in the past. Perhaps because of the greater availability of careers and the range of choices, women with a particular pattern of problems have been seen recently with greater frequency. Some examples follow.

One woman was a successful lawyer. She came because of dissatisfaction with her work and with her relationship with a young man who was also successfully climbing a career ladder toward success. Her central complaint was that he became irrationally angry, and she then felt demeaned. In the course of therapeutic work, memories emerged in which, during her mother's depression and hospitalization, she had spent time with her father, who in his alcoholic periods would shout at her, and whom she never felt she could reach. The successful career she had embarked upon was meant both to finally win his approval and also to identify with him. Her lover was in part also chosen for his resemblance to her father; her hope was that in quelling his outbursts, she would master the painful experiences of the past. In therapy she was able to sort out past goals and wishes from present possibilities to realize and, to some extent, give up her expectations of her father and her disappointment with her lover. She was able to pursue her work more for its own sake and find gratification in it, and then to choose another man. Disappointment that the career success had not made possible the fulfillment of a childhood wish had initially been experienced as disappointment with the career choice itself. In helping women deal with impediments to productive work and relationships, understanding of these latent meanings and agendas become important.

Another young woman was fairly successful in a business career in a larger organization. She had been the youngest of three children. Her two brothers were considerably older and she always felt that she had been an afterthought. Although admired for her prettiness, she was left alone for long periods of time and was often depressed and lonely as a child. Her parents were socially prominent, her father a successful lawyer. She married and found herself bitterly resenting her father's interest in her husband, a relationship from which she felt excluded. Her mother had had a period during which she too had been depressed, though not to the point of hospitalization, but had been remote, sad, preoccupied. This coincided with the illness of her own parents. The mother's depression took place when this young woman was about 9 or 10; she remembered that there would be long periods of being with her mother while she was uncommunicative and seemed not to notice much about her. She too had worked very hard to achieve and to please. The daughter was bitterly competitive and resentful and eventually separated from her husband, who seemed to offer nothing more than the reflected status and prestige of his success, but little warmth. Although in her mid-30s and functioning fully as an adult, she still was driven to fury by her father's inability or refusal to listen to her seriously.

Although one could go into considerable detail about the individual histories of these women, one part of the pattern seems to stand out. These are women who have had a mother who was either severely or moderately and chronically depressed, and who, whether employed or in a traditional housewife role, was emotionally unavailable to the girl growing up. The father was turned to for support and also identification, and there was a wish for the father's admiration, some closeness to him, or some sense of relatedness and attention. This became incorporated into a life pattern involving effort, achievement, and success, with at least one goal being to finally "make it" in forming the desired relationship.

One important aspect of this constellation is that the disappointment felt by these young women seemed on the surface to be due to the fact that the career for which they had worked so hard and had been successful in was not fulfilling its promise. The central wish they had was not expressed in terms of "femininity" or realizing the traditional role of mother or marriage, but had to do with a long-standing wish to achieve some special relationship to their fathers. We have known through the work of many child developmentalists, particularly in recent years, how important the father is for the development of the self-esteem of the girl and even for her sense of "femininity." In these cases the fathers were especially important by contrast to the depressed and unavailable mothers. The success in the achieving and mastery aspect of these women's careers was considerable and real, as were the gratifications. However, the importance of the unfulfilled part of the wishes went unrecognized until further explored.

This syndrome appears to be occurring more frequently, and raises questions about the effects of a mother's depression on a daughter's directions and identifications. In the cases cited, a choice that seemed to lead to fulfillment still had some components missing. Perhaps a family constellation of a mother who is depressed and a father who is clearly more successful. interesting, available to some degree—although not really making the girl feel valued and supported—may be a spur for her toward achievement. This spur can result in very consider-

ble and genuine accomplishment on the part of the daughter, even if
here is disappointment at not winning her father's approval or close-
ess. This discontent should not be seen as simply due to the problems
f choosing a life-style that might be nontraditional; one must clearly
nderstand the meanings of the relationships and strivings involved.

Another example is worth considering, that of a woman who is a
uccessful physician. As a young girl, she had been shy. Her mother, a
choolteacher, seemed to be able to do anything—to run the family,
ook, be an admired professional, and maintain a marriage. Her father
vas a scientist. She herself was bright in school but avoided all the areas
n which her mother excelled. One day she hesitantly talked with her
nother about her vague future plans. To her surprise, her mother sup-
orted an interest in medicine, saying she herself would have wanted to
o this but had no talent for science. Her mother's admission of a weak-
ess and, at the same time, her support seemed amazing to the girl. She
elt less intimidated, explored the possibilities, and eventually went to
nedical school. At another point of indecision she sought counseling.
he female therapist also felt it was an appropriate and possible goal, an
nportant factor in her decision. Later, when she was in her 30s and
vorrying whether there was still time for childbearing, her mother said
n a visit to her city, "Why not?" Eventually, not only did she become a
nother but her career tended in an academic direction and she too
ecame a teacher, completing an identification with her mother that had
n some ways previously been conflicted because of her perception of
er mother's greater strength, and her own competitiveness and ambi-
on.

We may expect mothers to play an increasingly positive role in the
ves, accomplishments, and well-being of their daughters, and thera-
ists' attention to patterns of needs, fulfillments, and relationships of
omen certainly must occur in the context of full awareness of new life
atterns, new solutions, and new options. These may help us find ways
o support the strengthening of women's self-esteem without relying on
utmoded views of appropriate behavior or "femininity."

EFERENCES

pplegarth, A. Some observations on work inhibitions in women. *Journal of the American Psychoanalytic Association*, 1976, *24*, 251–268.
rnard, J. *Perspectives on marriage*. Paper presented at the Radcliffe College Precentennial Conference on Perspectives on the Patterns of an Era, 1978.
adelson, C., Notman, M., Miller, J., and Zilbach, J. Aggression in women: Conceptual issues and clinical implications. In M. Notman and C. Nadelson (Eds.), *The woman patient* (Vol. 3). New York: Plenum Press, 1982.
ott, J. The mechanization of women's work. *Scientific American*, 1982, *247*, 167–187.

exuality and the Middle-Aged Voman

ELLA LURIA AND ROBERT G. MEADE

ENOPAUSE: THE WRONG QUESTION

overnment-funded research on sexual behavior is usually about one of o groups: adolescents or those over age 60. For the former group, the al is to stop, or regulate, the behavior; for the older group, the aim is document the potential lifelong availability of a God-given sexual gift, iven by the rule "Use it or lose it." As the proportion of older citizens the population increases, their political clout sparks research on the nditions that maintain sexual behavior after age 60. Lost in the push e aged) and pull (back the young) are the middle-aged, those roughly -60 years old.

Middle age, like other life stages, is not pure biology. Its onset and ration depend on self-image, life events, presumed life-span, and the eraction among these factors. Our notion of the life cycle may be tically related to particular milestones and to our reference groups. nder, class, education, and occupation undoubtedly influence our ws of middle age and life's course. Female sexuality is intimately ated to a woman's life-cycle concepts.

Insistence on reproductive capacity as the key to women's sexuality s in the face of available evidence. In Neugarten's study (1963) of 100 men aged 43–53, only one-sixth of the women thought that sexual ations became less important with menopause; the rest rated sex the ne as before menopause, or even better now that pregnancy was

LA LURIA AND ROBERT G. MEADE • Psychology Department, Tufts University, Med-l, Massachusetts 02155

impossible. There were no personality differences among premenopau
sal, menopausal, and postmenopausal women. In fact, only 4% of th
women saw menopause as a principal concern. These middle-age
women feared losing their husbands, getting older, and cancer—nc
menopause. A volunteer "opportunity" sample of 484 women of mixe
ages had similar results: no significant grief accompanying the passin
of menses and reproduction (Boston Women's Health Book Collective
1976). Rossi (1980) suggests that menopause is a private event bu
postmenopausal signs are public: "grey hair, wrinkles, dentures, drow
siness, age spots, thickening of the waistline, sagging of abdomen an
breasts, and biofocal glasses."

Recent changes in women's sexual behavior belie the notion tha
female sexuality exists only as an adjunct to romantic love, yet we kno
remarkably little about the meanings of specific sexual acts in women
lives. The almost total absence of such information in our culture
unlikely to continue, however. Anthropological studies of other culture
are already providing us with knowledge that we lack about our ow
society (Ortner and Whitehead, 1981). What we do know about wom
en's experience of being sexual in midlife depends on the women's ag
cohort, their marital status, and the measure of being sexual.

Middle-Aged Women in Kinsey's Time

Information about what middle-aged women's sex lives were like
the relatively recent past comes from the Kinsey, Pomeroy, Martin, ar
Gebhard volume on women (1953). Those data are based on small ar
selected samples. Middle-aged women are reluctant to talk about the
sexual experiences; in Kinsey's day, they were even more so. Howeve
without this basis for comparison with the past, current data on tl
middle-aged woman's sex life fall into a vacuum.

Kinsey's sample of middle-aged women came from the birth c
horts of 1880 to 1910. Those cohorts are not entirely homogeneous wi
respect to sexual histories. Women born after 1900 were likely to ha
had more premarital intercourse and more petting to orgasm than d
the earlier cohorts. The liberal sexuality of the post-World War I won
had a much greater impact on women born after 1900 than it did
those born before the turn of the century. In spite of these difference
some clear-cut findings emerged from the data of these mixed cohor

Married women had more frequent intercourse as well as oth
forms of sexual "outlets" (Kinsey's term) than women of the same a
who were not married. Unmarried middle-aged women showed lc
levels of all forms of sexual activity, but no lower than younger unma
ried women!

Among women who were born before 1900 and had never married ged 50–69), one-third never had any overt sexual activity beyond sim- e petting; they experienced little sexual arousal during petting, and no gasm ever. The other two-thirds of these never-married women had ore sexual experience; 62% of them had had intercourse, 16% had had tensive homosexual relations. The rest had engaged in other forms of xual behavior (Christenson and Johnson, 1973). While these relatively rren sexual histories may seem ascetic to modern readers, these wom- were not so unusual in their day. Theirs was a culture in which there ere substantial numbers of unmarried women. Sex went with marriage was an exchange made just before marriage. Most women had one xual partner in their lives—their husband. Given that framework, the terosexually active and the homosexually active groups are extremely teresting.

Overall, availability of a partner predicted how much sex a woman d. But even stably married women reported age-related changes in eir sex lives. As a group, married women over 40 experienced a steady op in incidence (do you ever . . . ?) of intercourse (Pfeiffer and Davis, 72). Current knowledge bears out Kinsey's intuition about the cause the decline; often, erectile difficulties lead husbands to discontinue xual intercourse.

How often a middle-aged married woman experienced intercourse is related to her age and to her husband's age, too. But age and rtner availability are not the only factors leading to declines in married xual behavior. A striking decline in sexual activity occurs among ung married pairs. A large urban sample of recently married young men, all under 30, showed a decline of about 25% in frequency of ual intercourse as early as the first 4 years of marriage (Udry, 1980). ese are especially important findings because they are based on longi- dinal data, which are in short supply in the sexual behavior literature. ven that declines in sexual behavior can be found in both the middle- d and the young, we must attend to the multiple sources other than that feed into coital decision-making by couples.

Kinsey viewed the decline in frequency of intercourse as due to les. He saw the age-related testosterone decrement in men as the logical basis for the lower levels of sexual behavior seen with increas- age. The behavioral decline is doubtlessly real; it occurs in study er study (Kinsey, Pomeroy, and Martin, 1948; Kinsey et al., 1953; ry, 1980; Westoff, 1974). Age-related declines in both circulating tes- terone levels and sexual behavior are characteristic of the male in all mmalian species studied. However, low hormone levels do not ac- nt in any simpleminded way for all of the behavioral decrements, at st in the human male, since the decrease in behavior antedates the

hormonal decline. Hormone–behavior relationships are typically de
scribed with arrows (of causality) going from hormone to behavior. Ye
evidence supports the arrow going in the other direction, too. Testoster
one in men goes up following sexual behavior, at least in some studie
(e.g., Kraemer, Becker, Brodie, Doering, Moos, and Hamburg, 1976)
Our hunch is that habituation in marriage and competing family ir
terests (especially children) help to lower the rate of sexual turn-on
(accounting for the early drop in marital coital frequencies). Diminishe
sexual behavior and slowly decreasing hormone levels conspire to fur
ther lower levels of sexual behavior in men. Testosterone levels in won
en are about 10% of those in men, and they do not decline with age. Th
role that testosterone plays in female libido is unknown. Recent work i
stumptail macaque monkeys indicates that, at least in this species, se
steroids are not required for the maintenance of sexual attractivenes
receptivity, or proceptivity by females (Baum, Koos Slob, de Jong, an
Westbrook, 1978).

About half of a small sample of middle-aged men and women,
Kinsey-study vintage, report a decrease in sexual interest and activity
age 45. By 55, 75–80% of the sample report declines. More women tha
men are aware of declines in sexual interest (Pfeiffer, Verwoerdt, ar
Davis, 1972).

For middle-aged women from the birth cohort 1900–1925, marit
status alone predicted sexual enjoyment, sexual frequency, and sexu
interest. Health, subjective or objective, was the predictor for men. B
health did not account for the variance among women. A partner mea
stability and the sanction of the law to these women (Pfeiffer and Dav
1972). Is all this work a belabored discovery of the double standar
Studies of women aged 40–60 in the 1980s would reflect an ailing, but
no means dead, double standard. Again, one searches for the meanin
of women's sexual acts.

WHAT CAUSES THE AGE-RELATED DECLINE IN SEXUAL BEHAVIOR?

For every married man who decided that his active sex life was ov
because of erectile problems, at least one woman has shared the co
Recent research leads to the counsel to men that erectile dysfunction
less likely and appears later when men eat well and exercise to contr
high blood pressure and to maintain weight. Lots of early sexual practi
also serves to forestall the onset of erectile difficulties (Martin, 197
Given the dependence of the sacral-mediated erectile reflex on the va
cular and peripheral neural systems, the current generation of regu
joggers and exercise devotees may well be the group to watch in th
middle and Medicare years. Pfeiffer and Davis's correlation of m

ood health and frequency of marital coitus fits well with Martin's find-
gs. The sexual rule for men is: Stay well. For women, it is: Stay mar-
ed. For both, the implicit rule is: Stay sexually active.

The search for the causes of the decline in marital sex with age
iterests endocrinologists, survey researchers, and developmental psy-
hologists alike. Kinsey found that wives typically reported higher fre-
uencies of intercourse than husbands. He reasoned that the actual
equencies seemed higher to wives because they were having more sex
ian they wanted. He thought that husbands were apt to underestimate
ie frequency of intercourse because they would have preferred a higher
ite. Thirty years later, Hunt's (1974) admittedly selective sample sug-
ests that husband–wife views on what constitutes "enough" have
:ached parity.

Using large-scale survey data on samples aged 44 and younger,
'dry and Morris (1978) examined the relative contributions of males'
nd females' ages to the decline in the frequency of marital coitus. They
llculated the mean decline in monthly coital frequency across succes-
ve 5-year age intervals. By holding the age of one spouse constant,
iey were able to examine the contribution of the age of the other spouse
) the decline. That portion of the decline attributable to male age is
naller in each successive sample. The contribution of female age to the
lean decline shows a complementary increase, starting low in 1965,
icking up substantially in 1970, and again in 1974. This finding should
ot be interpreted as indicating that wives today are depressing the
uantity of marital coitus more than they did in Kinsey's time. Today's
oung marrieds are having intercourse more often than did their coun-
·rparts in previous generations. Udry and Morris's data most likely
:flect the increased role played by wives' sexual appetites or wishes in
)ital decisionmaking. Such coital decisions by women can be based on
onsexual reasons.

Degler (1980) provides an exciting array of reasons for the sexual
ioices of 19th-century women. The reasons given do not add up to a
mple lack of sexual interest by women. There is independent evidence
om medical books and from purity-movement documents that sexual
:lations were important to women. But it was to be a qualitatively
ifferent relationship: gentler, more slowly paced, affectional, and less
equent.

Degler's summary suggests that 19th-century women were using
:x to change power relations in the Victorian family, to prevent recur-
·nt pregnancies, and to provide sufficient postpartum abstention so
iat women could nurse children through the dangers of early child-
ood. Demographic statistics from the late 19th century suggest that
iese women succeeded in their nonsexual motives by sexual means. Of

course, some men helped them, convinced by the arguments of th
various purity movements and of their wives.

A Drop in Female Libido

On the basis of a sample of about 900 adults, aged 18 to 60, Eysenc
(1976) reported that "the libido of older subjects [is] weaker than that c
younger subjects." His measure of sexual libido is based on scores from
50 self-report scales that examine the degree of pleasure derived from
sexual thought and action, as well as attitudes toward many sexua
issues (i.e., polygamy, masturbation, prostitution). Eysenck (1976
holds that genetic/hormonal contributions drive the reported libido c
males. Data on females appear to fit a cultural-pressures model instead
All told, however, the sources of female libido are yet to be convincingl
specified.

Do Gay Women Show Age-Related Decline?

The primary source of information about social sexual behavior :
data describing heterosexual acts. Thus, conclusions drawn about th
behavior of one sex are, of necessity, confounded by the contribution o
the other sex. Heterosexual acts bring together people who differ no
only in genital morphology and brain/hormone organization but also i
cultural socialization. What happens to sexual behavior with age whe
the sexual pair have not been socialized in different directions? Ga
people have no other-sex partner who can account for age-relate
changes in sexuality. The largest study of gay men and women finc
that sexual interest is not age-related for gay men, but that it is for ga
white women (Bell and Weinberg, 1978). ("Interest" is based on tw
interview items concerning thinking about sex and the importance of se
to the respondent.) In fact, across all ages, gay white men report signif
cantly higher sexual interest than do gay white women. This sex di
ference is also reflected in behavior patterns, with gay white male
showing higher frequencies of sexual interactions than their gay fema
counterparts. Both gay men and gay women show declines in the fr
quencies of actual sexual encounters with age, however.

The difficulty in making any general predictions about female sexu
ality from the data on gay women is that gay women are far fro
homogeneous. Black gay women do not report lower sexual intere
than do black gay men, nor do they show any age-related decline :
sexual interest. They are not like their white gay counterparts in th
respect. In addition, while black gay males show overall higher freque
cies of sexual behavior than their white counterparts, this racial patte

oes not exist among gay women. Results like this explain (but do not
istify) why many researchers preferred single-sex studies.

olor and Sexual Subculture

Black and white cultures differ markedly in their acceptance of
·male sexuality (see Angelou, 1981, pp. 66–67). As white cultural pro-
:riptions against female sexuality are relaxed, we may see patterns of
·xual behavior among white women moving toward those associated
·ith the behavior of black populations. Some shifts in sexual behavior
·nong young women suggest that this may be so, i.e., earlier age at first
·ital experience, greater acceptance of premarital sex.

EEKING OUT SEX: KINSEY TO ERICA JONG

What determined the likelihood of a middle-aged woman of Kinsey-
·imple vintage seeking out sexual relations? A woman's past orgasmic
·xperience makes seeking further sexual opportunities more likely when
·ie is postmarried (Christenson and Gagnon, 1965). This accords with
·ore recent findings that, in married women, past sexual enjoyment
·as significantly correlated with sexual functioning in middle age
·feiffer and Davis, 1972). Past enjoyment alone predicts sexual func-
·ning in middle age for women; for men, past sexual frequency, enjoy-
·ent, and interest predict sexual functioning in middle age. Sexual ac-
·vity, once encountered and enjoyed by women (and men too), tends to
·ntinue. Good sex begets good sex later.

Even though they lacked easy access to sexual partners after their
·arriages ended, 37% of the postmarried women in the Christenson
·id Gagnon study reported having intercourse at age 50. At 55, 29%
·ere doing so, and at 60, 12% were. By 65 and older, none reported
·itus. At 55, the frequencies of intercourse were only two-thirds that of
·arried women their age, but double that of sexually active never-mar-
·ed women (Christenson and Johnson, 1973). Given the birth cohort of
·iese postmarried women, these results are striking evidence of the
·iddle-aged woman's capacity to seek out and maintain sexual relations
·ice she has already had steady sexual experience with a marital part-
·r. But they also emphasize the fact that marital status goes with the
·ghest incidences and frequencies of sexual intercourse. The married
·ed negotiate less than any other subgroup in order to have sex. And
·eir partners are built in.

Gebhard (1971) extended and refined the data cited above by inter-
·ewing divorced and widowed women in the sample. Interviews of 632
·hite women led him to conclude that, even with ages matched, di-

vorced women are almost twice as likely as widowed women to have postmarital coitus (82% vs. 43%). Beyond age 50, this difference in sexual activity diminishes. At that point, a woman's age was a more salient factor in her sexual behavior than was the cause of the end of her marriage. Obviously, the way a marriage ends provides different sexual contexts for the divorced woman and for the widow. Although both situations surely involve loss, cultural stereotypes have the divorcee freely moving into an easygoing postmarried life-style, while the widow bravely shoulders her grief. How a marriage functioned affects its aftermath too: 8% of the widows had had extramarital relations during the marriage, while a third of the divorced women had had the experience often during the last year of the marriage, the year of *de facto* divorce. Fewer widows than divorced women remarried—27% and 47%, respectively. Among many factors, the grief and the continuing attachment of the widow to her dead spouse delay her reentry into sexual relations.

Nonetheless, even in the Kinsey cohort, most women who are sexually active postmaritally (whether widowed or divorced) have more than one sexual partner. Once a woman reenters the sexual scene, she has acknowledged her motivation for sex—and, probably, marriage—and it is unlikely that her first partner will fulfill all her expectations. For most postmarried women, the sexual marketplace is much different from what it was in their premarital days. Entry into that new marketplace involves learning new gender-role values and new negotiation skills (Hunt, 1966). Having acquired these new skills, the postmarital woman who has one sexual partner is more likely to move on to another.

To what extent do postmarital women use masturbation as a compensation for decreased sexual intercourse? It would seem to be as close a physiological substitute as possible. Kinsey surely conceived of masturbation as an "outlet" of just that sort. Masters and Johnson (1966) provide data that support masturbation as being more orgasmically efficient than coitus. When postmarried women are age-matched with married women, a markedly higher incidence of masturbation occurs among the former—almost double at age 50, 1 ½ times greater at 55 (Christenson and Johnson, 1973). All the masturbation episodes of the postmarried women do not add up to the frequencies of coitus plus masturbation of their married counterparts of like age.

Reading these studies, one is impelled to ask what masturbation stands for in relation to coitus among women. We wonder if a woman researcher would have conceived of sexual behaviors as "outlets," with masturbation and coitus as simple variants of sexual expression. The concept carries with it the image of a well of undifferentiated sexual energy waiting to be discharged—a concept not unfamiliar to Freudian theory. It is dubious whether women experience their sexual needs of vishes in this way. In truth, Kinsey, and Freud too, were well aware of the psychological differences in the experiences of masturbation and coitus. The difference between the two experiences seems to us to be potentially greater among women than among men because of gender-role differences. Coitus is a relational act and masturbation is not (except in fantasy). The female gender scripts embeds sexual acts in personal, emotional relationships. The "zipless fuck" violates that script; it titil-ates, but is finally doomed by its woman author (Jong, 1973).

SEXUAL MOTIVATION, AROUSAL, AND GENDER SCRIPTS

Current efforts to legitimize female masturbation contribute to the sexual development of women who often lack feelings of sexual entitle-ment (Barbach, 1975). The relational context of sex in the female gender script leads to a predominantly incentive theory view of female sexu-ality. An available social sexual object helps to produce sexual drive. Such sexuality is not driven by deprivation (as much of male sex drive in thought to be) (Luria and Rose, 1979). Incentive theory does not fit the masturbation data on women, however. Again, we need to know more about what masturbation means to women.

Arousal Is Simpler for Males

There may be some biological reasons that make more probable the separation of sexual arousal from relational issues in males than in females. The penis is a well-engineered biofeedback device. In addition to providing pubescent males with information about where their minds/genitals are, it permits the ready labeling of discrete objects and events as sexual turn-ons. Obviously, females have the potential for such biofeedback of their arousal state, but it is more subtle and requires more learning. Unlike the male, the female requires prior sexual experi-ence to identify arousal. Geer and Morokoff (1974) find clear physiologi-cal evidence of vaginal vasocongestion in women shown arousing stim-uli. But the sexually inexperienced women in the sample do not report arousal; the sexually experienced women do. Even among orgasmic, sexually experienced women, the correlation between subjective arousal and the most reliable physiological indicator of arousal (vaginal color change due to vasocongestion) is lower and less sure than it is for men (Steinman, Wincze, Sakheim, Barlow, and Maussakalian, 1981). Nature has arranged the penis to be visible and handy. While both males and females learn the culturally defined classes of events and persons to whom one may respond sexually, females must also learn to discrimi-nate subtle changes in their own state of sexual arousal. Pubertal in-

creases in testosterone in males assure many visible erections, henc
many opportunities to learn sequences of behavior that lead to pleasur
able outcomes. Males who do not discover ejaculation through con
scious effort are initiated by nocturnal emissions. No equivalent exist
for the pubescent female's orgasm. Female nocturnal orgasm, if it i
experienced, tends to occur later in life, among the sexually experi
enced.

Penetration Makes a Difference

Sexual intercourse is an act that violates female body space, lik
violent acts. Acts that pierce body space—i.e., force feeding, prizefigh
ing, inoculations—are typically regulated by authorities. While societie
regulate sexual acts in all cultures, females must also monitor any poter
tially violent acts against them. This issue will occur only in societie
where females are victims of such violent acts, especially forcible rape
The sorting out of violence and sex requires some knowledge of th
space violator. Our surmise would be that this alone would assure wom
en's concern with relationships. Even nonhuman females do not mat
randomly. Obviously, one could construct a world that would severel
mute the sex difference in awareness of arousal and concern with rela
tionships. With respect to the latter, there is some evidence of mergin
of the two gender scripts—with males moving closer to the femal
script—among the educated young (Finger, 1975). It is conceivable tha
in a world with no double standard, women would have more oppo
tunities to learn about sexual arousal, especially through the removal c
mislabelings and misattributions of female arousal (Barbach, 1975). Bu
there is no Rousseau-esque world where male and female sexuality ar
the same in the "natural" state. Even in cultures where sexual pleasu
is equally expected (and realized) by males and females, teaching abou
how to make love is tailored to each sex separately (Marshall, 1971).

UPDATING KINSEY: THE 1970s AND EARLY 1980s

Kinsey's pioneering work made it easier for researchers followir
him to study sexual behavior. However, current studies have a narrow
focus than did Kinsey's work. Nowhere do we find a recent study wit
the same breadth of population sampled and behaviors surveyed. Ve
few studies permit the luxury of Kinsey's comparisons across birth c
horts. Kinsey's work virtually ended the era of studies with very lor
data-collection periods and with mounds of data on each individu
studied. Funding agency policies assured the demise of such high-ri
enterprises. Instead, we have more sharply-focused studies with small

amples and fewer measures. The group least likely to be studied is the middle-aged.

The studies described so far are based on earlier cohorts than those that furnish our current popular view of middle age. Alice Rossi (1980) has described the special conditions encountered by the cohort born during the years 1920–1932: a lowered birthrate during the late 1920s, which made for a small birth cohort; the experience of the Great Depression in adolescence or younger; participation in World War II and/or the Korean War; the postwar economic boom, complete with significant and stable financial rewards (especially in comparison with those of their parents).

Rossi describes life for many women of this cohort: the pioneering and isolating settlement of suburbia, large families, and rising incomes. These families were members of that "lucky generation who came closer than any other to the ideal of American domesticity: a nice suburban home; a breadwinner husband and a homemaker wife; dedication to childrearing; and status gained from a high level of consumption of housing, automobiles, appliances and other consumer goods" (Masnick and Bane, 1980, pp. 1–2). Ironically, the net outcome of this is a squeeze in income when three, four, or five children reach adolescence and college age. In many cases, family income cannot keep pace with education costs and felt consumer needs.

The gap between expenses and income has largely been filled by middle-aged, married women's entry into paid work. The working mother changed family life-styles as much as, if not more than, the escape to the suburbs. It has also had the effect of making work of special importance to the sense of self-worth of many middle-aged women (Baruch and Barnett, 1981). Middle age is their time for themselves.

More Sex and More Variety

Because the Playboy Foundation wanted an early 1970s study to compare with Kinsey's two volumes, Hunt (1974) included middle-aged respondents in his "replication." While his sample is flawed, it is valuable because it surveys many sexual behaviors and it includes people's feelings. When median weekly frequency of marital intercourse was studied, Hunt found increases for every age category compared to Kinsey's. Thus, middle-aged married couples in the 1970s were having more sex together than earlier cohorts at a similar time in their lives.

Since the extent of sexual functioning in middle age is highly dependent on early experience and enjoyment of sex, the trend toward more marital sex is hardly surprising. Remember, the middle-aged generation of Hunt's study was the young generation studied by Kinsey *et al.* Kinsey found consistent differences between the younger and older subsets of the female sample, always with greater sexual freedom among the young. (That is still true in every Western country studied today.) Fully 20% more of Kinsey's young married women were having orgasms than were their older counterparts. The young experienced more nudity, variation in coital positions, and variety in foreplay. Younger married women were more likely than older married women to experience stimulation from oral–genital, manual–genital, and mouth–breast contacts.

Given this increase in the variety of coital techniques and types of foreplay used, it requires no great leap of imagination to infer that marital sex among the more recent birth cohort was generally more pleasurable and hence would be practiced more often. Inferences about the relative contributions of the husbands and the wives to the increase in frequency are somewhat more speculative. In comparing the Kinsey data with his own, Hunt consistently found that, in both sexual attitudes and behavior, the magnitude of liberalization was greater for females than for males. (Females were farther away than males from ceiling on most measures. Thus, they had more room for increases.) Hunt argues that the social emancipation of women of this generation removed many cultural inhibitions surrounding sexuality. This, in turn, led to a general increase in wives' desire for marital coitus.

Hunt assumes that part of the new freedom for women is the freedom to tell their partners their sexual wishes. Lest the reader be reassured that modern women readily communicate their sexual wishes to their partners, Hite (1976) notes that two out of three women in a feminist sample find it difficult indeed. This is not so when a male communicates to a female (Pietropinto and Simenauer, 1977). Pietropinto and Simenauer found that although men insist that they want their lovers to communicate their sexual desires, women believe that men don't want to know their wishes.

While we have no data that directly support the assertion that it is wives who are responsible for the general increase in the frequency of marital coitus, a recent study seems to support that conclusion. Large-scale National Fertility Surveys of married couples showed, at all ages, an increase in average 4-week coital frequency in 1970 as compared to 1965—up 2.46 for women under 25, up 2.06 for women 25–34, and up .43 for women 35–44 (Westoff, 1974). The rate of increase is lower for the older than for the younger women, but at all ages Westoff found increased frequencies. This sexualization of all ages is considered a major sociological event. Some investigators are dubious that the trend will continue (Udry and Morris, 1978), but that the sexualizing events have occurred is universally acknowledged. Westoff (1974) saw some of the trend as due to a subset of educated women with "modern" gender views. Later work changed his mind (see p. 389).

The influence of marital status on middle-aged sexuality is less clear-cut for the post-World War I birth cohort than for the previous one. Its limitations notwithstanding, the Kinsey study did provide comparable information on married, postmarried, and never-married men and women in convenient 5-year age intervals across the adult life-span. No directly comparable data exist for the more recent cohort. The only current information we have on sexual behavior among postmarried women is that of Hunt. His survey of postmarrieds is limited to the divorced and never-married; unfortunately, the samples are too small to permit reasonable analysis by age. For the purpose of cross-cohort comparisons, the closest match to Hunt's data on divorced women is the divorced subset of the Gebhard sample, a comparison across 30 years. These women were all under age 55 at the time of the interview. Hunt found that 90% of the divorced women in his sample were coitally active, compared to Gebhard's 70%. Among the coitally active women in the Hunt study, the median weekly frequency of coitus is twice per week as compared to Gebhard's report of a mean frequency of slightly over once per week. Women in both studies reported high rates of orgasm and satisfaction with postmarital coitus. A majority of divorced women in the Gebhard sample reported that they had more orgasms in postmarital than in marital sex. While Hunt provides no directly comparable data, his sample reported that their postmarital sex was generally more liberated than their marital sex had been, and over 90% of the women rated postmarital coitus as very or mostly pleasurable. But we can't be sure that the samples are comparable across the 30 years.

Hunt supplies no information about never-married middle-aged women; in fact, only 5% of the 1970s population of women had never married. Hunt's never-married are all under age 35. The only current information that we have on middle-aged single women comes from a recent study of 60 women, aged 35 to 65 years (Lowenstein, Block, Campion, Epstein, Gale, and Salvatore, 1981). The criterion for being single in this "snowball" sample was that the women defined themselves as single, rather than viewing lack of a partner as transitional. In actual fact, only 38 of the women had never married; the balance were widowed, divorced, or separated. None of these women had children under 18 living at home. The sample overrepresented highly educated and professional women. Of the 38 never-married women, 1 provided no data concerning sexuality, and 22 (60%) reported that they had never engaged in coitus. The frequency of coital (or other) activity among the remaining 15 women is not reported. For the group as a whole, current sexual gratification bore no relation to life satisfaction. (This finding is replicated in a *Consumer Reports* study, cited just below.) Approximately half of Lowenstein's women expressed no sexual needs. The provocative contents of this study make one wish to know more. What about masturbation? Is sex really a take-it-or-leave-it matter for women without stable male partners? Are sexual partners important only when women have them?

In a recent, as yet unpublished, survey of 1845 middle- and upper-class women readers over age 50, the magazine *Consumer Reports* finds 91%% of the women expressing some degree of interest in sex and 84% coitally active. In a sample in which almost one-third of the women are never-married, widowed, or divorced, 84% represents a high incidence of sexual activity. Selective sampling may increase the figures for sexual interest somewhat since the sample is solidly middle class and highly educated (Corby and Brecher, 1984). Nonetheless, it is of interest that any class of women over 50 is found with such high coital incidences, given the rest of the literature. On the other hand, incidence figures always follow the rule "A swallow makes a spring." It takes only one coital act to be counted among the coitally active. The story of the coital decline with age shows up first in frequency statistics and is subsequently corroborated by lowered incidence figures.

Masturbation

Current data describing masturbatory patterns among middle-aged women are nonexistent. Hite's book (1976) is not organized so that one can extract reliable data by age. Hunt reports that, by their late 20s and early 30s, over 80% of single women and 70% of married women are masturbating. No one has ever shown that females stop masturbating once they have begun, Freud's "On the Anatomical Distinction between the Sexes" notwithstanding. Even if one assumes that Hunt's figures are inflated by his selected sample, these figures suggest an increase in the incidence of masturbation among women since the time of Kinsey when one-half of single and one-third of married women reported that they masturbated. Women have found their genitals, even though culture and morphology made it somewhat difficult for them to do so.

Wholesale modifications of sexuality during middle age are relatively rare, even during the recent sexualization of our society. For most people, their sexual self-concept ripens during the earlier, more formative periods of preadolescence, adolescence, and young adulthood. Pfeiffer and Davis cite the high correlation between levels of sexual functioning in young adulthood and in middle age. Important factors characterizing one's personality tend to display relatively consistent pat erns throughout adult life. Pfeiffer and Davis call this "continuity of life-style." Most of the middle-aged women that Hunt interviewed reported that while the "sexual revolution" of the 1960s had liberalized their attitudes, their marital sexual patterns were too well established to undergo much change. Some expressed regret. Middle-aged women differ from young women not only in biology but also in the different scripts they learned for sexual experience and initiation. Among divorced women (middle-aged and younger) some reschooling in the new sexuality occurs. Many of the middle-aged women in the Rubin (1979) study reported that their marital sex had improved over time, but some bemoaned their inability to be sexually liberated like the younger generation—"too many years of repression and too many lessions learned too well."

The Baby Boom in Middle Age

Any extrapolation from the Kinsey data to the middle age of the women born from 1945 to 1960 (the baby boom) would be an error. The Kinsey sample was a mixture of cohorts, viewed by Kinsey as pre- and post-1900 births. Kinsey documented the sexual revolution that came with the adolescents of the post-World War I world, those born 1900 and after. One part of that post-World War I birth cohort is the 1920–1932 group described by Rossi. That post-1920 birth cohort produced the children who are the upcoming middle-aged of 1985 and thereafter. The post-World War II cohort, called the baby boom, grew up with economic prosperity, many jobs, high consumption, extended education, widespread travel, and high occupational aspirations. They hit their 20s at the time of shifting cultural views of the double standard, premarital sex, and oral sex.

While the 1960s represent the period of shifting sexual views, the 1970s represent the period of changed sexual behavior (Reiss, 1972). Although some women still marry as virgins, the norm has shifted toward "premarital intercourse with love." In many Western countries (France, Germany, United States), the sexual experience that women once acquired first in marriage is now far more likely to be gained premaritally. The changes include (a) relatively speedy climbing of the scaled steps from the French kiss to intercourse, (b) becoming reliably orgasmic in oral sex and/or intercourse before marriage, (c) greater acceptance of initiation of sexual invitations by women, (d) greater availability and use of reliable contraception by women, (e) greater probability of having more than one premarital sexual partner, (f) having premarital sex in stable relationships more frequently, hence having more sexual practice premaritally.

Predicting the Sexual Future

All of these factors lead to the prediction that, on average, women of the baby boom cohort are going to have more sex and more orgasms than their grandmothers did. Since the predictors of continued incidence of sex and frequency of sex are previous experience and enjoyment of sex, the baby boom cohort should be a relatively sexually active group in middle age. Permissive and abundant sex in a woman's teens and 20s should predict more sex later.

What happens when one goes beyond the correlational data just cited and asks: What are the concurrent social factors most likely to influence the sexuality of the next generation of middle-aged women? We see three main factors exerting a change: greater social acceptance of women as sexual beings throughout life; the growing absence of stable male sexual partners for many women, due to high rates of divorce and the shorter life expectancy of males than females; and women's changing role in the paid work force. Predicting how these factors will affect the sexuality of middle-aged women is a matter of data and conjecture.

We would expect that the middle-aged woman will be seen as asexual far less often than she is today. Better health and longer life-spans should help to convince older people that sexuality is a life-span process. But middle age, with its skewed sex ratio, means that more women than men will be without stable sex partners. Current data on young women suggest that there will continue to be lesser salience of genital sex for women in comparison with relational aspects of sex. This lesser salience in a context of significant proportions of male-absent, late-middle-age households will probably continue to depress the social sexual activity of women for reasons that will be as valid in the future as they were in the past: the absence of a stable sexual partner with whom a woman has a relationship.

As the base rate for early female masturbation goes up (as it has), a safe prediction is that tomorrow's divorced, widowed, or never-married middle-aged women will enjoy solitary sex more often than did her older sister or mother in like circumstances. It is unlikely to be a simple substitution for social sex. Short- or long-term sexual relationships outside of legal marriages are already on the increase—a trend likely to continue. Our society has begun to accept the Scandinavian model of cohabitation as an aspect of courtship. The Swedes came to that model from a rural history where cohabitation tested a woman's fertility: we have come to the model as a test of interpersonal/sexual compatibility. Such a test is as important for the middle-aged woman as it is for her younger counterpart.

Extramarital sex will frequently be in the context of transition out of marriage into new sexual and/or marital arrangements. Demographers see the future life-span being divided into more married and unmarried sequences than has been customary heretofore. Social sexual sequences will probably show the same on/off timing, with social sex on for a period of time, then off.

Among middle-aged women of the recent past, an extramarital affair was predicted by marital unhappiness. This isn't as true for women now beginning to push middle age; they are somewhat more likely to be seeking variety. These are younger women with more premarital sexual experience than middle-aged women of the past had. Their appestats, experience, sexual values, and knowledge of scripts for sexual solicitation may be higher.

INFLUENCE OF LABOR FORCE PARTICIPATION ON SEXUALITY

How will being in the paid labor force affect women's sexual lives? Masnick and Bane (1981) describe three revolutions—already realized or potential—in women's work patterns. The first, a dramatic increase in participation in the paid labor force by women, especially married women, has already occurred. The second revolution, in the nature of women's attachment to the labor force, is just under way. The shift is toward full-time, permanent attachment to the labor force. Government projections show about 80% of the women aged 35 and over remaining stably in the labor force by 1990. Part, but not all, of the steady attachment to the labor force is caused by increasing numbers of women with college education. As women invest more in preparing for careers, they are less willing to stay out of the labor force. Married women who are permanently and full time in the labor market differ from both women who do not work and women who work part time or sporadically. Women and their families who come to expect wives' earnings regularly and predictably are likely to change in economic and noneconomic ways: Wives' incomes will be required in the family budget; the amount of time devoted to responsibilities related to home and family is likely to change; pressure not to bear children is likely to be higher than we have seen in the post-World War II period; and where children are born, they are likely to be few and to be born when mothers are older. As we write, Massachusetts has reported a record high proportion of first births to women over 30. The strategy of entering the labor market after an early birth typically founders when the husband's higher earning ability sets up the traditional role pattern, ending with a wife at home, rather than in the labor market (LaRassa and LaRassa, 1981).

Masnick and Bane (1981) surmise that a quiet third revolution may be starting because of women's increasing relative contribution to family

income. Working women under 24 in two-worker families are providing
a somewhat larger portion of family income than did older women
Although the number of two-worker families in which women earr
more than men is still low (< 10%), it is well known that women's
earnings often bring their families' incomes over the poverty line. The
obvious mutual protection against unemployment in two-earner house
holds is also well known. Should earnings approach parity, real shifts ir
power can be expected, and power in negotiating sex may move sexua
activity up or down.

Not only are more women working, but for increasing numbers o
them—married and unmarried—working represents a way of life. The
picture of the breadwinner husband with a homemaker wife who peri
odically drops in and out of the paid work force to provide the family
with "luxuries" is being rapidly replaced by a scenario in which it take:
two full-time salaries to achieve even a minimal desired level of materia
comfort. For most families, breadwinning now requires the full-time
efforts of two people outside the home. A new revolution—akin to the
Industrial Revolution—is taking women of all ages into the labor mar
ket. It is emptying homes of women, just as the Industrial Revolution
pulled workers out of the countryside and into the cities.

Only among women who never marry will these changes have little
effect. Without the economic advantage of a working husband, these
women have traditionally engaged in lifelong work (their career spar
averaging 45 years). Widowed, separated, and divorced women have
also been overrepresented in long-term attachment to the labor force
when compared to women in general. Loss or absence of a stably pre
sent working partner represents not only loss of companionship and, o
course, social sex, but also loss of income (Cherlin, 1981). All of these
losses are important, but at least partial substitutes for male companion
ship and sex are available; substitutes for the kind of money that mer
earn are the most difficult to come by.

In past generations, commitment to family-building, loyalty to on
man, and an elastic commitment to the labor market characterized wom
en's lives. Women's occupational training was once likened to a mat
tress: something to fall back on. Women's first commitment was to
family; men's first commitment was to work.

While both men and women today report that their greatest gratifications come from family ties (Gurin, Veroff, and Feld, 1960), som
major pushes and pulls are coming from the world of work. Thes
pushes and pulls do not stop at the bedroom door. Women who marr
late, who have entered the labor force well before marriage, and wh
know that they will remain in the labor force throughout marriage ar
likely to experience themselves as more equal partners in marriage tha

lid their mothers and grandmothers. In matters sexual, this may mean that the presumed sexual rate-setting prerogative of the male will be muted, in cohabitation as well as in marriage.

It is an open question whether stably working women will negotiate sexual activity in marriage up or down. A West German survey found working women reporting that they are so tired after work that marital sex is less often desired by them than by nonworking women (John Gagnon, personal communication, 1979). The Udry and Morris (1978) survey data show nonworking wives having intercourse more often than working wives. Estimates of coital frequency have recently been called into question as a measure. Follow-ups of continuously married women revealed that coital frequencies were "unlikely to be associated with socioeconomic, demographic, or even attitudinal variables" (Trussell and Westoff, 1980, p. 249). Social scientists are rarely treated to such a thorough housecleaning of all classes of their most trusted variables. Only reliable contraception or sterilization has dependable effects on coital frequency.

More women of the future will probably spend part of their adult lives without spouses. This does not mean that they will never marry. They will probably marry more often, but they will also divorce more frequently. Thus, for many adult women, life patterns will include periods with spouses and periods without. Permanent attachment to the work force might make divorce a somewhat less traumatic event than it has been in the past, when the inevitable losses of divorce were confounded by the economic and emotional dilemma of the displaced homemaker. The fatigue and lack of time engendered by full-time work, especially in the case of single mothers, may place even more constraints on the sex lives of postmarried women than on these of their married counterparts. Single parents (often with teenaged children) must shoulder the same responsibilities that were shared by two people when they were married. For a woman with no live-in, stable sexual partner, sex requires more negotiation, time, and effort, as well as social skills and economic resources. Some women will consider the effort worthwhile; others will join the take-it-or-leave-it group.

Exposure to the paid work world may promote the maintenance of social skills that are useful in the sexual marketplace when women reenter it after marriage. Additionally, the shared work world of men and women gives more women independent access to a pool of potentially available sexual and marriage partners.

Any attempt to predict what sexuality will be like among tomorrow's middle-aged women is filled with hazard. Adult women do not constitute a homogeneous group. If marriage continues to be the popular choice it has been since World War II (with 95% of Americans marrying at some time in their lives), then one set of predictions would fit the large married group. There, the major issue would be: To what extent do the variables that predicted sexual behavior in middle-age in the past apply to this new group?

If current divorce trends do not attenuate radically, middle-aged women will constitute many subgroups: long-term marrieds (10 or more years), short-term or long-term remarrieds, divorced or widowed but not remarried, and never-marrieds. We have not even tried to make predictions about gay women because of the paucity of life-cycle data on gay women (even Bell and Weinberg provide few data on older gay women). While many of the same forces that operate on heterosexual women also operate on gays, there are special problems related to marriage and divorce that gay women do not share with straight women. These are problems related to changing sex ratios in middle and old age and to the different views held by straight *men* and gay *women* about youth, age, and sexual attractiveness. Data on remarriage underline the salience of age in the heterosexual marketplace.

NEW FAMILIES, SEX, AND THE MIDDLE-AGED WOMAN

The lower rates of remarriage by women compared to men are age graded: Divorced women aged 35–44 remarry at 75% the rates of their former husbands; divorced women 45–54 remarry at 62% of their former husbands' rates. For all women over 44, the remarriage ratio of divorced women to divorced men is 56:100. The 1980 U.S. census counts 8,870,000 divorced or separated women versus 5,915,000 men of that status. The female:male ratio for widowhood is even more ominous—245:100. The latter figure reflects both the earlier age of male versus female death, plus the custom of women marrying men older than themselves (Cherlin 1981). On average, men die 7–8 years younger than do women; on average, first marriages find women 2–3 years younger than their mates. This makes a substantial period of widowhood highly likely for most women. Where middle-aged men divorce and remarry, their second wives are, on average, 9 to 10 years younger than they are. These women will be widowed for an even longer time than first wives, if they do not remarry.

Some factors will affect the sexuality of all three groups: never marrieds, marrieds, and postmarrieds. These include widespread acceptance of nonmarital sexuality, widespread knowledge of female capacity to enjoy sex, and increased permission for the expression of female sexuality, as reflected in bestsellers from *The Total Woman* to *The Joy of Sex*.

Beyond that, the sexual patterns of the three groups are likely to differ. The single factor that made the most difference in the past for

iddle-aged women was availability of a sexual partner. A major reason
·r that effect in the past came from operation of the double standard.
ttenuation of that standard has meant that more divorced, widowed,
ıd never-married women of all ages are sharing quarters, and sex, with
.en of all statuses, marital and nonmarital. While the popular literature
Iunt, 1966) on the formerly married suggests fast entry and exit from
·xual relationships, we know of no solid study of the nature and course
 such relationships where female age is followed as a variable. Remar-
ıge rates by age suggest that the scene of the formerly married is
ıything but age-blind.

   When marriage meant breadwinning for men and child-rearing for
omen, the age relations of husbands and wives made good sense. A
ɑn better equipped to earn (more experience at work, an established
ade or profession) traded his earning capacity for sexual favors, family
ıd personal care, and fertility in a woman. In the years of the Feminine
'ystique, the ideology behind that division of labor persisted, but some
 the objective conditons that had supported the trade-off were chang-
g. Maximum fertility was no longer so highly valued; women's educa-
ɔn was no longer so different from that of men; family care became less
ıerous as the incidence of life-threatening diseases in children de-
·eased; and sex was no longer something that women reluctantly
ʒave" men—rather, it had become a feminine pleasure. Betty Friedan's
'963) rage caught on because she challenged the already obsolete trade-
·f that kept women dependent.

   Today, women trade attractiveness for the advantages of marriage.
ιe social psychological literature makes it clear that physical attractive-
ɔss is the single most powerful variable determining men's choices in
.e dating and sexual scene. For women, that would be a careless lux-
·y. Women look for men who do well in life. (Woody Allen catches the
fference in The Front when he tells one woman in a resort hotel that he
 a writer, and another woman that he is a dentist. Only the latter
oman finds him attractive.)

   If divorce becomes more common and more men must share their
ιrnings with earlier families, the earning capacity of the middle-aged
oman may expand the choices available to her. Some remarriages by
·en occur because their new wives have earning capacity, i.e., "I could
ıly marry a woman who earns a lot." Men who wish to work at jobs
ith financial uncertainty (e.g., writing, art, politics) may seek out part-
ɔrs who can share the economic risk. Trade-offs such as this imply that
·me women will be able to shed the old division of gender roles, which
·ctated that the husband be older, a better earner, and more powerful
ιan the wife. Such roles work against middle-aged women.

   Regardless of strategies, there are fewer men than women. Humans
ιrt life with more male than female conceptions, more male than

female births, but by middle age, the higher vulnerability of males to accidents and disease leaves more females than males. What are middle aged women to do if they want sexual relationships? So long as we are not a polygynous society, it is clear that some women will not have husbands during their middle years. The number of possible solutions is finite: (1) Women can marry younger men; (2) women can have sexual relationships stably or sporadically with married men; (3) women can have relationships with men who are between marriages; (4) more than one woman can have sexual relationships with the same man; (5) women can have homosexual relationships on a stable or a sporadic basis.

All of the above five alternatives are occurring. The alternative that we have not cited is that suggested by the Lowenstein sample: Opt out of sexual relationships altogether. It is possible that the take-it-or-leave it position is an adaptation to a sex ratio that is unfavorable to middle aged women. No man or woman ever died of sexual deprivation. It is our hunch, however, that young women sexualized during the 1960 and 1970s will not lightly give up sexual relationships. It is possible that the five alternatives cited above will be chosen more often. A recent sampling of just three 1982 issues of *Cosmopolitan* leads us to believe that the outrage that some of today's older women express toward the alternatives cited above may not be true in the future, given the wide-ranging social sexualization occurring in popular magazines for younger women. In August, *Cosmopolitan* told their readers how to be a mistress to a married man while being independent. It also offered advice on how to have sex at conventions and how to marry older men. The September issue contained a complete (and quite explicit) "guide to lovelier (lustier) sex," while in October, readers were offered some insights into lesbianism and a lyrical, well-written essay on fellatio.

Almost all of the alternatives violate some of our gender rules. Some violate widely held beliefs. We all "know" that men can be turned on only by youth, that families will be destroyed by extramarital liaisons, and that people are not able to perform homosexually if they are hetero sexual in orientation. We can all think of instances that challenge each of these beliefs, too. Our purpose in citing these beliefs is to show what barriers exist to middle-aged women implementing any of the above choices. It is our guess that there will be some surprises in the future

Once upon a time, the third alternative—sex with a man between marriages—was unthinkable because "good" women stayed away from divorced men. Today, this alternative gives no offense. There will be fewer men than women in the unmarried pool. Moreover, these men will remarry down in age. It may well be that the middle-aged woman's sexual life will often be a matter of temporary liaisons with men *en rout*

) marriage with younger women. In considering all these alternatives, 'e do not recommend any in particular. An examination of the alterna- ves may make it easier to understand the women in Lowenstein's ımple who opt out of the search for sex.

Despite our optimistic predictions concerning the sexual pleasure of ıe next group of middle-aged, the baby boom cohort, caution is in rder. More of the next group of middle-aged women will work than ver before. Work and other responsibilities, especially family respon- bilities, compete with sex for time. Life with a stable sexual partner is lled with more than sexual feelings and goals. Gagnon (1982) suggests ıat couples may have to decide how important sex is to them in com- arison with other goals; tired people don't have a lot of sex whether ıey are older married couples or young medical students. People who alue careers over personal commitments are likely to defer sex. Cou- les who are married for long periods are more likely to develop ac- vities that compete with their sexual time. Gagnon believes that the ecrease in frequencies of sexual intercourse seen in married couples flects this competition for time, rather than a biological decrease. The xplanation may well be a combination of biological and social factors.

Being in the labor force may produce competition for time but it ıay also render a woman a more interesting partner. She knows more ɔout the world of paid work and brings home the wisdom, the mores, ıe peopled quality of her workplace. To the extent that this "new" ıput is a turn-on, sex may become more—rather than less—interesting ı a dual-job or dual-career family.

Similarly, new postdivorce couples would be expected to start their ›xual relations with higher rates of coitus, if only because they haven't :cumulated competing demands for time together. In all couples, chil- ren present enormous competing needs. Rubin (1979) reports that ɔme of the women that she interviewed were hypersensitive to the ›arby presence of children during intercourse. The women reported ıat their partners were unconcerned.

Marital sex has built-in gratifications as well as problems. Sex is ıere upon request in marriage. The forms of request are personally orked out, from the direct to the indirect; they are the couple's forms. Iarital sex lacks some of the elements of the nonmarital sexual search. nce one is married, the partner has said "yes" to sex. While partners ın be tired, they cannot routinely say "no" without violating the mari- l contract. Eliciting a "yes" during early erotic attraction carries a sexu- confirmation of self that marital sex probably loses after the first few ›ars. We believe that this factor operates to reduce the frequency of arital sex over time.

Tomorrow's middle-aged women have had their sexual appestats set higher than did previous generations. They are likely to have en joyed their early sex and to expect to enjoy their latter, middle-aged sex The context for their sexual lives will determine how much sex they have, as well as how they feel about that sex. Married sex is regular relatively frequent, but goes down with age. Middle-aged women wh had positive starts to their sex lives are likely to experience higher coit frequencies and higher orgasmic rates in marriage than did earlier gen erations. Smaller families will produce less competition for time, bu paid work will increase competition for time. Where the interactio comes out probably depends on the couples' valuation of sex. Move ment in and out of marriage is associated with less stable sexual relation ships, but with more partners. Middle-aged women are likely to have difficult time (as compared with younger women) in the postmarrie sexual milieu as they are less frequently chosen from among sexu partners for the middle-aged man's marital intimacy. While marital sex ual intimacy is not the only form of sustained sexual intimacy, it is th most common form that commits men to stable sex.

The never-married middle-aged group will probably bear little r semblance to the Kinsey group with those characteristics. These wome will be sexually experienced in youth and are likely to remain sexual active in some form during middle age, much more so than previou generations in their situations. The defining characteristic of this grou of women is their decision to postpone marriage, to give higher priori to paid work and education and lower priority to childbearing. In pas generations, some opprobrium attached to women neither marrying n bearing children. This group of women is likely to have greater acce tance; they will be less likely seen as asexual. Their stability in the lab force may make them economically advantaged, too.

THE FRAMEWORK FOR SEXUALITY: A SEARCH FOR MEANINGS

Any statement about any group's sexuality based on a single cultu requires some qualification. The cross-cultural story underlines the vie of male sexuality as more often urgent and of female sexuality as mo "discretionary" (Ford and Beach, 1951). However, our anthropologic colleagues tell us that there are some cultures where that definition sexual appetite is not accepted. Mangaian women (and men) seek o sex. Tshambuli women want sex more than do Tshambuli men (Mea 1935). Some cultural arrangements sanction older husbands taking ma sexual partners while no sexual arrangements are made for wives wl have had their complement of babies, a presumption that men "nee sex and women (at least older women) don't. A culture's conceptio bout sexuality are not independent of the general *Weltanschauung* held y that culture. Sexuality requires some such framework to make sense ithin a culture (Davenport, 1977).

In our society, men and women share a decline in sexual perfor-ance with age. Couples who are stably paired show a slow decline ith age, perhaps reflecting the danger of routine, the ultimate anaph-disiac. "He's turned on by our bed, not me; he only touches me in ed," says the intimacy-seeking 40-year-old wife. Few couples can af-rd restorative sex in hotel rooms away from children. Family experi-nces other than having sex take on greater legitimacy since they ex-ude fewer family members. Nonsexual issues drive decisions in the xual area.

The view that men are sex-driven without wifely provocation surely opposite to that which motivated the writing of *The Total Woman* Morgan, 1973). The syndicated newspaper columnist, Abigail Van Bu-n, tried to find out, in her own way, whether or not women over 50 ked sex (Van Buren, 1981). She asked older readers of her "Dear Abby" lumn. Half of her respondents wanted out; one wrote, "Even a hook-: gets to retire." The other half invented tricks, à la Marabelle Morgan, entice their sexually dormant husbands. While the *Consumer Reports* rvey required answering a long questionnaire, Dear Abby required nly that her readers write a short note. Moreover, Dear Abby's re-ondents probably represent a wider sample of middle-aged women.

Dear Abby's survey results raise many questions. National maga-nes, e.g., *McCall's*, run columns quoting psychiatrists on sex, love, mmitment, and intimacy. *McCall's* is flooded with letters from trou-ed women responding to the helping and self-help nature of the arti-es. Women readers ask how to get husbands to interact, pay attention, xpress affection. Their letters reflect a world in which many men feel at it is enough if they support their families economically. The women arch for affection, sex, and intimacy. Sex is often the only—and infre-uent—intimacy, and many women feel that coitus is less sexual outside a broader context of expressed affection.

We have stayed fairly close to the few existing sets of survey data on e sexuality of women in middle age. The big question for the soon-to--middle-aged centers around how the two gender scripts will fuse and ange. What will be most interesting and hardest to predict is how ose changes will be experienced by tomorrow's middle-aged women. he only certainty is that the range of their sexual choices will be greater an it was for their mothers and grandmothers. We wonder whether e choices will satisfy the heightened expectations of the upcoming iddle-aged cohort.

REFERENCES

Angelou, M. *The heart of a woman*. New York: Random House, 1981.

Baum, M. J., Koos Slob, A., de Jong, F. H., and Westbrook, D. L. Persistence of sexual behavior in ovariectomized stumptail macaques following dexamethasone treatment or adrenalectomy. *Hormones and Behavior*, 1978, 2, 323–347.

Barbach, L. *For yourself: The fulfillment of female sexuality*. Garden City, N.Y.: Doubleday, 1975.

Baruch, G. K., and Barnett, R. *Who has multiple role strain? The "woman in the middle" revisited*. Paper presented at the Meeting of the Gerontological Society, Toronto, 1981.

Bell, A. P., and Weinberg, M. S. *Homosexuality: A study of diversity among men and women*. New York: Simon & Schuster, 1978.

Boston Women's Health Book Collective. *Our bodies, ourselves*. (2nd ed.). New York: Simon & Schuster, 1976. Pp. 327–336.

Cherlin, A. J. *Marriage, divorce, remarriage*. Cambridge, Mass.: Harvard University Press, 1981.

Christenson, C. V., and Gagnon, J. H. Sexual behavior in a group of older women. *Journal of Gerontology*, 1965, 20, 351–356.

Christenson, C. V., and Johnson, A. B. Sexual patterns in a group of older never-married women. *Journal of Geriatric Psychiatry*, 1973, 6, 80–98.

Corby, N., and Brecher, E. *Love, sex, aging*. Mt. Vernon, N.Y.: Consumers Union, 1984.

Davenport, W. H. Sex in cross-cultural perspective. In F. A. Beach, *Human sexuality in four perspectives*. Baltimore: Johns Hopkins University Press, 1977.

Degler, C. *At odds*. New York: Oxford University Press, 1980.

Eysenck, H. J. *Sex and personality*. Austin: University of Texas Press, 1976.

Finger, F. W. Changes in sex practices and beliefs of male college students over 30 years. *Journal of Sex Research*, 1975, 11, 304–317.

Ford, C. S., and Beach, F. A. *Patterns of sexual behavior*. New York: Harper & Row, 1951.

Friedan, B. *The feminine mystique*. New York: Dell, 1963.

Gagnon, J. Are you really too tired for sex? *Working Mother*, 1982, January, 53–55.

Gebhard, P. Postmarital coitus among widows and divorcees. In P. Bohannan (Ed.), *Divorce and after*. Garden City, N.Y.: Doubleday, 1971.

Geer, J., Morokoff, P., and Greenwood, P. Sexual arousal in women. The development of a measurement device for vaginal blood volume. *Archives of Sexual Behavior*, 1974, 4, 559–564.

Gurin, G., Veroff, J., and Feld, S. *Americans view their mental health*. New York: Basic Books, 1960.

Hite, S. *The Hite report*. New York: Macmillan, 1976.

Hunt, M. *The world of the formerly married*. New York: McGraw-Hill, 1966.

Hunt, M. *Sexual behavior in the 1970's*. Chicago: Playboy Press, 1974.

Jong, E. *Fear of flying*. New York: New American Library, 1973.

Kinsey, A. C., Pomeroy, W. B., and Martin, C. E. *Sexual behavior in the human male*. Philadelphia: Saunders, 1948.

Kinsey, A. C., Pomeroy, W. B., Martin, C. E., and Gebhard, P. *Sexual behavior in the human female*. Philadelphia: Saunders, 1953.

Kraemer, H. C., Becker, H. B., Brodie, H. K. H., Doering, C. H. Moos, R. H., and Hamburg, D. A. Orgasmic frequency and plasma testosterone levels in normal human males. *Archives of Sexual Behavior*, 1976, 5, 125–132.

LaRassa, R., and LaRassa, M. M. *Transition to parenthood: How infants change families*. Beverly Hills: Sage, 1981.

ewenstein, S. F., Bloch, N. E., Campion, J., Epstein, J. S., Gale, P., and Salvatore, M. A study of satisfactions and stresses of single women in midlife. *Sex Roles*, 1981, *11*, 1127–1141.

ria, Z., and Rose, M. D. *The psychology of human sexuality*. New York: Wiley, 1979.

arshall, D. S. Sexual behavior in Mangaia. In D. S. Marshall and R. C. Suggs (Eds.), *Human sexual behavior*. Englewood Cliffs, N.J.: Prentice-Hall, 1971.

artin, C. E. Sexual activity in the aging male. In J. Money and H. Musaph (Eds.), *Handbook of sexology*. Elsevier/North Holland Biomedical Press, 1977.

asnick, G., and Bane, M. J. *The nation's families: 1960–1990*. Boston: Auburn House, 1981.

asters, W. H. and Johnson, V. *Human sexual response*. Boston: Little, Brown, 1966.

ead, M. *Sex and temperament in three primitive societies*. New York: Morrow, 1935.

organ, M. *The total woman*. Old Tappan, N.J.: F. H. Rovell, 1973.

eugarten, B. L. Women's attitudes towards the menopause. *Vita Humana*, 1963, *6*, 140–146.

tner, S., and Whitehead, H. *Sexual meanings*. Cambridge, England: Cambridge University Press, 1981.

eiffer, E., and Davis, G. C. Determinants of sexual behavior in middle and old age. *Journal of the American Geriatric Society*, 1972, *20*, 151–188.

eiffer, E., Verwoerdt, A., and Davis, G. C. Sexual behavior in middle life. *American Journal of Psychiatry*, 1972, *128*, 1262–1267.

tropinto, A., and Simenauer, J. *Beyond the male myth*. New York: New York Times Books, 1977.

iss, I. L. Premarital sexuality: Past, present, and future. In I. L. Reiss (Ed.), *Readings on the family system*. New York: Hall, 1972.

ssi, A. Lifespan theories and women's lives. *Signs*, 1980, *6*, 4–32.

bin, L. *Women of a certain age*. New York: Harper & Row, 1979.

inman, D. L., Wincze, J. P., Sakheim, D. K., Barlow, D. H., and Maussakalian, M. A comparison of male and female patterns of sexual arousal. *Archives of Sexual Behavior*, 1981, *10*, 529–547.

ssell, J. and Westoff, C. F. Contraceptive practice and trends in coital frequency. *Family Planning Perspectives*, 1980, *12*, 246–249.

ry, J. R. Changes in the frequency of marital intercourse from panel data. *Archives of Sexual Behavior*, 1980, *9*, 319–325.

ry, J. R., and Morris, N. M. Relative contribution of male and female age to the frequency of marital intercourse. *Social Biology*, 1978, *25*, 128–134.

n Buren, A. *The best of Dear Abby*. Kansas City, Kansas: Andrews McMeel, 1981.

roff, J., and Feld, S. *Marriage and work in America*. New York: Van Nostrand, 1970.

stoff, C. F. Coital frequency and contraception. *Family Planning Perspectives*, 1974, *6*, 136–141.